Effective Practices for Mental Health Promotion in Education

Louiza Ioannidou
European University Cyprus, Cyprus

Agathi Argyriadi
Frederick University, Cyprus

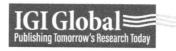

Published in the United States of America by
    IGI Global
    701 E. Chocolate Avenue
    Hershey PA, USA 17033
    Tel: 717-533-8845
    Fax: 717-533-8661
    E-mail: cust@igi-global.com
    Web site: https://www.igi-global.com

Library of Congress Cataloging-in-Publication Data

CIP Pending
ISBN:979-8-3693-5325-7
EISBN: 979-8-3693-5327-1

British Cataloguing in Publication Data
A Cataloguing in Publication record for this book is available from the British Library.

All work contributed to this book is new, previously-unpublished material.
The views expressed in this book are those of the authors, but not necessarily of the publisher.

This book is dedicated
to our beloved family and children,
whose love and support are the foundation of everything we do.
And to all the educators, counselors, and mental health professionals
who tirelessly work to nurture the minds and hearts of students.

Table of Contents

Detailed Table of Contents

Lefki Kourea, University of Nicosia, Cyprus
Argyro Fella, University of Nicosia, Cyprus

Students get to learn and flourish in school environments where the school climate
is positive, the staff is consistent in their support, and caring relationships with all
students are promoted. School climate is a complex and multifaceted construct
that has drawn the attention of several scholars who have extensively explored its
theoretical and conceptual definition. Changing the school climate is not an easy task.
Nonetheless, research findings have shown that when whole-school approaches are
designed and implemented, student and teacher perceptions of school climate change
positively. The purpose of this chapter is to describe the example of the School-Wide
Positive Behavioral Interventions and Supports (SWPBIS) framework, its critical
features, and pedagogical philosophy as a targeted solution for cultivating a safe
school climate and empowering students and staff psycho-emotional well-being.
Further, the chapter will provide an overview of the empirical basis of the impact
of SWPBIS on student academic achievement and well-being and conclude with
implications for practice.

Chapter 2

Sarah Holmes, Liverpool Hope University, UK
Vicky Sinclair, Liverpool Hope University, UK

Informed by our professional experience and empirical research in the UK, we highlight principles and approaches which could be integrated into the development of strategies of primary schools seeking to support children's mental health and wellbeing. We consider the challenges and opportunities of implementing research-informed approaches in schools, and the balance between maintaining individuality and context specific support in each school, whilst collaborating with other schools to share resources, training opportunities and expertise. Our research findings revealed the need for bespoke and context-specific strategies, rather than using externally produced frameworks or curricula. However, the staff interviews also showed the value of groups of schools working together to support and equip one another in shaping their vision and ethos. Approaches which were implemented holistically across the school were more effective and valuable, and communication across the whole staff body further supported the implementation and effectiveness within the whole school community.

Chapter 3

Lefki Kourea, University of Nicosia, Cyprus
Fotini Lytra, University of Nicosia, Cyprus

Student mental health has received increased attention over the last years, with researchers and governments trying to identify the best ways to support students and adolescents (e.g., Johns Hopkins Bloomberg School of Public Health & United Nations Children's Fund, 2022). Efforts have concentrated on initiating mental health services and increasing school-and program-based mental health supports to address student needs at individual and school levels. Recently, some researchers have suggested teaching social-emotional skills within a prevention-focused school-wide tiered model because simply adopting a socio-emotional curriculum does not lead to adequate implementation or improved student outcomes (Greenberg et al., 2017). This chapter describes the mental health challenges at-risk students face and suggests strengthening their socio-emotional skills within the tiered continuum of supports of the School-wide Positive Behavioral Interventions and Supports framework.

Chapter 4

Efi Glymitsa, National and Kapodistrian University of Athens, Greece
Eleni Zafiriadou, National and Kapodistrian University of Athens,
   Greece
Maria Zafiropoulou, Thessaly University, Greece
Evangelia Galanaki, National and Kapodistrian University of Athens,
   Greece

This chapter presents strategies that teachers can use for preventing and dealing with students' behavior problems in the school community. These strategies are based on behavioral, cognitive behavioral, ecosystemic, and humanistic approaches. The basic premise of this chapter is that the effectiveness of prevention and intervention is enhanced when strategies from all these approaches are used by educators. The basic principles of behavioral, cognitive behavioral, ecosystemic, and humanistic models are briefly presented based on which, management strategies are described that teachers can implement to prevent and deal with children's behaviour problems as well as to increase desirable behaviours. These prevention and intervention programs are delivered at the individual, classroom, whole school, and family levels. Specific examples are given for all these strategies. Finally, two case studies or scenarios are presented with the aim of illuminating the effective use of these strategies in real situations within the school community.

This chapter will not only delve into the rising interest in mental health among children and adolescents but also provide a comprehensive examination of school-based mental health programs and interventions, providing practical guidance for stakeholders.The aim is to assess their effectiveness in supporting students facing mental health challenges. Importantly, this chapter will offer practical strategies and evidence-based solutions that are readily applicable in helping school districts implement effective mental health interventions tailored to the diverse needs of students. By targeting prevalent challenges such as anxiety, depression, ADHD, trauma, and others, school communities can advocate for the well-being and safety of their students. Educators, mental health practitioners, and policymakers can benefit from understanding the most effective programs and areas for improvement in current interventions. Ultimately, this discussion will contribute to enhancing the efficacy and future implementation of school-based mental health interventions

Recent trends in educational research underscore the significance of cultivating mental flow to enhance well-being, especially for health-vulnerable individuals. Scholars have delved into the nuances of creating conducive learning environments that cater to the unique needs of students facing health vulnerabilities. Adopting a systematic review approach, this chapter synthesizes findings from diverse studies published over the past decade. The examination of empirical research, intervention strategies, and case studies aims to provide a comprehensive understanding of the ways in which mental flow can be nurtured to support the well-being of health-vulnerable students in educational settings. The synthesis of literature highlights the positive impact of tailored learning experiences on the mental flow and overall well-being of health-vulnerable students. From inclusive teaching practices to adaptive curriculum design, the findings emphasize the importance of creating environments that prioritize the unique needs of these individuals.

In recent years there has been an increasing amount of research on the practice of mindfulness in education. There are several studies that examine the practice of mindfulness and its effectiveness in various aspects of the lives of both students and teachers. The purpose of the chapter is to mention the different practices that have already been implemented in different educational levels, either in pupils/ students or teachers/ tutors and their effectiveness in different aspects of their lives, through literature. It is also discussed mindfulness as a quite promising practice, which is likely to be a pedagogical practice that serves educational purposes that have long been part of the tradition of education.

Cultivating mental resilience to manage stressful situations strengthens children's mental health and well-being. Preventive intervention programs to enhance resilience have been implemented internationally in learning settings involving schools, communities, parents, and children. Regarding Cyprus, the research preventive program "We.R.Stars" has been developed and implemented in schools to promote children's resilience and well-being. The program is oriented around five key factors: personal empowerment, social skills, self-regulation, good links with the school, and positive parental involvement. The program refers to children aged 9 to 12. The program consists of ten sessions with the children conducted within the school and three meetings with the parents. The program's results indicated that children developed higher self-esteem, self-efficacy, and resilience after implementing the program. Research results highlighted that applying resilient programs in education prevents student difficulties at school and empowers children's positive emotions, strengths, and well-being.

Alexandros Argyriadis, Frederick University, Cyprus
Dimitra V. Katsarou, University of the Aegean, Greece
Olga Drakopoulou, Ministry of Education, Religious Affairs, and Sports,
*   Greece*
Agathi Argyriadi, Frederick University, Cyprus

Recent research trends highlight an increasing recognition of the need for specialized attention to students with chronic health problems. Adopting a systematic review approach, this chapter synthesizes findings from diverse studies published over the past decade. The synthesis of literature underscores the significance of tailored support systems and compassionate care in promoting resilience among students with chronic health problems. The findings emphasize the multifaceted nature of resilience-building strategies, ranging from school-based interventions to collaborative efforts involving educators, healthcare professionals, and families. In conclusion, this review advocates for a compassionate and holistic approach to supporting students with chronic health conditions. Understanding and addressing the unique needs of this student population are crucial for fostering resilience, ensuring their academic success, and enhancing overall well-being.

Chapter 10

Agathi Argyriadi, Frederick University, Cyprus
Louiza Ioannidou, European University Cyprus, Cyprus
Olga Drakopoulou, Ministry of Education, Religious Affairs, and Sports,
*   Greece*
Alexandros Argyriadis, Frederick University, Cyprus

The recent surge in research on mental health and cultural diversity in schools reflects a growing awareness of the multifaceted nature of students' experiences. Scholars have explored cultural influences on stressors, coping mechanisms, and help-seeking behaviors, contributing to a nuanced understanding of the interplay between cultural diversity and mental health outcomes. This literature review adopts a systematic approach, synthesizing findings from a diverse range of studies published over the past decade. By analyzing empirical research, theoretical frameworks, and practical interventions, this review aims to provide a comprehensive overview of the current state of knowledge in the field. The synthesis of literature reveals that cultural diversity significantly influences students' mental health experiences, affecting aspects such as stressors, resilience factors, and access to mental health resources. In conclusion, this review highlights the intricate relationship between mental health and cultural diversity in schools.

Chapter 11

Asteropi Polykandrioti, University of Athens, Greece
Maria Malikiosi, University of Athens, Greece

The aim of this study was to examine depressive symptoms in typically developing children and in children with dyslexia, attention deficit/hyperactive disorder, and autism spectrum disorder. Participants were 120 children; 60 of them were diagnosed with these disorders and attended inclusive classrooms, whereas 60 were typically developing children. All children completed the Children's Depression Inventory as developed by Kovacs. Results indicated that children with dyslexia, attention deficit/hyperactive disorder, and autism spectrum disorder had significantly higher scores on depression than typically developing children. The strongest differences were found in anhedonia, interpersonal problems, negative self-esteem, ineffectiveness, and negative mood. These findings underline the need for teachers and parents to provide emotional and social support to children with specific learning difficulties and developmental disorders to reduce the negative impact of these disorders and enhance children's resilience.

Chapter 12

Potheini Vaiouli, University of Luxembourg, Luxembourg & University
of Cyprus, Cyprus
Marios Theodorou, Frederick University, Cyprus & University of
Cyprus, Cyprus
Georgia Panayiotou, University of Cyprus, Cyprus

The success of Higher Education as an effective learning environment rests on establishing an inclusive context that promotes life-long learning opportunities. Psycho-social skills are considered fundamental competencies for youth development: crucial for individuals' academic achievement, mental health, and life success. Although universal skills development programs have produced promising findings, there are several challenges in effectively providing such services to the wide student population. There is growing literature indicating the potential of incorporating music strategies and music-based intervention as an effective medium for these programs integrated into the universal academic pathway. This chapter presents the rationale and the development pathway of an enhanced (standard + music) classroom-based Emotion Regulation skills training to meet the diverse needs of university students. Through a multiphase method, we present data from three pilot single-arm studies on the acceptability and preliminary effectiveness of the program on students' adaptive emotion regulation.

Chapter 13
Giulia Perasso, University of Genoa, Italy
Carmela Lillo, Fondazione Patrizio Paoletti, Italy
Sandro Anella, Fondazione Patrizio Paoletti, Italy
Giulia Viviano, University of Genoa, Italy
Matilde Pisano, University of Genoa, Italy
Elena Vigogna, University of Genoa, Italy
Erika Salemi, University of Genoa, Italy
Tania Di Giuseppe, Fondazione Patrizio Paoletti, Italy

This scoping review emphasizes the importance of understanding children's cognitive and socio-emotional capacities in navigating discussions about war and peace. Tailoring communication strategies to these developmental nuances enables meaningful dialogues between adults and children, fostering empathy and conflict resolution skills. Additionally, pedagogical interventions highlighted in the review aim to nurture peacebuilding skills among children, empowering them to contribute positively to their communities. In conclusion, by considering children's developmental needs and implementing effective communication and educational strategies, adults can play a crucial role in cultivating peaceful mindsets and behaviors in future generations.

Preface

In today's fast-paced and increasingly complex world, the mental health and well-being of students have never been more critical. Schools are not only places of academic learning but also pivotal environments where students develop the emotional and psychological resilience needed to navigate life's challenges. As editors of this volume, "Effective Practices for Mental Health Promotion in Education," we are deeply committed to exploring and disseminating the most effective strategies for fostering mental well-being within educational settings.

Drawing on research and real-world examples, "Effective Practices for Mental Health Promotion in Education" bridges the gap between theory and practice, empowering readers to implement effective mental health promotion initiatives. The book guides educators in creating inclusive environments and prioritizing mental well-being by offering insights into fostering a sense of belonging, reducing stigma, and supporting students with diverse needs. Its focus on practical solutions and evidence-based practices not only guides educators and mental health professionals but also underscores the importance of collaboration between schools, families, and communities in enhancing mental health support systems and promoting a holistic approach to student well-being.

"Effective Practices for Mental Health Promotion in Education" is a comprehensive guide that covers a wide range of topics related to mental health in educational settings. Our contributors delve into a wide range of topics, from promoting resilience and a sense of belonging to addressing stigma and implementing mindfulness practices. Each chapter offers evidence-based insights and actionable strategies designed to create a supportive environment where students can thrive emotionally and psychologically.

CHAPTER OVERVIEW

In chapter 1, the authors explore the critical role of a positive school climate in fostering student and staff well-being. Recognizing the complexity of school climate as a multifaceted construct, the chapter delves into the School-Wide Positive Behavioral Interventions and Supports (SWPBIS) framework as an evidence-based approach to creating safer and more supportive school environments. The chapter outlines the key features and pedagogical philosophy of SWPBIS, illustrating how whole-school approaches can transform perceptions of school climate. Additionally, the chapter reviews empirical evidence linking SWPBIS to improvements in academic achievement and well-being, providing practical implications for educators and administrators committed to enhancing school climate.

Drawing from professional experience and empirical research conducted in the UK, chapter 2 highlights the importance of context-specific strategies for supporting children's mental health and well-being in primary schools. The authors argue against a one-size-fits-all approach, emphasizing the need for tailored interventions that respect the individuality of each school. By exploring the challenges and opportunities of implementing research-informed practices, the chapter demonstrates the value of collaboration among schools for sharing resources, training, and expertise. The findings underscore the effectiveness of holistic approaches that engage the entire school community, offering valuable insights for educators and policymakers alike.

Chapter 3 addresses the pressing issue of student mental health, with a focus on at-risk students. The authors advocate for the integration of social-emotional skills training within a prevention-focused, school-wide tiered model of support, specifically within the SWPBIS framework. Recognizing that a simple adoption of socio-emotional curricula is insufficient, the chapter emphasizes the need for a systematic approach to strengthen the socio-emotional competencies of students. By highlighting the mental health challenges faced by at-risk students, the chapter provides a comprehensive guide for educators to effectively implement and sustain these supports within the school environment.

In chapter 4, the authors present a comprehensive array of strategies for preventing and managing student behavior problems, grounded in behavioral, cognitive behavioral, ecosystemic, and humanistic approaches. The chapter outlines the basic principles of each model and offers practical strategies that educators can apply at the individual, classroom, whole school, and family levels. Through detailed descriptions and real-life case studies, the chapter demonstrates how these integrated strategies can enhance the effectiveness of prevention and intervention efforts, ultimately fostering a more positive school environment.

Chapter 5 offers a thorough examination of school-based mental health programs and interventions, with a focus on their effectiveness in supporting students facing mental health challenges. The authors provide practical guidance for stakeholders, including educators, mental health practitioners, and policymakers, on how to implement these programs effectively. By addressing common mental health issues such as anxiety, depression, ADHD, and trauma, the chapter equips school communities with the tools needed to advocate for student well-being and safety. The discussion also highlights areas for improvement in current interventions, contributing to the ongoing enhancement of school-based mental health support.

Chapter 6 synthesizes recent educational research on cultivating mental flow as a means of enhancing well-being, particularly for health-vulnerable students. Through a systematic review of studies published over the past decade, the authors explore how tailored learning environments can support the unique needs of these students. The chapter emphasizes the importance of inclusive teaching practices and adaptive curriculum design in fostering mental flow, ultimately contributing to the overall well-being of health-vulnerable students. By highlighting successful intervention strategies, the chapter offers valuable insights for educators seeking to create supportive and empowering learning environments.

Mindfulness has gained significant attention in educational research, and chapter 7 explores its application and effectiveness in both students' and teachers' lives. Through a review of existing literature, the authors discuss the various mindfulness practices that have been implemented across different educational levels and their impact on various aspects of participants' lives. The chapter positions mindfulness as a promising pedagogical practice that aligns with long-standing educational traditions, offering a balanced perspective on its potential to enhance mental health and well-being in educational settings.

Focusing on the importance of resilience in children's mental health, chapter 8 presents the 'We.R.Stars' program, a research-based preventive intervention developed and implemented in Cypriot schools. Targeting children aged 9 to 12, the program aims to enhance personal empowerment, social skills, self-regulation, school engagement, and positive parental involvement. The chapter details the program's structure, including its ten sessions with children and three meetings with parents, and presents empirical findings that demonstrate significant improvements in self-esteem, self-efficacy, and resilience. The chapter underscores the value of resilience-building programs in preventing student difficulties and promoting well-being.

Chapter 9 underscores the critical need for specialized support systems for students with chronic health problems. Through a systematic review of recent research, the authors highlight the multifaceted strategies required to build resilience in this vulnerable population. The chapter advocates for a compassionate and holistic approach that involves collaboration between educators, healthcare professionals, and families. By addressing the unique challenges faced by students with chronic health conditions, the chapter provides practical recommendations for fostering resilience, ensuring academic success, and enhancing overall well-being.

Chapter 10 synthesizes a decade of research on the intersection of mental health and cultural diversity in educational settings. The authors explore how cultural factors influence stressors, coping mechanisms, and help-seeking behaviors among students, providing a nuanced understanding of the relationship between cultural diversity and mental health outcomes. The chapter offers a comprehensive overview of empirical research, theoretical frameworks, and practical interventions, highlighting the importance of culturally sensitive approaches to mental health promotion in schools.

Chapter 11 presents a study examining depressive symptoms in children with dyslexia, ADHD, and autism spectrum disorder, compared to typically developing children. The findings reveal significantly higher levels of depression among children with these disorders, particularly in areas such as anhedonia, interpersonal problems, and negative self-esteem. The chapter emphasizes the importance of providing emotional and social support to students with specific learning and developmental disorders, offering strategies for educators and parents to reduce the negative impact of these conditions and enhance resilience.

Focusing on the role of psycho-social skills in youth development, chapter 12 explores the potential of music-based interventions in enhancing emotion regulation among university students. The authors present the development and pilot testing of an enhanced classroom-based Emotion Regulation skills training program that integrates music strategies. Through data from three pilot studies, the chapter demonstrates the acceptability and preliminary effectiveness of this approach, offering a novel pathway for addressing the diverse emotional needs of students in higher education.

Chapter 13 emphasizes the importance of understanding children's cognitive and socio-emotional capacities when discussing sensitive topics like war and peace. Through a scoping review, the authors explore how tailored communication strategies can facilitate meaningful dialogues between adults and children, fostering empathy and conflict resolution skills. The chapter also highlights pedagogical interventions designed to nurture peacebuilding skills, empowering children to contribute positively to their communities. By considering developmental needs and effective communication strategies, the chapter offers valuable insights for cultivating peaceful mindsets and behaviors in future generations.

CONCLUSION

We recognize that the challenges faced by students are diverse and multifaceted, and therefore, the approaches to promoting mental health must be equally varied and adaptable. This book provides a rich resource for educators, school counselors, psychologists, and other professionals working in educational settings. It offers practical guidance for implementing mental health promotion initiatives and serves as a bridge between research and practice.

Our hope is that this volume will not only equip readers with the tools needed to support students' mental health but also inspire further research and collaboration in this vital area. By fostering a community of practice around mental health promotion in education, we can collectively contribute to students' well-being and help shape a future where every student has the opportunity to flourish.

We would like to express our deepest gratitude to the contributors who have shared their expertise and insights in this volume. Their work is a testament to the importance of collaboration and interdisciplinary approaches in addressing the complex issues of mental health in education. We also extend our thanks to the educators, counselors, administrators, and mental health professionals who are on the front lines, working tirelessly to support students every day. Your dedication and commitment are the foundation upon which this book is built.

As you explore the chapters of this book, we hope you find not only valuable knowledge but also inspiration and encouragement. Together, we can make a meaningful difference in students' lives and create educational environments where mental health is prioritized, supported, and celebrated.

Sincerely,

Louiza Ioannidou
European University Cyprus, Cyprus

Agathi Argyriadi
Frederick University, Cyprus

Chapter 1
Whole–School Approaches and Their Impact on School Climate and Student Psycho–Emotional Being:
The Example of School–Wide Positive Behavioral Interventions and Supports (SWPBIS) Framework

Lefki Kourea
https://orcid.org/0000-0003-4572-6377
University of Nicosia, Cyprus

Argyro Fella
University of Nicosia, Cyprus

ABSTRACT

Students get to learn and flourish in school environments where the school climate is positive, the staff is consistent in their support, and caring relationships with all students are promoted. School climate is a complex and multifaceted construct that has drawn the attention of several scholars who have extensively explored its theoretical and conceptual definition. Changing the school climate is not an easy task. Nonetheless, research findings have shown that when whole-school approaches are designed and implemented, student and teacher perceptions of school climate change positively. The purpose of this chapter is to describe the example of the School-Wide

DOI: 10.4018/979-8-3693-5325-7.ch001

Positive Behavioral Interventions and Supports (SWPBIS) framework, its critical features, and pedagogical philosophy as a targeted solution for cultivating a safe school climate and empowering students and staff psycho-emotional well-being. Further, the chapter will provide an overview of the empirical basis of the impact of SWPBIS on student academic achievement and well-being and conclude with implications for practice.

WHOLE-SCHOOL APPROACHES AND THEIR IMPACT ON SCHOOL CLIMATE AND STUDENT PSYCHO-EMOTIONAL BEING: THE EXAMPLE OF SCHOOL-WIDE POSITIVE BEHAVIORAL INTERVENTIONS AND SUPPORTS (SWPBIS) FRAMEWORK

School climate is a complex and multifaceted construct that has drawn the attention of several scholars who have extensively explored its theoretical and conceptual definition (e.g., Rudasill et al., 2018). Although the importance of school climate in providing high-quality learning environments to students was recognized by Arthur Perry as early as 1908 (Perry, 1919), there is still a lack of consensus on its definition (Lee et al., 2017). Some researchers introduced the concept of an abstract definition, and they described school climate as "the quality and character of school life" (Cohen et al., 2009, p. 182), "the school's spirit or character" (Klik et al., 2023, p. 807) or "the heart and soul of the school" (Freiberg & Stein 1999, p.11). At the same time, some others suggested a more concrete and tangible definition of school climate (see Wang & Degol, 2016). For example, Haynes et al. (1997) suggested that school climate refers to the quality and consistency of interpersonal relationships within (e.g., student interactions, student-teacher interactions) and outside of the school community (i.e., home-school interactions). The National School Climate Council (2007) introduced a broader definition of school climate, which is a reflection of norms, objectives, interpersonal interactions, instructional strategies, and organizational structures and is based on patterns of people's experiences with school life. More recently, the relevant definitions have been expanded to include the feeling of safety (e.g., Thapa et al., 2013) and the importance of a supportive and caring environment (National Center on Safe Supportive Learning Environments [NCSSLE], n.d.).

From the beginning of this chapter, it is pointed out that school climate and school culture do not have the same connotation; however, they are often used interchangeably as they intend to capture the school character. When comparing both variables, Van Houtte (2005) concludes that school climate emphasizes shared perceptions of students, families, and school staff within the organization, while school culture focuses on shared assumptions, beliefs, and meanings about the organization. School climate is evaluated via perceptual measurement, whereby school members (i.e., students, staff, and administrators) perceive what their colleagues believe or assume (Grazia & Molinari, 2020). School culture measures are based on what school members believe or assume themselves. Nonetheless, both variables are critical in school improvement efforts. In this chapter, the emphasis is placed only on school climate, as the title suggests.

School Climate and its Contextual Dimensions

According to Wang and colleagues (2014), perceptions are important not just for evaluating school climate but also for determining how the climate dimensions affect the expected outcomes. Much of this type of correlational research has indicated that *students' and staff perceptions* of school climate appear to be a meaningful measure as it has been associated with multiple student outcomes, including:

(1) academic achievement (e.g., Bear et al., 2011; Brand et al., 2008; Maxwell et al., 2017; Saputra et al., 2020),
(2) school engagement and burnout (e.g., Molinari & Grazia, 2023),
(3) school attendance (e.g., Maxwell, 2016),
(4) mental health (e.g., Aldridge & McChesney, 2018),
(5) sense of resilience (Aldridge et al., 2016), and
(6) bullying (e.g., Beaudoin & Roberge, 2015).

Furthermore, positive teacher perceptions of school climate were associated with teacher well-being (e.g., Yang et al., 2022), job satisfaction (e.g., Collie et al., 2012; Malinen & Savolainen, 2016), self-efficacy (e.g., Aldridge & Fraser, 2016), teaching approaches (Oder & Eisenschmidt, 2018), and motivation (e.g., Reaves & Cozzens, 2018).

Over the last four decades, there have been several notable attempts to explain the multi-faceted concept of school climate and its core elements (e.g., Kutsyuruba et al., 2015). For example, in the late 1970s, Moos (1979) proposed three major and broad dimensions of school climate: (a) *relationships*, or the extent to which people in the environment assist and encourage each other (i.e., friendships among students, bonding between teachers and students); (b) *personal development*, or the extent to which self-enhancement can occur (i.e., whether the school's overarching objective prioritizes carrying out task plans, if it values student performance, whether it recognizes achievement, etc.); and (c) *maintenance and system change*, or the extent to which the environment is structured, and capable of altering (i.e., if there are clear policies and procedures, whether teachers have appropriate control over their actions, etc.).

Subsequent research suggested that four key components define the climate within schools (e.g., Cohen, 2006; Cohen et al., 2009): (a) *safety* (i.e., physical and socio-emotional), (b) *relationships* (i.e., respect for diversity, school community and collaboration, morale and "connectedness"), (c) *teaching and learning* (i.e., quality of instruction, social, emotional, and ethical learning, professional development and leadership), and (d) *environmental-structural arrangement* (i.e., cleanliness, curricular and extracurricular offerings). More recently, Thapa et al. (2013), in a review study, pinpointed five essential dimensions of school climate: (a) *safety* (e.g., rules and norms, physical safety, emotional safety), (b) *relationships* (e.g., respect for diversity, social support, leadership, and students' race and ethnicity and their perceptions of school climate), (c) *teaching and learning* (e.g., social, emotional, civic and ethical education, service learning, support for academic learning, support for professional relationships, teachers' and students' perceptions), (d) *institutional environment* (e.g., school connectedness/engagement, physical layout and surroundings of school, resources, supplies), and (e) *the school improvement process* (e.g., professional capacity, order, safety and norms, parent community ties, instructional guidance).

To summarize, the consistent pattern evident across independent research investigations is that school climate is a cluster of interconnected and intertwined variables (e.g., relationships, safety, teaching, and learning) that significantly impact student and teacher outcomes. Examining closely the relationship between school climate and student outcomes would allow stakeholders to analyze further actions for school change.

School Climate and Student Academic and Behavioral Outcomes

A substantial body of empirical evidence has shown that school climate is significant in promoting positive student well-being and academic outcomes (e.g., Daily et al., 2019). Specifically, researchers have long suggested that a positive school climate is positively associated with a variety of academic-related measures, including student achievement (e.g., Benbenishty et al., 2016; Jones & Shindler, 2016; Wang et al., 2014), student engagement in school activities (e.g., Lombardi et al., 2019), school motivation (e.g., Dincer, 2021), and student perceived quality of life satisfaction (e.g., Zullig et al., 2018).

For the academic domain, Daily and colleagues (2019) focused on middle and high-school students to explore the relationship between school climate and academic achievement. Their findings suggest that under a positive school climate, both student populations felt content with the amount of work received, confident in completing required assignments, and showed overall academic satisfaction. What was interesting in their study, but not tested statistically, was the fact that positive levels of school climate had a stronger effect on middle-school students' academic performance than among high-school students. Researchers concluded that a positive school climate seemed an important factor in student academic achievement at the middle school level.

For the socio-emotional and behavioral domain, research findings show that a sustained positive school climate promotes student social, mental, and emotional well-being (e.g., Lester & Cross, 2015) and thus, it is associated with reduced violence, aggression, and antisocial behavior (Konold et al., 2017; Li et al., 2021; Manzano-Sánchez et al., 2021), fewer sexual harassment experiences (e.g., Crowley et al., 2021), and reduced bully victimization and delinquency (e.g., Aldridge et al., 2018; Wang et al., 2013). For example, Thapa et al. (2013), in their review study, examined 206 records and, among others, reported a positive relationship between school climate and lower levels of drug use and school suspensions, as well as enhanced psychological well-being. Similarly, Aldridge and McChesney (2018) highlighted the importance of school climate in influencing adolescents' mental health, such as their psychosocial well-being (e.g., self-esteem, self-efficacy, positive mental health) and their preventative and prosocial behaviors (e.g., resilience, positive coping strategies). In another study, Aldridge et al. (2018) found that aspects of positive school climate, such as school connectedness, rule clarity, and teacher support, were negatively associated with bully victimization and delinquency, suggesting that by modifying school climate variables, safety-related behaviors can be increased (e.g., Zacharia & Yablon, 2021).

To sum up, school climate plays a central role in impacting student academic and behavioral learning in schools. Changes to school climate affect student outcomes. In the era of raising student academic achievement and promoting 21st-century skills to students, educational stakeholders should consider regulating school policies and introducing empirically-based educational innovations (e.g., whole-school approaches) that alter school climate positively.

School Climate and International Policies

Given the growing body of research documenting a strong association between school climate and academic and socio-emotional well-being, policymakers have considered such findings in their action planning and school initiatives. For example, the NCSSLE, funded by the United States (U.S.) Office of Safe and Healthy Students (OSHS, 2016) has developed a theoretical framework, training packages, and improvement tools (e.g., action guides, online modules, etc.) for guiding school staff to understand and improve school climate and its associated conditions. The NCSSLE has made its resources publicly available, encouraging school districts to invest in school climate improvement by assessing, intervening, and monitoring its progress. Recently, the Council of European Union (2022) prioritized early school leaving and low achievement in education by providing recommendations to member states on promoting a positive learning climate and whole-school approaches. According to the Pupils' Well-Being Policy Framework (Schola Europaea/Office of the Secretary-General, 2022), European schools are devoted to providing a safe and secure academic environment to all members. The European framework encourages schools to address ongoing and upcoming difficulties (e.g., child protection, anti-bullying, good behavior, anti-substance use, and safety) by developing and implementing local policies to protect, promote, and fulfill the rights of their students.

Consequently, extant research suggests that school climate is a fundamental collective measure that strongly impacts student outcomes. If students are to thrive academically and socially in schools, researchers and educational stakeholders should closely examine the relationship between school climate, school safety, and student outcomes.

School Climate, School Safety, and Student Outcomes

In this section, we examine the relationships between school climate and school safety and school safety with student learning outcomes.

School safety is defined as the level of physical and emotional security offered by the school, as well as the existence of effective, consistent, and fair school "rules and norms" (Thapa et al., 2013; Wang & Degol, 2016). School safety and climate are correlated concepts (e.g., Cornell & Huang, 2019). Promoting a positive school climate may be a key factor in enhancing school safety (e.g., Zacharia & Yablon, 2021). Specifically, when students perceive the school climate as positive and the school personnel as supportive and caring, they are more likely to follow school safety rules and improve their social behaviors (e.g., NCSSLE, n.d.; Wang et al., 2013). On the other hand, when students perceive school climate as negative, unjust, and unsupportive, then such school environment provides the social context for negative behaviors to flourish (see Wang et al., 2013).

A safe school environment strongly impacts students' emotional well-being, academic performance, and social outcomes (see Kutsyuruba et al., 2015). For example, in a meta-analysis of social and emotional learning interventions aiming at increasing school safety and reducing problem behaviors, Durlak et al. (2011) reported improvements in social and emotional skills, attitudes toward self and school, and social behaviors. Similarly, Côté-Lussier and Fitzpatrick (2016), in a longitudinal study with 1,234 adolescents, investigated the relationship between students' feelings of safety and their tendency to follow directions, finish their work on time, and work effortfully and autonomously in the classroom. Their results revealed that students who felt safer were more engaged in the classroom, demonstrated fewer depressive symptoms, and reported less victimization. Conversely, feeling physically or emotionally unsafe in school may be a significant barrier to academic and socio-emotional well-being (e.g., Thapa et al., 2013). In schools lacking supporting norms, structures, and connections, students are more likely to face violence, peer victimization, and harsh disciplinary measures, leading to increased absenteeism and poor academic success (e.g., Astor et al., 2010; Lacoe, 2020).

In a nutshell, any school improvement efforts to support student academic and socio-emotional learning and staff well-being should consider the strong associations between school climate and safety as well as student safety and learning outcomes.

Research-Based Approaches for Improving School Climate

A safe, predictable, and positive school climate is critical to building effective school environments. When whole-school approaches are designed and implemented in schools, student and teacher perceptions of school climate change positively (e.g., Charlton et al., 2021). Specifically, Bradshaw and colleagues (2021), in their literature review on school climate, proposed three predominant types of research-based strategies or frameworks for improving school climate. The first framework aims to improve the whole-school environment through comprehensive approaches that establish a common set of behavioral expectations across the school context and involve all relevant stakeholders in prevention. For example, the Olweus Bullying Prevention Program (OBPP; Olweus et al., 2007) is one approach of a whole-school strategy aiming to improve school climate and prevent non-safety related behaviors, such as bullying. The OBPP is not a circumscribed program but instead a set of principles, procedures, and mechanisms designed to create a safe and positive school climate (e.g., student activities supervision, meetings, school-wide anti-bullying rules, school-wide Bullying Prevention Coordinating Committee, school-community partnerships). The program's outcomes have shown reductions in students' reports of bullying-related behaviors, decreases in students' antisocial behaviors, and improvements in school climate (see Olweus 2005). Recently, Olweus et al. (2020) have highlighted the favorable long-term effects of the program, suggesting the importance of creating a safe and positive school climate where bullying-related problems are systematically addressed and prevented. Another whole-school example is the

School-Wide Positive Behavioral Interventions and Supports (SWPBIS), which is the focus of this chapter and will be presented in the next section.

The second framework that enhances school climate focuses on interventions designed to strengthen students' socio-emotional and cognitive development in ways that potentially impact the school's climate (Bradshaw et al., 2021). For example, social and emotional learning (SEL) programming aims to create a safe and supportive learning environment through the development of five core social and emotional competencies: self-awareness, self-management, social awareness, relationship-building skills, and responsible decision-making (CASEL, 2015; Weissberg et al., 2015). A recent meta-analysis found that SEL interventions that encourage the development of social and emotional assets through school-based interventions yielded significant improvement in SEL skills, positive attitudes, prosocial behavior, and academic performance at follow-up periods ranging from 56 to 195 weeks (Taylor et al., 2017). However, regarding school climate outcomes, not all programs and approaches to SEL are effective, as they rarely improve all school climate dimensions (see Bradshaw et al., 2021). Recent efforts have incorporated SEL program implementation within a whole-school approach to create an equitable and positive school climate (Mahoney et al., 2021) (for further analysis, readers may check the chapter *"Strengthening the Socio-Emotional Skills of Students at Risk for Mental Health Issues Within School-Wide Positive Behavioral Interventions and Supports"*).

The third framework emphasizes the role of the physical environment in enhancing school climate (e.g., Bradshaw et al., 2021). In some studies, aspects of the physical environment of the schools, including general cleanliness and security measures, were associated with school climate and specifically with its safety dimension. For instance, in Plank et al.'s (2009) study, the physical characteristics of the school, such as the absence of broken windows, were related to increased perceived safety among students. Similarly, Lindstrom Johnson et al. (2012) highlighted the role of the physical environment (e.g., security cameras) in preventing school violence. However, Voight and Nation (2016) provided moderate evidence for the effectiveness of the school's physical characteristics (i.e., cleanliness and maintenance, natural surveillance, number of custodians) on students' achievement, attendance, and safety perceptions.

As presented thus far, research has been clear that any educational changes to student learning outcomes should take into account school-wide changes (namely physical environment, school systems and procedures, practices, school climate, etc). Changing the school's organizational framework requires an orchestrated effort with substantial planning, technical assistance support and strong theoretical foundations. The section below describes in detail such efforts to improve school climate and student outcomes.

School-Wide Positive Behavioral Interventions and Supports (SWPBIS): An Empirically-Validated Whole-School Framework

School-wide Positive Behavioral Interventions and Supports (SWPBIS) is a well-established implementation framework for maximizing the selection and use of evidence-based prevention and intervention practices within a multi-tiered continuum to support the academic, social, emotional, and behavioral competence of all students (Center on Positive Behavioral Interventions and Supports, 2024). An extensive research knowledge base has been established in the U.S. (e.g., Santiago-Rosario et al., 2023) and across the world (e.g., Kourea & Phtiaka, 2023; Kubiszewski & Carrizales, 2024; Närhi, Kiiski, Peits, & Savolainen, 2015; Ogden et al., 2012; Willemse et al., 2022), documenting the SWPBIS effectiveness in improving school and student outcomes for more than three decades.

SWPBIS was conceptualized originally in the U.S. during the mid-90s by a group of practitioners and researchers who worked together to develop, implement, and evaluate school practices and procedures for establishing a safe, positive, and predictable school environment for all students and with specific emphasis on the ones with disabilities (Horner & Sugai, 2015; Sugai & Horner, 2020). Incorporating scientific knowledge from the implementation and systems logic (Fixsen et al., 2005), SWPBIS expanded with large-scale implementations (e.g., Sadler, 2000; Simonsen et al., 2010) and has been widely adopted by all 50 states of U.S. Specifically, in the 2022-2023 school year, more than 27,500 schools across the 50 states of the U.S. implemented SWPBIS with local state support (Center on PBIS, 2024). In Europe, SWPBIS cultural adaptations and initial explorations began approximately a decade later (e.g., Sørlie, & Ogden, 2007; Kourea et al., 2016; Närhi et al., 2013; Nelen et al., 2020). Soon enough, SWPBIS efforts expanded in Europe, which led to the establishment of the Positive Behavior Support-Europe Network (Goei & Kourea, 2017), attracting initially more than 19 European countries (Kourea & Goei, 2018). Concurrently, implementation efforts continued in other parts of the world, such as Australia (Barker et al., 2023; Hepburn, 2022), Canada (Kelm et al., 2014), Japan (Ohkubo et al., 2022; Otsui et al., 2022), etc.

Research on SWPBIS expands from systematic reviews (e.g., Horner et al., 2010; Lee & Gage, 2020), exploratory (e.g., Ross et al., 2012), quasi-experimental (e.g., Colvin & Fernandez, 2000; McIntosh et al., 2013; Deltour et al., 2021), experimental single-case design studies (e.g., Gladney et al., 2021) to large-scale randomized trials (e.g., Bradshaw et al., 2009, 2012; Weist et al., 2022). SWPBIS has been implemented across elementary (e.g., Horner et al., 2009; Kelm et al., 2014), middle (e.g., Sprague et al., 2017), and high school (e.g., Bradshaw et al., 2021; Estrapala et al., 2021), with the latter school level requiring more time for the SWPBIS implementation to start and grow. Noteworthy, SPWBIS framework has been adopted in alternative settings (for further review see Grasley-Boy et al., 2021) such as special schools (e.g., Simonsen et al., 2010), juvenile system structures (e.g., Kumm et al., 2020; Lopez et al., 2015), residential facilities for students with disabilities (e.g., Ennis et al., 2012), and family environments (e.g., Center on PBIS & Center for Parent Information & Resources, 2020).

Evidence from this plethora of research methodology and implementation sites has demonstrated that it is important to invest in SWPBIS because both students and teachers benefit substantially. Specifically, improved student outcomes include problem behavior reductions (Horner et al., 2009; Kelm et al., 2014), increases in student social competencies (e.g., Bradshaw et al., 2012, 2015; McIntosh et al., 2011), reduced rates of bullying and peer rejection (Ross et al., 2009; Waasdorp et al., 2012), increased attendance (Freeman et al., 2016), lowered rates of externalizing problem behaviors (Benner et al., 2012), and improved academic achievement (e.g., Angus et al., 2021; Madigan et al., 2016). For instance, Angus and colleagues analyzed archival data from eight middle schools (n=8515 students) of an urban American school district where SWPBIS was mandated. Their results demonstrated that the SWPBIS implementation positively impacted student academic scores, and this association was stronger as schools implemented the SWPBIS fully and with fidelity. Previously, McIntosh et al. (2011) evaluated 11 elementary schools and one secondary school (n=3800 students) over a five-year period to determine the effects of SWPBIS on academic achievement. Comparing schools that implemented SWPBIS with high fidelity and those with low fidelity, data showed that student academic achievement scores exceeded the district's average for the school cohort that SWPBIS implementation maintained high fidelity. Interestingly, the latter school cohort included a higher rate of families from low socioeconomic status compared to the school cohort that SWPBIS implementation was with low fidelity.

SWPBIS investigations have also demonstrated improved teacher outcomes on positive school climate (Bradshaw et al., 2008; Elrod et al., 2022; McIntosh et al., 2021) and school safety perceptions (e.g., Bradshaw et al., 2021; Horner et al., 2009), improved school organizational health perceptions (Bradshaw et al., 2008; Flannery et al., 2014), decreased rates of office discipline referrals and suspensions (Bradshaw et al., 2010) and increased teacher well-being and efficacy (Ross et al., 2012). Interpreting the above findings further, it is evident that when teachers feel supported and safe in a school environment, their perceptions of school climate and safety shift. For instance, longitudinal findings indicate that teachers' perceptions of school climate increased after multiple years of SWPBIS implementation for elementary (see Bradshaw et al., 2008) and middle school teachers (see Caldarella et al., 2011). In their group randomized control study, Bradshaw and her colleagues collected data from 2,596 elementary teachers on school climate over a five-year period of SWPBIS implementation. Their findings suggest that school climate (as measured by collegial leadership and institutional integrity) was impacted positively when SWPBIS practices were in place and were implemented with fidelity. Recently, Elrod et al. (2021) concurred with previous findings showing that additional years of SWPBIS implementation were associated with higher fidelity and stronger school climate, as measured by 204,701 students in 288 middle and high schools.

The recent work by Rutherford and colleagues (2022) sheds light on identifying specific SWPBIS elements that may contribute to improvements in school climate. After controlling for demographic variables (e.g., gender, race, years of teaching experience) among 490 teachers, they found that explicit teaching of schoolwide behavioral expectations and a well-defined hierarchy of strategies for discouraging unexpected behaviors positively predicted staff perceptions of school climate. On the contrary, a strong reinforcement system and district support negatively predicted staff school climate perceptions. Such findings are interpreted within the urban school context, where most students came from ethnically diverse backgrounds and the majority of teachers were White. Identifying explicit behavioral teaching as a strong predictor of positive teacher perceptions of school climate suggests that this strategy allowed teachers to be more positive, clear, and fair to their diverse learners so students felt respected. Rutherford's findings provide several implications for teacher professional development as listed in the last section.

SWPBIS has expanded and sustained over the years compared to other initiatives because it is not a curriculum program or a packaged social skill intervention (Gion et al., 2020; Sugai & Horner, 2020). Instead, it is a collection of empirically-based practices orchestrated in a continuum using the implementation framework logic, which permits school stakeholders to progress in the stages of implementation based on internal and external resources available.

SWPBIS Three-tiered Continuum and Its Core Elements

SWPBIS aims to establish an inclusive, non-discriminatory social culture and necessary socio-emotional and behavioral support for all students in a school. It is a systems-change approach that enhances the capacity of schools, families, and communities to design effective and efficient learning environments that (a) address student needs by providing a continuum of supports; (b) regularly monitor the implementation of evidence-based practices (EBPs) and outcomes, and (c) follow data-based decision making through continuous data-collection process (Horner, Sugai, & Lewis, 2015). This systems-change approach requires at least a 3-to-5-year investment to efficiently differentiate behavioral instruction for all students across three tiers, as presented in Figure 1 (Center on PBIS, 2024) (for further analysis, readers may check the chapter "Strengthening the Socio-Emotional Skills of Students at Risk for Mental Health Issues Within School-Wide Positive Behavioral Interventions and Supports").

Figure 1. SWPBIS Three-tiered Continuum of Supports

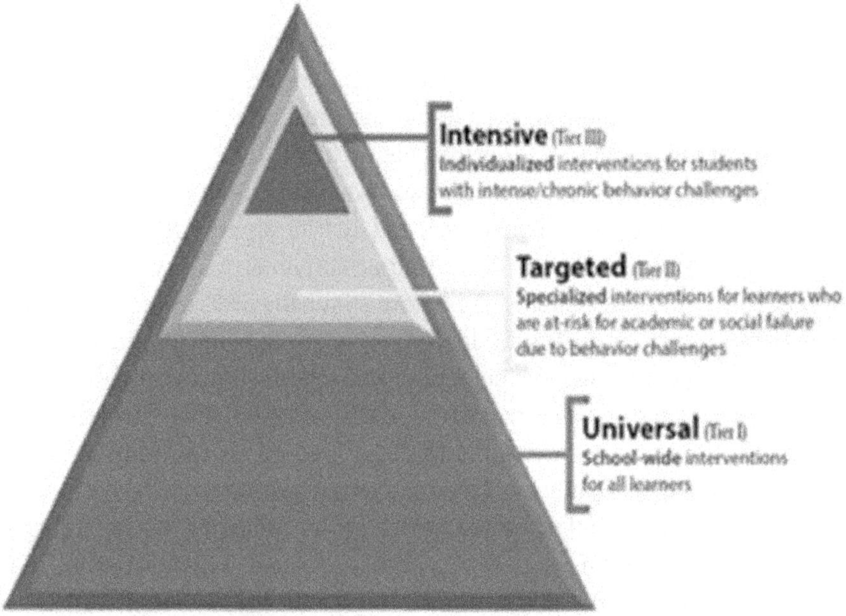

Intensive (Tier III)
Individualized interventions for students with intense/chronic behavior challenges

Targeted (Tier II)
Specialized interventions for learners who are at-risk for academic or social failure due to behavior challenges

Universal (Tier I)
School-wide interventions for all learners

Tier 1 support (Universal/Primary prevention) is built on the assumption that all students can exhibit appropriate behavior. As a result, school staff is trained, coached, and supported to assess the contextual setting events and environmental conditions and incorporate evidence-based practices and resources to increase the probability of appropriate behavior. Teachers work to effectively teach, encourage, and model school-wide expectations (e.g., respect, safety, responsibility) and appropriate behaviors (e.g., respect means using kind words and actions) to all students across all school areas (e.g., classroom, hallways, playground). The staff engages families and students in developing a universally positive and inclusive language about the school's vision and mission, identifying schoolwide expectations, teaching explicitly expected behaviors and routines, recognizing student and teacher positive behaviors, and providing specific positive feedback on student social errors inside and outside of classrooms. Teachers are trained and supported through an active SWPBIS leadership team and an external SWPBIS coach. Families are encouraged to use the common language and schoolwide expectations at home. Tier 1 support is critical because it sets the structural framework of each school that shifts from reactive, exclusionary negative approaches and moves to proactive systems where the emphasis is relational building. This effort cohesively unites all the adults using 1) common language, 2) common practices, and 3) common procedures. Current research evidence on Tier 1 points out the importance of implementing Tier 1 with fidelity before moving to Tiers 2 and 3 (Horner & Sugai, 2015). Doing so produces the maximum behavioral and academic outcomes for students.

Tier 2 supports (Secondary Prevention) are for those students whose social and academic needs are more intense and who would benefit from additional layers of instructional support. Interventions are usually of low intensity and can be administered by school personnel with high efficiency. A Tier 2 school team is established to coordinate intervention efforts. Family members become involved by providing consent to their child's receiving support and becoming involved, where applicable, in the intervention. Moving to Tier 2 means that the school has already met the readiness criteria for Tier 2 participation and has been implementing Tier 1 with more than 80% fidelity (Bruhn & McDaniel, 2021).

Tier 3 supports (Tertiary prevention) are provided to non-responders to Tiers 1 and 2 and focus on individual students who exhibit chronic behavioral difficulties. For these students, schools would need to provide intensive individual support. At this stage, the collaboration between school and family is continuous for designing and implementing an individualized student support plan (Sugai et al., 2000).

For each prevention tier, SWPBIS incorporates five essential interconnected elements: equity, systems, data, practices, and outcomes. Table 1 describes in detail how each core element is integrated into each level of support.

Table 1. SWPBIS Core Elements for Each Prevention Tier

Prevention Tier	Core Elements	
Tier 1 (Primary)	Equity:	Assessing and incorporating aspects of student and teacher culture in school decisions and procedures.
	Systems:	Tier 1 leadership team
	Practices:	School vision and schoolwide expectations defined, explicit teaching of schoolwide expectations, schoolwide acknowledgement system, continuum of consequences for problem behaviors
	Data:	Data collection on academic and behavioral student performance, data analysis for decision making
	Outcomes:	Student improvement of academic and social behaviors School climate improvement

continued on following page

Table 1. Continued

Prevention Tier		Core Elements
Tier II (Secondary)	*Equity:*	Assessing and incorporating aspects of student and teacher culture in school decisions and procedures.
	Systems:	Tier 2 leadership team
	Practices:	Universal screening, system for increasing structure and predictability, system for increasing contingent adult feedback, system for linking academic and behavioral performance, system for increasing family-school communication
	Data:	Progress monitoring of student performance, data analysis for decision making
	Outcomes:	Student improvement of academic and social behaviors Minimizing the number of students with at-risk status
Tier III (Tertiary)	*Equity:*	Assessing and incorporating aspects of student and teacher culture in school decisions and procedures.
	Systems:	Tier 3 leadership team
	Practices:	Functional behavioral assessment, system for connecting academic and behavioral supports, wraparound services provisions, individualized intervention plans based on: (a) prevention of problem contexts, (b) instruction on functionally equivalent skills, and instruction on desired performance skills, (c) strategies for placing problem behavior on extinction, (d) strategies for enhancing contingent reward of desired behavior, and (e) use of negative or safety consequences if needed.
	Data:	Team-based comprehensive assessment, student progress monitoring, data analysis for decision making
	Outcomes:	Minimizing the chronic impact of behavioral and/or academic difficulties on student performance

Equity is a newly added core element in the tiered logic to ensure that all learners, regardless of diverse backgrounds, have their individual needs met and are held to high expectations. It is placed at the center of all elements as the emphasis is on supporting teachers in adapting practices to ensure success for everyone. *Systems* are the procedures that school staff use to receive support, be trained, and be coached. For each level of prevention, leadership is established to ensure that teachers are guided in implementing evidence-based practices and are supported to meet student needs. *Data* are gathered to determine student progress and implementation fidelity at each tier. Depending on the school context, teachers collect academic and behavioral data that should analyze and make effective decisions about student outcomes and SWPBIS implementation. *Practices* are empirically-validated strategies and tools incorporated during instruction to support student academic and socio-emotional needs. Whatever instructional decisions teachers make at each tier should be supported with empirical evidence. *Outcomes* are the overall school goal in which data, systems, practices, and equity are included. School, student, and family needs define outcomes. Both school staff and families work together to meet identified outcomes.

The core elements of SWPBIS are integrated within organizational systems in which teams, working with administrators and behavior specialists, provide the training, policy and organizational supports needed for (a) initial implementation, (b) active application, and (c) sustained use of the core elements (Sugai & Horner, 2020).

SWPBIS Implementation Fidelity and School Climate

Students get to learn and grow in school environments where the school climate is positive, the staff is consistent in their instructional support, and caring relationships with all students are promoted. To establish a positive school climate, school staff should ensure that SWPBIS is implemented with high fidelity. When schools implement the SWPBIS framework with fidelity, students flourish academically and socio-emotionally (e.g., Bradshaw et al., 2008; Ellis et al., 2022; Elrod et al., 2021; McIntosh et al., 2021).

In a major data analysis, La Salle-Finley (2024) compared elementary (n=184,940), middle (n=130,867), and high (n=100,041) school students on their school climate perceptions based on the level of SWPBIS implementation fidelity (low, approaching, at fidelity). Her findings demonstrated that students attending elementary and middle schools with fidelity had significantly higher perceptions of school climate than their peers from SWPBIS schools with lower levels of fidelity. No significant impact of SWPBIS fidelity was documented on student perceptions of school climate at the high school level. However, the relationship between perceptions of school climate and SWPBIS implementation fidelity was significant for culturally and linguistically diverse students across all school levels. La Salle-Finley's findings lend support to previous research (e.g., Bradshaw et al., 2008), stating that SWPBIS can positively impact the school climate when systems and practices are implemented with fidelity. Moreover, her findings demonstrate that SWPBIS can create a safe and positive learning environment for diverse learners regardless of age. Charlton et al.'s (2021) systematic review of the impact of schoolwide intervention programs on student and teacher perceptions of school climate concluded that the way SWPBIS is carefully and systematically implemented produced large effect sizes on teacher ($d=1.03$) and student ($d=1.93$) perceptions of school climate compared to other schoolwide intervention programs. The authors recommended that systematic and rigorous fidelity measures should be taken into account when schoolwide intervention programs are implemented, and those fidelity tools need to be aligned with the emphasis that the schoolwide intervention gives. In the SWPBIS example, the fidelity measures incorporated consider staff efforts on aspects of school climate (e.g., relationships, safety). Such alignment allows researchers and staff to develop targeted efforts in sustaining SWPBIS systems and practices.

SWPBIS Implementation Sustainability

As stated earlier, SWPBIS is a widely adopted framework worldwide for enhancing student socio-emotional, behavioral, and academic outcomes. The degree to which schools produce positive student outcomes depends greatly on the degree to which school staff implements SWPBIS procedures with fidelity and consistently over time (Center on PBIS, 2024). Interestingly enough, SWPBIS implementation has sustained over the decades compared to other educational initiatives, and part of the reason is the fact that SWPBIS was designed not to be a predefined curriculum but an organizational framework that is adjusted to the needs and capacities of every organization in different countries (Gion et al., 2020; Sugai & Horner, 2020). In their recent systematic review, Fox and his colleagues (2021) identified 22 variables among 29 research studies that may be facilitators or barriers to a successful and sustainable SWPBIS implementation. Specifically, the identified *facilitators* included access to resources to support implementation (e.g., time, materials, funding), effective leadership team, effective use of data, consistent implementation with fidelity, supportive leadership, access to ongoing training, staff buy-in to SWPBIS, school characteristics, access to external expertise and support, contextually relevant adaptation of SWPBIS, effective communication about the purpose and outcomes of SWPBIS implementation efforts, and district characteristics.

The most commonly identified *barriers* included staff beliefs that conflict with SWPBIS philosophy, low fidelity implementation, lack of access to necessary resources, school characteristics (e.g., school size, school level), lack of supportive leadership, lack of staff buy-in, lack of staff understanding about the purpose and principles of SWPBIS implementation, lack of student and family involvement, school climate, and high levels of staff turnover. When prioritizing the above factors with respect to their importance, Fox et al. listed four important facilitators to sustained implementation: adequate resources, strong fidelity of implementation, effective leadership team, and meaningful data collection and use (McIntosh et al., 2013). The successors for a sustainable SWPBIS framework highlight some implications for practice concerning policy stakeholders, teacher training, and family involvement.

Implications for Practice

Policy stakeholders are in a position to define and mandate educational initiatives to schools. However, whatever it is asked from schools to become involved needs to align with existing school needs and expected outcomes. If a mismatch occurs between school goals and policy stakeholders' decisions, then the educational initiative is deemed to fail. Thus, SWPBIS is designed in a way that allows schools to meet their identified needs (i.e., improving student social competencies, improving school climate). Its framework sets the foundation for school staff to organize their practices and procedures, and SWPBIS, when implemented with fidelity, provides opportunities for improving school climate and school safety.

To increase initial staff buy-in, school administrators present to staff the rationale for SWPBIS implementation and explain how SWPBIS will address school needs. Data and other forms (e.g., student attendance, problem behaviors recorded, low academic achievement, diverse ethnic student population) of evidence are presented to teachers to justify school needs. Administrators initiate individual and group conversations with teachers about the importance of the whole-school approach, teacher gains obtained, and student behavioral changes acquired. During the initial exploration phase, school leaders may contact other schools with more experience in SWPBIS implementation and exchange perspectives on how the school-wide approach has impacted students, teachers, and families. Having open and honest conversations about the "why" allows for a smooth transition to the implementation phase.

When a school decides to implement the SWPBIS framework, teachers are the driving force for change. They are asked to work with colleagues, discuss and agree on universal practices, and follow similar implementation procedures. For teachers with many years of teaching experience, this change does not come easy. It is imperative to incorporate systematic coaching and short professional development trainings to enhance teacher efforts in implementing schoolwide practices successfully and with fidelity. School administration should be mindful of the number of school initiatives introduced to staff. When teachers are asked to make a change in their daily practices, administrators must provide the time and space for the change to happen. Introducing several educational initiatives and asking for teacher involvement increases the risk of low-quality of SWPBIS implementation or teacher resistance to SWPBIS practices. Conversely, when teachers commit and become actively involved in the SWPBIS, student behaviors change. With SWPBIS, teachers' consistency in teaching, providing practice, and acknowledging positive behaviors lays the foundation for teaching with respect and care. These values are important for all students, but more so for the ones who experience social and academic hardships.

Finally, schoolwide intervention approaches that are carefully designed and implemented with fidelity, such as SWPBIS, produce positive teacher and student socio-emotional and behavioral outcomes. However, families and community members play a significant role in incorporating schoolwide practices and expectations in non-school settings, thus increasing the likelihood of creating holistic, safe, predictable, and positive learning environments for all.

REFERENCES

Aldridge, J. M., & Fraser, B. J. (2016). Teachers' views of their school climate and its relationship with teacher self-efficacy and job satisfaction. *Learning Environments Research*, 19(2), 291–307. DOI: 10.1007/s10984-015-9198-x

Aldridge, J. M., Fraser, B. J., Fozdar, F., Ala'i, K., Earnest, J., & Afari, E. (2016). Students' perceptions of school climate as determinants of wellbeing, resilience and identity. *Improving Schools*, 19(1), 5–26. DOI: 10.1177/1365480215612616

Aldridge, J. M., & McChesney, K. (2018). The relationships between school climate and adolescent mental health and wellbeing: A systematic literature review. *International Journal of Educational Research*, 88, 121–145. DOI: 10.1016/j.ijer.2018.01.012

Aldridge, J. M., McChesney, K., & Afari, E. (2018). Relationships between school climate, bullying and delinquent behaviours. *Learning Environments Research*, 21(2), 153–172. DOI: 10.1007/s10984-017-9249-6

Angus, G., & Nelson, R. B. (2021). School-Wide Positive Behavior Interventions and Supports and student academic achievement. *Contemporary School Psychology*, 25(4), 443–465. DOI: 10.1007/s40688-019-00245-0

Astor, R. A., Guerra, N., & Van Acker, R. (2010). How can we improve school safety research? *Educational Researcher*, 39(1), 69–78. DOI: 10.3102/0013189X09357619

Barker, K., Poed, S., & Whitefield, P. (2023). *School-wide Positive Behaviour Support: The Australian handbook*. Routledge.

Bear, G. G., Gaskins, C., Blank, J., & Chen, F. F. (2011). Delaware school climate survey–student: Its factor structure, concurrent validity, and reliability. *Journal of School Psychology*, 49(2), 157–174. DOI: 10.1016/j.jsp.2011.01.001 PMID: 21530762

Beaudoin, H., & Roberge, G. (2015). Student perceptions of school climate and lived bullying behaviours. *Procedia: Social and Behavioral Sciences*, 174, 213–330. DOI: 10.1016/j.sbspro.2015.01.667

Benbenishty, R., Astor, R. A., Roziner, I., & Wrabel, S. L. (2016). Testing the causal links between school climate, school violence, and school academic performance: A cross-lagged panel autoregressive model. *Educational Researcher*, 45(3), 197–206. DOI: 10.3102/0013189X16644603

Benner, G. J., Nelson, J. R., Sanders, E. A., & Ralston, N. C. (2012). Behavior intervention for students with externalizing behavior problems: Primary-level standard protocol. *Exceptional Children*, 78(2), 181–198. DOI: 10.1177/001440291207800203

Bradshaw, C., Waasdorp, T., & Leaf, P. (2012). Examining the variation in the impact of School-wide Positive Behavioral Interventions and Supports. *Pediatrics*, 10(5), 1136–1145. DOI: 10.1542/peds.2012-0243

Bradshaw, C. P., Cohen, J., Espelage, D. L., & Nation, M. (2021). Addressing school safety through comprehensive school climate approaches. *School Psychology Review*, 50(2–3), 221–236. DOI: 10.1080/2372966X.2021.1926321

Bradshaw, C. P., Koth, C. W., Bevans, K. B., Ialongo, N., & Leaf, P. J. (2008). The impact of school-wide positive behavioral interventions and supports (PBIS) on the organizational health of elementary schools. *School Psychology Quarterly*, 23(4), 462–473. DOI: 10.1037/a0012883

Bradshaw, C. P., Koth, C. W., Thornton, L. A., & Leaf, P. J. (2009). Altering school climate through school-wide positive behavioral interventions and supports: Findings from a group-randomized effectiveness trial. *Prevention Science*, 10(2), 100–115. DOI: 10.1007/s11121-008-0114-9 PMID: 19011963

Bradshaw, C. P., Mitchell, M. M., & Leaf, P. J. (2010). Examining the effects of Schoolwide Positive Behavioral Interventions and Supports on student outcomes: Results from a randomized controlled effectiveness trial in elementary schools. *Journal of Positive Behavior Interventions*, 12(3), 133–148. DOI: 10.1177/1098300709334798

Bradshaw, C. P., Pas, E. T., Debnam, K. J., & Johnson, S. L. (2021). A randomized controlled trial of MTSS-B in high schools: Improving classroom management to prevent EBDs. *Remedial and Special Education*, 42(1), 44–59. DOI: 10.1177/0741932520966727

Bradshaw, C. P., Waasdorp, T. E., & Leaf, P. J. (2015). Examining variation in the impact of school-wide positive behavioral interventions and supports: Findings from a randomized controlled effectiveness trial. *Journal of Educational Psychology*, 107(2), 546–557. DOI: 10.1037/a0037630

Brand, S., Felner, R. D., Seitsinger, A., Burns, A., & Bolton, N. (2008). A large-scale study of the assessment of the social environment of middle and secondary schools: The validity and utility of teachers' ratings of school climate, cultural pluralism, and safety problems for understanding school effects and school improvement. *Journal of School Psychology*, 46(5), 507–535. DOI: 10.1016/j.jsp.2007.12.001 PMID: 19083370

Bruhn, A. L., & McDaniel, S. C. (2021). Tier 2: Critical issues in systems, practices, and data. *Journal of Emotional and Behavioral Disorders*, 29(1), 34–43. DOI: 10.1177/1063426620949859

Caldarella, P., Shatzer, R. H., Gray, K. M., Young, R. K., & Young, E. L. (2011). The effects of School-wide Positive Behavior Support on middle school climate and student outcomes. *RMLE Online: Research in Middle Level Education*, 35(4), 1–14. DOI: 10.1080/19404476.2011.11462087

CASEL. (2015). *Effective social and emotional learning programs: Middle and high school education*. Author.

Center on Positive Behavioral Interventions and Supports. (2024). *PBIS: An evidence-based framework for making schools safe, positive, predictable, and equitable*. Center on PBIS, University of Oregon. www.pbis.org

Center on Positive Behavioral Interventions and Supports & Center for Parent Information & Resources. (2020). *Supporting families with PBIS at home*. University of Oregon. www.pbis.org

Charlton, C. T., Moulton, S., Sabey, C. V., & West, R. (2021). A systematic review of the effects of schoolwide intervention programs on student and teacher perceptions of school climate. *Journal of Positive Behavior Interventions*, 23(3), 185–200. DOI: 10.1177/1098300720940168

Cohen, J. (2006). Social, emotional, ethical, and academic education: Creating a climate for learning, participation in democracy, and well-being. *Harvard Educational Review*, 76(2), 201–237. DOI: 10.17763/haer.76.2.j44854x1524644vn

Cohen, J., McCabe, E. M., Michelli, N. M., & Pickeral, T. (2009). School climate: Research, policy, practice, and teacher education. *Teachers College Record*, 111(1), 180–213. DOI: 10.1177/016146810911100108

Collie, R. J., Shapka, J. D., & Perry, N. E. (2012). School climate and social–emotional learning: Predicting teacher stress, job satisfaction, and teaching efficacy. *Journal of Educational Psychology*, 104(4), 1189–1204. DOI: 10.1037/a0029356

Colvin, G., & Fernandez, E. (2000). Sustaining effective behavior support systems in an elementary school. *Journal of Positive Behavior Interventions*, 2(4), 251–253. DOI: 10.1177/109830070000200414

Cornell, D., & Huang, F. (2019). Collecting and analyzing local school safety and climate data. In Mayer, M. J., & Jimerson, S. R. (Eds.), *School safety and violence prevention: Science, practice, policy* (pp. 151–175). American Psychological Association. DOI: 10.1037/0000106-007

Côté-Lussier, C., & Fitzpatrick, C. (2016). Feelings of safety at school, socioemotional functioning, and classroom engagement. *The Journal of adolescent health: official publication of the Society for Adolescent Medicine, 58*(5), 543–550.

Council of the European Union. (2022). *Council recommendation of 28 November 2022 on pathways to school success and replacing the council Recommendation of 28 June 2011 on policies to reduce early school leaving.*https://eur-lex.europa.eu/legal-content/EN/TXT/PDF/?uri=CELEX:32022H1209(01)

Crowley, B. Z., Cornell, D., & Konold, T. (2021). School climate moderates the association between sexual harassment and student well-being. *School Mental Health*, 13(4), 695–706. DOI: 10.1007/s12310-021-09449-3

Daily, S. M., Mann, M. J., Kristjansson, A. L., Smith, M. L., & Zullig, K. J. (2019). School climate and academic achievement in middle and high school students. *The Journal of School Health*, 89(3), 173–180. DOI: 10.1111/josh.12726 PMID: 30680750

Deltour, C., Dachet, D., Monseur, C., & Baye, A. (2021). Does SWPBIS increase teachers' collective efficacy? Evidence from a quasi-experiment. *Frontiers in Education*, 6, 720065. DOI: 10.3389/feduc.2021.720065

Dincer, B. (2021). Investigating the school climate perceptions and school motivations of middle school students. *International Journal of Educational Methodology*, 7(2), 361–372. DOI: 10.12973/ijem.7.2.361

Durlak, J. A., Weissberg, R. P., Dymnicki, A. B., Taylor, R. D., & Schellinger, K. B. (2011). The impact of enhancing students' social and emotional learning: A meta-analysis of school-based universal interventions. *Child Development*, 82(1), 405–432. DOI: 10.1111/j.1467-8624.2010.01564.x PMID: 21291449

Ellis, K., Gage, N. A., Kramer, D., Baton, E., & Angelosante, C. (2022). School climate in rural and urban schools and the impact of SWPBIS. *Rural Special Education Quarterly*, 41(2), 73–83. DOI: 10.1177/87568705221098031

Elrod, B. G., Rice, K. G., & Meyers, J. (2022). PBIS fidelity, school climate, and student discipline: A longitudinal study of secondary schools. *Psychology in the Schools*, 59(2), 376–397. DOI: 10.1002/pits.22614

Ennis, R. P., Jolivette, K., Swoszowski, N. C., & Johnson, M. L. (2012). Secondary prevention efforts at a residential facility for students with emotional and behavioral disorders: Function-based check-in, check-out. *Residential Treatment for Children & Youth*, 29(2), 79–102. DOI: 10.1080/0886571X.2012.669250

Estrapala, S., Rila, A., & Bruhn, A. L. (2021). A systematic review of tier 1 PBIS implementation in high schools. *Journal of Positive Behavior Interventions*, 23(4), 288–302. DOI: 10.1177/1098300720929684

European Council. (2022). Pathways to school success. *Official Journal of the European Union, C*, 496, 1–15. https://eur-lex.europa.eu/legal content/EN/TXT/PDF/?uri=CELEX:32022H1209(01)

Falcon, S., Izzard, S., & Bastable, E. (2021). Effects of an equity-focused PBIS approach to school improvement on exclusionary discipline and school climate. *Preventing School Failure*, 65(4), 354–361. DOI: 10.1080/1045988X.2021.1937027

Fixsen, D. L., Naoom, S. F., Blase, K. A., Friedman, R. M., & Wallace, F. (2005). *Implementation research: A synthesis of the literature* (FMHI Publication No. 231). University of South Florida, Louis de la Parte Florida Mental Health Institute, National Implementation Research Network.

Flannery, K. B., Fenning, P., Kato, M. M., & McIntosh, K. (2014). Effects of school-wide positive behavioral interventions and supports and fidelity of implementation on problem behavior in high schools. *School Psychology Quarterly*, 29(2), 111–124. DOI: 10.1037/spq0000039 PMID: 24188290

Fox, R. A., Leif, E. S., Moore, D. W., Furlonger, B., Anderson, A., & Sharma, U. (2022). A systematic review of the facilitators and barriers to the sustained implementation of school-wide positive behavioral interventions and supports. *Education & Treatment of Children*, 45(1), 105–126. DOI: 10.1007/s43494-021-00056-0

Freeman, J., Simonsen, B., McCoach, D. B., Sugai, G., Lombardi, A., & Horner, R. (2016). Relationship between school-wide positive behavior interventions and supports and academic, attendance, and behavior outcomes in high schools. *Journal of Positive Behavior Interventions*, 18(1), 41–51. DOI: 10.1177/1098300715580992

Freiberg, H. J., & Stein, T. A. (1999). Measuring, improving and sustaining healthy learning environments. In Freiberg, H. J. (Ed.), *School climate: Measuring, improving and sustaining healthy learning environments* (pp. 11–29). Falmer Press.

Gion, C., Peshak George, H., Nese, R., McGrath Kato, M., Massar, M., & McIntosh, K. (2020). School-wide Positive Behavioral Interventions and Supports. In Reschly, A. L., Pohl, A. J., & Christenson, S. L. (Eds.), *Student engagement: Effective academic, behavioral, cognitive, and affective interventions at school* (pp. 171–184). Springer. DOI: 10.1007/978-3-030-37285-9_10

Gladney, D., Lo, Y.-y., Kourea, L., & Johnson, H. N. (2021). Using multilevel coaching to improve general education teachers' implementation fidelity of culturally responsive social skill instruction. *Preventing School Failure*, 65(2), 175–184. Advance online publication. DOI: 10.1080/1045988X.2020.1864715

Goei, S. L., & Kourea, L. (2017). Positive Behaviour Support Europe Network. *Remediaal*, 17(4-5), 5–8.

Grasley-Boy, N. M., Reichow, B., van Dijk, W., & Gage, N. (2021). A systematic review of tier 1 PBIS implementation in alternative education settings. *Behavioral Disorders*, 46(4), 199–213. DOI: 10.1177/0198742920915648

Grazia, V., & Molinari, L. (2020). School climate multidimensionality and measurement: A systematic literature review. *Research Papers in Education*, 36(5), 561–587. DOI: 10.1080/02671522.2019.1697735

Haynes, N. M., Emmons, C., & Ben-Avie, M. (1997). School climate as a factor in student adjustment and achievement. *Journal of Educational & Psychological Consultation*, 8(3), 321–329. DOI: 10.1207/s1532768xjepc0803_4

Hepburn, L. (2022). Installation of school-wide positive behaviour support in government schools: Queensland experiences. *International Journal of Positive Behavioural Support*, 12(1), 13–20.

Horner, R., Sugai, G., Smolkowski, K., Todd, A., Nakasato, J., & Esperanza, J. (2009). A randomized control trial of School-wide Positive Behavior Support in elementary schools. *Journal of Positive Behavior Interventions*, 11(3), 113–144. DOI: 10.1177/1098300709332067

Horner, R. H., & Sugai, G. (2015). School-wide PBIS: An example of Applied Behavior Analysis implemented at a scale of social importance. *Behavior Analysis in Practice*, 8(1), 80–85. DOI: 10.1007/s40617-015-0045-4 PMID: 27703887

Horner, R. H., Sugai, G., & Anderson, C. M. (2010). Examining the evidence base for school-wide positive behavior support. *Focus on Exceptional Children*, 42(8). Advance online publication. DOI: 10.17161/foec.v42i8.6906

Horner, R. H., Sugai, G., & Lewis, T. (2015). *Is school-wide positive behavior support an evidence-based practice?* Center on PBIS.

Jones, A., & Shindler, J. (2016). Exploring the school climate-student achievement connection: Making sense of why the first precedes the second. *Educational Leadership and Administration*, 27, 35–51.

Kelm, J. L., McIntosh, K., & Cooley, S. (2014). Effects of implementing school-wide positive behavioural interventions and supports on problem behaviour and academic achievement in a Canadian elementary school. *Canadian Journal of School Psychology*, 29(3), 195–212. DOI: 10.1177/0829573514540266

Klik, K. A., Cárdenas, D., & Reynolds, K. J. (2023). School climate, school identification and student outcomes: A longitudinal investigation of student well-being. *The British Journal of Educational Psychology*, 93(3), 806–824. DOI: 10.1111/bjep.12597 PMID: 37068920

Konold, T., Cornell, D., Shukla, K., & Huang, F. (2017). Racial/ethnic differences in perceptions of school climate and its association with student engagement and peer aggression. *Journal of Youth and Adolescence*, 46(6), 1289–1303. DOI: 10.1007/s10964-016-0576-1 PMID: 27663576

Kourea, L., & Goei, S. (2018). *Developing network efforts in PBS across Europe*. Poster presentation at the 15th International Conference of the Association for Positive Behavior Support (APBS), Denver, CO.

Kourea, L., Lo, Y.-y., Scardina, T., & Phtiaka, H. (2016). Implementing schoolwide positive behavior support across diverse elementary schools in the United States and in Cyprus. [University of Nevada-Las Vegas & University of Nicosia.]. *Proceedings of the Building Bridges Among Researchers and Practitioners: Special Education Conference*, II, 16–24.

Kourea, L., & Phtiaka, H. (2023). Initial exploration and implementation efforts of SWPBIS Tier 1 in Cyprus: Results from two model demonstration sites. *Exceptionality*, 31(5), 395–415. DOI: 10.1080/09362835.2023.2266534

Kubiszewski, V., & Carrizales, A. (2024). Effects of school-wide positive behavioral interventions and supports on students' perceptions of teachers' practices. *European Journal of Psychology of Education*. Advance online publication. DOI: 10.1007/s10212-024-00848-z

Kumm, S., Mathur, S. R., Cassavaugh, M., & Butts, E. (2020). Using the PBIS Framework to meet the mental health needs of youth in juvenile justice facilities. *Remedial and Special Education*, 41(2), 80–87. DOI: 10.1177/0741932519880336

Kutsyuruba, B., Klinger, D., & Hussain, A. (2015). Relationships among school climate, school safety, and student achievement and well-being: A review of the literature. *Review of Education*, 3(2), 103–135. DOI: 10.1002/rev3.3043

La Salle-Finley, T. (2024). *School climate and PBIS fidelity*. Center on PBIS, University of Oregon.

Lacoe, J. (2020). Too scared to learn? The academic consequences of feeling unsafe in the classroom. *Urban Education*, 55(10), 1385–1418. DOI: 10.1177/0042085916674059

Lee, A., & Gage, N. A. (2020). Updating and expanding systematic reviews and meta-analyses on the effects of school-wide positive behavior interventions and supports. *Psychology in the Schools*, 57(5), 783–804. DOI: 10.1002/pits.22336

Lee, E., Reynolds, K. J., Subasic, E., Bromhead, D., Lin, H., Marinov, V., & Smithson, M. (2017). Development of a dual school climate and school identification measure–student (SCASIM-St). *Contemporary Educational Psychology*, 49, 91–106. DOI: 10.1016/j.cedpsych.2017.01.003

Li, Z., Yu, C., & Nie, Y. (2021). The association between school climate and aggression: A moderated mediation model. *International Journal of Environmental Research and Public Health*, 18(16), 8709. DOI: 10.3390/ijerph18168709 PMID: 34444470

Lindstrom Johnson, S., Burke, J. G., & Gielen, A. C. (2012). Urban students' perceptions of the school environment's influence on school violence. *Children & Schools*, 34(2), 92–102. DOI: 10.1093/cs/cds016 PMID: 26726297

Lombardi, E., Traficante, D., Bettoni, R., Offredi, I., Giorgetti, M., & Vernice, M. (2019). The impact of school climate on well-being experience and school engagement: A study with high-school students. *Frontiers in Psychology*, 10, 2482. DOI: 10.3389/fpsyg.2019.02482 PMID: 31749747

Lopez, A., Williams, J. K., & Newsom, K. (2015). PBIS in Texas juvenile justice Department's division of education and state programs: Integrating programs and developing systems for sustained implementation. *Residential Treatment for Children & Youth*, 32(4), 344–353. DOI: 10.1080/0886571X.2015.1113460

Madigan, K., Cross, R. W., Smolkowski, K., & Strycker, L. A. (2016). Association between schoolwide positive behavioural interventions and supports and academic achievement: A 9-year evaluation. *Educational Research and Evaluation*, 22(7–8), 402–421. DOI: 10.1080/13803611.2016.1256783

Mahoney, J. L., Weissberg, R. P., Greenberg, M. T., Dusenbury, L., Jagers, R. J., Niemi, K., Schlinger, M., Schlund, J., Shriver, T. P., VanAusdal, K., & Yoder, N. (2021). Systemic social and emotional learning: Promoting educational success for all preschool to high school students. *The American Psychologist*, 76(7), 1128–1142. DOI: 10.1037/amp0000701 PMID: 33030926

Malinen, O.-P., & Savolainen, H. (2016). The effect of perceived school climate and teacher efficacy in behavior management on job satisfaction and burnout: A longitudinal study. *Teaching and Teacher Education*, 60, 144–152. DOI: 10.1016/j.tate.2016.08.012

Manzano-Sánchez, D., Gómez-Mármol, A., Valero-Valenzuela, A., & Jiménez-Parra, J. F. (2021). School climate and responsibility as predictors of antisocial and prosocial behaviors and violence: A study towards self-determination theory. *Behavioral Sciences (Basel, Switzerland)*, 11(3), 36. DOI: 10.3390/bs11030036 PMID: 33802667

Maxwell, L. E. (2016). School building condition, social climate, student attendance and academic achievement: A mediation model. *Journal of Environmental Psychology*, 46, 206–216. DOI: 10.1016/j.jenvp.2016.04.009

Maxwell, S., Reynolds, K. J., Lee, E., Subasic, E., & Bromhead, D. (2017). The impact of school climate and school identification on academic achievement: Multilevel modeling with student and teacher data. *Frontiers in Psychology*, 8, 2069. DOI: 10.3389/fpsyg.2017.02069 PMID: 29259564

McIntosh, K., Bennett, J. L., & Price, K. (2011). Evaluation of social and academic effects of School-wide Positive Behaviour Support in a Canadian school district. *Exceptionality Education International*, 21(1), 46–60. DOI: 10.5206/eei.v21i1.7669

McIntosh, K., Mercer, S., Hume, A., Frank, F., Turri, M., & Mathews, S. (2013). Factors relate to sustained implementation of schoolwide positive behavior support. *Exceptional Children*, 79(3), 293–311.

McIntosh, K., Girvan, E. J., McDaniel, S. C., Santiago-Rosario, M. R., St. Joseph, S., Fairbanks Falcon, S., & Bastable, E. (2021). Effects of an equity-focused PBIS approach to school improvement on exclusionary discipline and school climate. *Preventing School Failure*, 65(4), 354–361.

Molinari, L., & Grazia, V. (2023). Students' school climate perceptions: Do engagement and burnout matter? *Learning Environments Research*, 26(1), 1–18. DOI: 10.1007/s10984-021-09384-9

Moos, R. H. (1979). *Evaluating educational environments: Procedures, measures, findings and policy implications*. Jossey-Bass.

Närhi, V., Kiiski, T., Peitso, S., & Savolainen, H. (2014). Reducing disruptive behaviours and improving learning climates with class-wide positive behaviour support in middle schools. *European Journal of Special Needs Education*, 30(2), 274–285. DOI: 10.1080/08856257.2014.986913

National Center on Safe Supportive Learning Environments. (n.d.). *School climate improvement*.https://safesupportivelearning.ed.gov/school-climate-improvement

National School Climate Council. (2007). *The school climate challenge: narrowing the gap between school climate research and school climate policy, practice guidelines and teacher education policy*.http://www.ecs. org/school-climate

Nelen, M. J., Willemse, T. M., van Oudheusden, M. A., & Goei, S. L. (2020). Cultural challenges in adapting SWPBIS to a Dutch context. *Journal of Positive Behavior Interventions*, 22(2), 105–115. DOI: 10.1177/1098300719876096

Oder, T., & Eisenschmidt, E. (2018). Teachers' perceptions of school climate as an indicator of their beliefs of effective teaching. *Cambridge Journal of Education*, 48(1), 3–20. DOI: 10.1080/0305764X.2016.1223837

Office of Safe and Healthy Students (OSHS). (2016). *Quick guide on making school climate improvements*. U.S. Department of Education. https://safesupportivelearning .ed.gov/SCIRP/Quick-Guide

Ogden, T., Sørlie, M.-A., Arnesen, A., & Meek-Hansen, W. (2012). The PALS School-Wide Positive Behaviour Support model in Norwegian primary schools – Implementation and evaluation. In J. Visser, H. Daniels, and T. Cole, (Ed.) *Transforming troubled lives: Strategies and interventions for children with social, emotional and behavioural difficulties* (*International Perspectives on Inclusive Education, Vol. 2*) (pp. 39-55). Emerald Group Publishing Limited. DOI: 10.1108/ S1479-3636(2012)0000002006

Ohkubo, K., Tsukimoto, H., Otsui, K., Tanaka, Y., Noda, W., & Niwayama, K. (2022). Effectiveness and social validity of Tier 1 intervention with school-wide positive behavioural support in a public elementary school in Japan. *International Journal of Positive Behavioural Support*, 12(2), 4–18.

Olweus, D. (2005). A useful evaluation design, and effects of the Olweus Bullying Prevention Program. *Psychology, Crime & Law*, 11(4), 389–402. DOI: 10.1080/10683160500255471

Olweus, D., Limber, S. P., Flerx, V. C., Mullin, N., Riese, J., & Snyder, M. (2007). *Olweus Bullying Prevention Program: Schoolwide guide*. Hazelden.

Olweus, D., Solberg, M. E., & Breivik, K. (2020). Long-term school-level effects of the Olweus Bullying Prevention Program (OBPP). *Scandinavian Journal of Psychology*, 61(1), 108–116. DOI: 10.1111/sjop.12486 PMID: 30277582

Otsui, K., Niwayama, K., Ohkubo, K., Tanaka, Y., & Noda, W. (2022). Introduction and development of school-wide positive behavioural support in Japan. *International Journal of Positive Behavioural Support*, 12(2), 19–28.

Perry, A. C. (1919). *The management of a city school*. The Macmillan Company.

Plank, S. B., Bradshaw, C. P., & Young, H. (2009). An application of "broken-windows" and related theories to the study of disorder, fear, and collective efficacy in schools. *American Journal of Education*, 115(2), 227–247. DOI: 10.1086/595669

Reaves, J. S., & Cozzens, J. A. (2018). Teacher perceptions of climate, motivation, and self-efficacy: Is there really a connection? *Journal of Education and Training Studies*, 6(12), 48–67. DOI: 10.11114/jets.v6i12.3566

Ross, S. W., Horner, R. H., & Higbee, T. (2009). Bully prevention in positive behavior support. *Journal of Applied Behavior Analysis*, 42(4), 747–759. DOI: 10.1901/jaba.2009.42-747 PMID: 20514181

Ross, S. W., Romer, N., & Horner, R. H. (2012). Teacher well-being and the implementation of school-wide positive behavior interventions and support. *Journal of Positive Behavior Interventions*, 14(2), 118–128. DOI: 10.1177/1098300711413820

Rudasill, K. M., Snyder, K. E., Levinson, H., & Adelson, L., J. (. (2018). Systems view of school climate: A theoretical framework for research. *Educational Psychology Review*, 30(1), 35–60. DOI: 10.1007/s10648-017-9401-y

Rutherford, L. E., Hier, B. O., McCurdy, B. L., Mautone, J. A., & Eiraldi, R. (2023). Aspects of School-wide Positive Behavioral Interventions and Supports that predict school climate in urban settings. *Contemporary School Psychology*, 27(3), 534–544. DOI: 10.1007/s40688-022-00417-5

Sadler, C. (2000). Effective behavior support implementation at the district level: Tigard-Tualatin school district. *Journal of Positive Behavior Interventions*, 2(4), 241–243. DOI: 10.1177/109830070000200411

Santiago-Rosario, M. R., McIntosh, K., Izzard, S., Cohen-Lissman, D., & Calhoun, T. E. (2023). *Is Positive Behavioral Interventions and Supports (PBIS) an evidence-based practice?* Center on PBIS. https://www.pbis.org/resource/is-school-wide-positive-behavior-support-an-evidence-based-practice

Saputra, W. N. E., Supriyanto, A., Astuti, B., Ayriza, Y., & Adiputra, S. (2020). The effect of student perception of negative school climate on poor academic performance of students in Indonesia. *International Journal of Learning. Teaching and Educational Research*, 19(2), 279–291.

Schola Europaea/Office of the Secretary-General. (2022). *Pupils' Well-Being Policy Framework of the European Schools.* https://www.eursc.eu/BasicTexts/2022-01-D-6-en-2.pdf

Simonsen, B., Britton, L., & Young, D. (2010). Schoolwide positive behavior support in an alternative school setting. *Journal of Positive Behavior Interventions*, 12(3), 180–191. DOI: 10.1177/1098300708330495

Sørlie, M.-A., & Ogden, T. (2007). Immediate impacts of PALS: A school-wide multi-level programme targeting behaviour problems in elementary school. *Scandinavian Journal of Educational Research*, 51(5), 471–492. DOI: 10.1080/00313830701576581

Sprague, J. R., Biglan, A., Rusby, J. C., Gau, J. M., & Vincent, C. G. (2017). Implementing school wide PBIS in middle schools: Results of a randomized trial. *Journal of Health Science & Education*, 1(2), 1–10.

Sugai, G., & Horner, R. H. (2020). Sustaining and scaling Positive Behavioral Interventions and Supports: Implementation drivers, outcomes, and considerations. *Exceptional Children*, 86(2), 120–136. DOI: 10.1177/0014402919855331

Sugai, G., Horner, R. H., Dunlap, G., Hieneman, M., Lewis, T. J., Nelson, C. M., Scott, T., Liaupsin, C., Sailor, W., Turnbull, A. P., Turnbull, H. R.III, Wickham, D., Wilcox, B., & Ruef, M. (2000). Applying positive behavior support and functional behavioral assessment in schools. *Journal of Positive Behavior Interventions*, 2(3), 131–143. DOI: 10.1177/109830070000200302

Tanner-Smith, E. E., Fisher, B. W., Addington, L. A., & Gardella, J. H. (2018). Adding security, but subtracting safety? Exploring schools' use of multiple visible security measures. *American Journal of Criminal Justice*, 43(1), 102–119. DOI: 10.1007/s12103-017-9409-3

Taylor, R. D., Oberle, E., Durlak, J. A., & Weissberg, R. P. (2017). Promoting positive youth development through school-based social and emotional learning interventions: A meta-analysis of follow-up effects. *Child Development*, 88(4), 1156–1171. DOI: 10.1111/cdev.12864 PMID: 28685826

Thapa, A., Cohen, J., Guffey, S., & Higgins-D'Alessandro, A. (2013). A review of school climate research. *Review of Educational Research*, 83(3), 357–385. DOI: 10.3102/0034654313483907

Van Houtte, M. (2005). Climate or culture? A plea for conceptual clarity in school effectiveness research. *School Effectiveness and School Improvement*, 16(1), 71–89. DOI: 10.1080/09243450500113977

Voight, A., & Nation, M. (2016). Practices for improving secondary school climate: A Systematic review of the research literature. *American Journal of Community Psychology*, 58(1-2), 174–191. DOI: 10.1002/ajcp.12074 PMID: 27535489

Waasdorp, T., Bradshaw, C., & Leaf, P. (2012). The impact of School-wide Positive Behavioral Interventions and Supports on bullying and peer rejection: A randomized controlled effectiveness trial. *Archives of Pediatrics & Adolescent Medicine*, 166(2), 149–156. DOI: 10.1001/archpediatrics.2011.755 PMID: 22312173

Wang, C., Berry, B., & Swearer, S. M. (2013). The critical role of school climate in effective bullying prevention. *Theory into Practice*, 52(4), 296–302. DOI: 10.1080/00405841.2013.829735

Wang, M.-T., & Degol, J. L. (2016). School climate: A review of the construct, measurement, and impact on student outcomes. *Educational Psychology Review*, 28(2), 315–352. DOI: 10.1007/s10648-015-9319-1

Wang, W., Vaillancourt, T., Brittain, H. L., McDougall, P., Krygsman, A., Smith, D., Cunningham, C. E., Haltigan, J. D., & Hymel, S. (2014). School climate, peer victimization, and academic achievement: Results from a multi-informant study. *School Psychology Quarterly: The Official Journal of the Division of School Psychology, American Psychological Association*, 29(3), 360–377. DOI: 10.1037/spq0000084 PMID: 25198617

Weissberg, R. P., Durlak, J. A., Domitrovich, C. E., & Gullotta, T. P. (2015). Social and emotional learning: Past, present, and future. In Durlak, J. A., Domitrovich, C. E., Weissberg, R. P., & Gullotta, T. P. (Eds.), *Handbook of social and emotional learning: Research and practice* (pp. 3–19). The Guilford Press.

Weist, M. D., Splett, J. W., Halliday, C. A., Gage, N. A., Seaman, M. A., Perkins, K. A., Perales, K., Miller, E., Collins, D., & DiStefano, C. (2022). A randomized controlled trial on the interconnected systems framework for school mental health and PBIS: Focus on proximal variables and school discipline. *Journal of School Psychology*, 94, 49–65. DOI: 10.1016/j.jsp.2022.08.002 PMID: 36064215

Willemse, T. M., Goei, S. L., Boei, F., & de Bruïne, E. J. (2022). School-wide positive behaviour interventions and support in Dutch schools for special education. *European Journal of Special Needs Education*, 38(3), 424–443. DOI: 10.1080/08856257.2022.2120331

Yang, C., Chan, M. K., Nickerson, A. B., Jenkins, L., Xie, J. S., & Fredrick, S. S. (2022). Teacher victimization and teachers' subjective well-being: Does school climate matter? *Aggressive Behavior*, 48(4), 379–392. DOI: 10.1002/ab.22030 PMID: 35383978

Zacharia, M. G., & Yablon, Y. B. (2021). School bullying and students' sense of safety in school: The moderating role of school climate. *European Journal of Psychology of Education*, 37(3), 903–919. DOI: 10.1007/s10212-021-00567-9

Zullig, K. J., Ward, R. M., Huebner, S. E., & Daily, S. M. (2018). Association between adolescent school climate and perceived quality of life. *Child Indicators Research*, 11(6), 1737–1753. DOI: 10.1007/s12187-017-9521-4

Chapter 2
Establishing Your Strategy:
How to Make Use of Shared Resources Whilst Tailoring to the Needs of Your School

Sarah Holmes
Liverpool Hope University, UK

Vicky Sinclair
Liverpool Hope University, UK

ABSTRACT

Informed by our professional experience and empirical research in the UK, we highlight principles and approaches which could be integrated into the development of strategies of primary schools seeking to support children's mental health and wellbeing. We consider the challenges and opportunities of implementing research-informed approaches in schools, and the balance between maintaining individuality and context specific support in each school, whilst collaborating with other schools to share resources, training opportunities and expertise. Our research findings revealed the need for bespoke and context-specific strategies, rather than using externally produced frameworks or curricula. However, the staff interviews also showed the value of groups of schools working together to support and equip one another in shaping their vision and ethos. Approaches which were implemented holistically across the school were more effective and valuable, and communication across the whole staff body further supported the implementation and effectiveness within the whole school community.

DOI: 10.4018/979-8-3693-5325-7.ch002

1. INTRODUCTION

Amongst discussion related to promotion of mental health in schools, it is key to focus on development of a context-specific strategy. Schools often express the value of promoting mental health and know what they would like to do but often struggle with knowing where to start as there are so many challenges and needs. Many schools pick up and implement ideas which they have seen elsewhere or curricula which are heavily promoted or incentivised, but these are often disparate and can lack direction in terms of meeting the needs of staff and children in their specific school. Others, perhaps, have a curricula imposed on them by their governance, partnership schools or similar. Many will be restricted from purchasing a scheme due to funding limitations, whilst others feel that they do not have the time or resources to focus on mental health at all since they are firefighting so many issues and situations on a daily basis. Therefore, formulating a strategy for individual schools is key, but this can be complex since schools often work in groups, such as Multi-Academy Trusts, educational groups or other permutations of partnerships and collaborations. Partnerships across schools, through either semi-formal formats such as supportive networks akin to 'critical friends' or formal regulated routes such as a Multi-Academy Trust are becoming more prevalent. Given the current funding limitations within schools, collaborative working can serve to produce the best outcomes for children by sharing resources, knowledge and best practice. Yet constructing a strategy for mental health and wellbeing to align with the needs of a broad range of schools is highly complex. This chapter therefore shares research-informed insights into how schools can establish their own bespoke approaches to support children's wellbeing, whilst simultaneously building and drawing upon wider support from partnership schools.

2. BACKGROUND

Vicky Sinclair has extensive experience teaching in UK primary schools (ages 3 to 11 years old), and more recently working as a teacher educator in Higher Education. This experience has been primarily in areas of deprivation in Northwest England. The combination of personal classroom experience, research and reading has supported the implementation of many new approaches, and has instigated changes to her own pedagogy and practice both in the classroom and across school. Having worked on many projects in school to support children and build partnerships, she can attest to the difference being 'research informed' can make.

Sarah Holmes has worked primarily in the third sector, always with a desire to support the development and holistic development of children. Working with children and families in community-based settings, she has learned first-hand the importance of listening to individuals and responding accordingly by reflecting on and adjusting practice to best meet the needs of those involved. Involvement over the past ten years in Higher Education, specifically research, have provided invaluable opportunities to work with schools, community provision and charities to refine and enhance their practice.

Together, they carried out empirical research in summer 2023, exploring the well-being approaches adopted in a group of schools in Northwest England. They were keen to find out what was working well and what was less effective, in addition to examining the extent to which these approaches were individual to each school context, or whether they could be implemented at a group level. The research findings are published elsewhere (Holmes and Sinclair, 2024 pending), but this chapter will illuminate how the findings could inform schools in establishing their strategy for supporting children's mental health and wellbeing.

3. HOW RESEARCH CAN INFORM YOUR STRATEGY

Research to underpin practice in the classroom has always been central to good educational approaches, although research into school mental health strategies has often been more difficult to apply (Lyon and Burns, 2019). Nevertheless, attentiveness to this has grown over many years, especially in Higher Educational settings in England, and is one of the key expectations of a 'professional'. The UK's Core Content Framework (CCF), which outlines the minimum expectations of teacher training, further demonstrates the drive to embed research to inform teaching practices, stating that research findings are independently assessed and endorsed by the Education Endowment Foundation (Department for Education, 2019). The scope of this framework was broadened in 2024, with an updated version published. Central to this framework is the drive for practitioners and teachers to focus on what research is saying and how to use best practice in classrooms. Further to this, in English education there has been a significant drive from statutory bodies such as the Department of Education and Office for Standards in Education, Children's Services and Skills (OfSTED)'s association with the Education Endowment Fund (EEF). This shows the importance of the role of research in support of teachers' ability to question and reflect on what they do, its impact and how it is fundamental to drive school improvement.

This chapter draws on findings from our own empirical research project, in conjunction with consideration of other published research findings in this field. Our empirical research occurred in a case study group of schools in England, with the aim of evaluating the approaches to children's well-being within the schools individually, but also as a collective of schools. The research comprised in-depth interviews with key staff members who were responsible for wellbeing at their school, with the aim of mapping the approaches to well-being intentionally embedded in the school, in addition to those which were more implicit. These interviews followed a semi-structured style so that we were able to focus on the approaches implemented within their specific school to promote wellbeing for their children and community. Crucial to our research was an exploration of how the schools made the choices they did and how the approaches and strategies were implemented. That is, how they varied or aligned across the group of schools, and the extent to which their choices reflected their local community needs and its social and economic context. Despite being within the same geographical region, the case study schools exhibited large differences in context, varying from affluent areas with many professional families to areas with social challenge and larger levels of need and unemployment. Our research sample was a group of seven primary schools, six of which are rated 'good' by Ofsted, and one as 'outstanding.' They worked together as a collective, with the overarching values of collaboration, respect and inspiration.

Participation of individual staff members was optional and voluntary, and participants were assured that their responses would be confidential. In order to mitigate against power relations from senior leadership, the invitation to participants was made by the research team, rather than school leadership. The project was approved by the ethics committee of Liverpool Hope University.

We utilised a qualitative comparative analysis as it enabled systematic and rigorous exploration of the complex and dynamic school contexts (Drozdova & Gaubatz, 2015) and facilitated the uncovering of reasons for change in the different school settings contexts. The comparative analysis was framed by the eight principles of a UK educational guidance document (Public Health England, 2021), to evaluate the effectiveness of each of the desired outcomes. Analysis of the dataset identified combination factors and patterns across the settings. Such an approach could be adopted by schools seeking to investigate and examine strategies for wider school improvement.

Our research findings ultimately highlighted the need for bespoke and context-specific strategies and approaches to be constructed and embedded within individual schools, rather than basing approaches on a framework or curricula which has been externally selected or imposed by an external body. However, we also identified from the data analysis the role which external bodies, such as a Multi-Academy Trust could serve, to scaffold, support and equip schools in the implementation of their bespoke vision and ethos. It was clear that approaches were much more effective and valuable when implemented holistically across the school rather than in individual curriculum elements, such as PHSE (Personal, Social and Health Education). Communication, collaboration, collegiality and investment across the whole staff team bespoke to each school but supported by a wider group of schools was seen to enhance the positive impact for the children and importantly their school community as a whole.

Drawing upon this empirical research base, this chapter presents our key reflections and insights into the processes and actions involved in formulating a research-informed strategy to enhance support for children's wellbeing in schools.

4. IDENTIFYING NEEDS

In the busy school environment, there are so many voices and needs which call out for attention. It can be hard, particularly with limited resources, to determine the hierarchy and importance of needs and how to respond to all needs appropriately, including perhaps those which are marginalised or quieter but indeed may be most pressing. Often those who are struggling most with their mental health may not be the ones shouting most loudly. This highlights why having an intentional approach to identify needs in your context is key to developing your overall strategy for supporting mental health and wellbeing.

Active and intentional listening. We all like to think that we are good at listening and hearing the needs of others. But making a choice to intentionally listen, in a methodical and active manner is so important as you are formulating your school's strategy for wellbeing (D'Alessandro et al., 2022). Schools often have bodies such as 'School Council' or interview children as part of the school Leadership Team's termly/yearly audit as 'child's voice.' These approaches are always well intentioned, although often the children selected are always those who are more erudite and more likely to be asked repeatedly, whereas the voices who struggle to be heard are those that we need to listen to the most. Equally, children are not always aware of what happens with this feedback and the impact that this might have on the school (Dolton et l., 2019). Alternative ways of achieving this may be to designate a set time and place and let it be known across the school that you want to hear about people's views and thoughts at this set time, in a very open manner. Perhaps, to aid ease of access for all pupils, you could rotate around each class every Tuesday afternoon for 30 minutes, visiting a different class each week and sitting listening to the children's views. It may be that many children find it hard to chat with you, akin to a formal interview, so you could try some play-based techniques, such as discussing the topic whilst playing with play doh or building blocks (Holmes, 2019). For example, you could ask the child to build their favourite part of school with the blocks and put in their favourite people (each person represented by a building block), and whilst the child is doing this, ask them about their favourite places and ask why. You could also ask which places they do not like and why. In this way, the child's focus is on the building blocks, releasing them to more freely explain their feelings and ideas to you. Similarly, you could use a hand puppet and ask the child to explain to the puppet the different feelings they have in different places around school and at different times of the school day. Again, this works well since it slightly takes the focus of the formal interaction of the child and teacher, and helps the child to feel more comfortable, telling the puppet about their views. Implementing these sorts of strategies of active and intentional listening will really help you to identify more clearly the pressing needs within your school community (Dolton et l., 2019).

Hearing the child's voice. Although primary schools have the child at the centre of all they do, it is often easy for the child's voice to be overlooked in the decision-making process. Some may feel that children do not know what is best for them or what their needs are when we ask about well-being or mental health. Others may simply be too busy or have such limited resources so feel that it is futile to ask children's suggestions, since the limitations will mean that the child's suggestions cannot happen, so there may be a feeling that it is not good to get the child's hopes up. Some may just never even think that children may have something to say on the subject. Indeed, in the five case study schools in our research, only one slightly involved children in decisions about mental health and wellbeing. Yet increasingly, the voice of children is being seen as fundamental to conversations and decisions regarding care and their environment (Dolton, Adams and & O'Reilly, 2020). So, listening to children's perspectives on what helps them to feel safe or their expectations of school staff are so key to capture as you are formulating a strategy to better meet the needs of children in your school.

Contextual conversations. It is so tempting to capture ideas which are working in other school settings, but simply because they are working in one context does not mean they will work elsewhere. Therefore, as you are developing a strategy for mental health which is specific to your setting, it is important that all of your conversations and deliberations are set in the context of your school, or relate to it directly and specifically. Huang et al. (2020) and Verhoog et al. (2022) emphasise the importance of applying specific tools and strategies in targeted and bespoke ways, in order to address the differing needs of each specific school context. This is particularly important if your school is working in collaboration with others - you can discuss common strategies and approaches but it is key that each strategy is then implemented in each school in context-specific ways. In order to do this, capturing input and feedback from different stakeholders is invaluable, such as a broad cross section of school staff, parents, and other professionals involved in the school community. In our research, it was evident that there were simultaneously opportunities and needs to work at both group and individual levels. Attentiveness to the uniqueness of children, families, schools and neighbourhoods of each school setting is key to identifying the needs and formulating a strategy for mental health and wellbeing.

Distinctiveness versus wider & universal approaches. With the expansion of online communication and the ability to share information and ideas so easily, there are more and more resources and curricula freely and easily available to schools around the world. However, often there is a temptation to pick up one of these such resources and use it as it has been written. Yet, this does not facilitate tailoring of the tool for your school context and the specific needs of your school community. Richter et al. (2022) highlighted the challenges of this. However, with the ever-present pressures upon modern-day teachers, we must be careful not to add further pressures and expectations, so as to negatively impact the mental health and wellbeing of teachers themselves. It is therefore key for you to be mindful of the need to balance your school's distinctiveness with universal approaches.

5. SOME FUNDAMENTAL PRINCIPLES

A common theme arising from our research project amongst the school conglomeration was the difficulty of having an overarching approach, vision and values to mental health and wellbeing, whilst meeting the needs of the diverse set of schools and settings within that group. Who should carry the responsibility for setting the values and why? The three group/trust values were collaboration, respect and inspiration, however the implementation of these differed across the individual schools, with some opting to retain these values and others establishing their own. This highlights the potential for the same words (school values) to be interpreted and implemented differently in different contexts. Careful choice of these words is key here as different words can carry different meaning for different people as found when initiating our own. There is also the possibility that these words may need to be altered in order to carry meaning for different ages of the children. Another question raised in the context of our research related to how these values reflected the importance of pupil mental health and wellbeing. Therefore, as you are starting to build your strategy, first it is key to consider some fundamental principles and values and think about how these will drive and shape the strategy for wellbeing in your school (Richter et al., 2022), but also, in our own experience, how this translates for families.

Basis of strategy. First consider intentionally what overall ethos you wish to build your school's strategy upon, for example Montessori, Froebel, or Maslow. Think about how these theoretical ideas can inform your school's strategy, and how pedagogy and different ways of learning dovetail with wellbeing approaches (Cavioni et al., 2020). School leaders are seasoned information-gatherers regarding what drives school improvement and what areas to focus on from year to year and cohort to cohort. Data is often context driven comprising areas such as number of children in the care system, number of unemployed families, number of children who would be classed as "summer born", children with SEND, or those new to the country. In my experience of using such an approach, starting from the information gathering stage, alongside more individualised methods such as taking time to watch children's developing patterns of behaviour and matching identified needs with approaches such as "creative" learning and "Possibility Thinking" based on the Craft, Cremin model can have a huge effect on children's engagement across the curriculum. Actual action will often sit alongside current areas of growth in academic research and this is true of the advancement in neuroscience and brain development. This has led to a flurry of research around self-regulation and metacognition in English education, which in turn has led to changes in pedagogical practices in schools. An example of this might be the recent growth in Nurture and Forest school-based pedagogy in schools. It is evident that school leaders are becoming more and more aware of the need to dovetail pedagogy across subject areas with research-informed wellbeing approaches and that a good sense of wellbeing leads to effective learning (Verhoog, 2022).

Reflection and evaluation. Embedding a reflective way of working from the start will enable you to gauge which parts of your strategy are working and which need refining. This should be an ongoing process, in order to continually develop and enhance your school's activity in this area (Huang, Edwards and Laurel-Wilson, 2020). This will enable you to ascertain the effectiveness of adding to staff workload, such as in one of our settings there was uncertainty about the value of having their 'worry monster,' and yet they continued with this despite the staff workload which it generated. Continuous evaluation should also consider the extent to which current strategies and approaches match the existing expertise of staff and whether the approaches either need to be tailored to maximise staff skills, or whether staff need further training to enable them to fully participate in the various details of your school's strategy.

Balancing universal and individual. Whilst developing your strategy, think carefully about different levels of support and intervention which are appropriate for your context, and reflect upon what can be implemented universally within the school, and what needs to be carried out on a small group or individual basis. There are advantages to implementing interventions or general practices universally - not least, the cost effectiveness and broad reach and impact (Verhoog et al., 2022). But universal preventive programs are also perceived to be less stigmatizing which contributes to the overall ethos of the whole school community and have been found to significantly reduce the internalizing of mental health problems such as stress, anxiety and depression symptoms (Cavioni et al., 2020). For example, having a whole-school (or MAT wide) approach to promoting and enhancing resilience in the children as a protective factor could lead to children in these schools being less prone to mental health problems such as depression and anxiety disorders. So, considering as a group of schools how specific targets, communications and activities could be implemented widely to foster and build resiliency amongst the children could be very impactful.

Collaboration. In shaping your strategy, there is a clear need to consider who and how you will collaborate within your approach to supporting mental health and wellbeing. This may be collaboration with other schools or external agencies. But it also may be enhanced involvement and engagement with families within the school community. Think about how policies within your school, or across your group of schools may facilitate or hinder collaboration. Policies such as safeguarding, building safety requirements and risk assessments all interact with the curriculum and overall school operation and ensure consistency is maintained across the schools and other schools. Yet schools still have the scope to adapt these approaches and policies in ways which best fit the needs of their own unique context. So think about what you want to achieve and which collaborations will foster this. What resources are already available? And what resource needs can you identify? What are the areas of expertise which already exist and how can these be nurtured, valued and used more? Knowing and valuing your workforce is key. What good links are already in place and what networks can be built on? Social support can serve as a highly effective protective factor (Huang et al., 2020), so think about building this into your emerging strategy.

Oversight and accountability. Whilst groups of schools can aid the sharing of resources or training opportunities, there is also significant value in a management or governing body providing healthy and constructive oversight of schools in their strategic work towards supporting children's mental health and wellbeing. This can be helpful in encouraging individual schools to keep on track with timelines and working towards targets (Lyon and Bruns, 2019). Such agencies serve schools well in keeping well-being on the agenda and ensuring that it is underpinning all of the ethos and activity of schools at individual and group level. Within this way of working though, it must be decided who will set the values, how they will be communicated and in what ways they will be implemented in bespoke and appropriate ways.

Value for money. This is undoubtedly one of the most challenging and most frustrating aspects of formulating a strategy. Limitations and restrictions are an ever-present reality for school leaders. So in forming and shaping your strategy, consider carefully how best value for money can be achieved as you support the children and families in your school community. External funding is sometimes available for groups of schools, so explore how this can be used best to invest across the whole school group and enhance opportunities (Lyon and Bruns, 2019). Examine how governing bodies or external agencies could support and facilitate the infrastructure which is needed. What is needed to boost the confidence of teachers in supporting children's wellbeing?

6. A FRAMEWORK FOR BUILDING YOUR STRATEGY

Our empirical research analysed the approaches of participant schools using a model devised for promoting a whole school approach to mental health and wellbeing (Public Health England, 2021), see figure 1. Overall, the schools unanimously raised frustration about limitations on their activity to support children's wellbeing due to funding restrictions. All of the staff reported substantial need for enhanced training, support and therapies for children in the school setting, more specialist staff within the school, more space within the school for calm or sensory zones, and greater access to external services for children on lengthy waiting lists. Participants also cited the challenges of time and space within the curriculum to be attentive to children's wellbeing, and also the challenges which often come from working with parents and carers.

Whilst we found that there were significant resourcing challenges expressed by the schools, we also discovered that there were many low cost but highly effective strategies utilised in some of these schools. It was surprising that many of these low cost ideas had not been shared across the other partnership schools. This highlighted the need for greater collaboration and communication across schools relating to children's wellbeing in order to enhance and embed an ethos of being supportive of children's wellbeing. We therefore offer our main research findings using this framework as a guide, since you can consider how these findings could inform your own strategy development.

Figure 1. Eight principles for promoting a whole school approach to mental health and wellbeing (Public Health England, 2021).

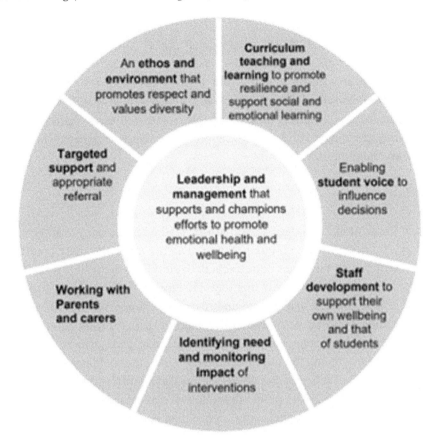

In this model, leadership and management is central to everything, yet our research revealed some ambiguity relating to the different layers of leadership and who would set the agenda and detail for each school's approaches to mental health and wellbeing. Leadership and management is therefore a helpful lens for considering how strategy can be devised and implemented in your school context.

All of the participant schools had a staff wellbeing team which sought to raise awareness and regularly promote activities to support staff wellbeing, as they expressed staff wellbeing to be key to ensuring children's wellbeing. Many explained explicit encouragement within their school for staff to take responsibility for their own wellbeing and to prioritise this. All of the schools also had staff wellbeing activities during the year. This ranged from counselling and advice services, to staff breakfasts, kindness projects and notes of encouragement. Some also gave staff time out of the classroom, specifically in response to traumatic or particularly challenging experiences which had occurred. Many of the respondents expressed that these efforts to support staff wellbeing were crucial since if staff morale is low, as it impacts upon the children.

All of the schools had staff allocated to a pastoral or wellbeing focus, and three schools had a child wellbeing team. This was made up of staff designated to work together to support specific children, but to also generally promote children's wellbeing across the school. This group usually comprised pastoral leads and often SENCO, since it was observed that SEND needs and wellbeing challenges often occurred simultaneously. This combined approach appeared to be highly beneficial in enhancing outcomes for the child.

Case Study

One of the schools had a designated pastoral lead who was present at the school gates every morning before children arrived. Parents knew that they could send this staff member text messages before school to alert the school staff if their child was struggling in a particular way that day. This meant that the pastoral lead was ready and able to provide appropriate and responsive support to the child as they arrived at school. This may be simple reassurance and support walking into school, or allowing the child to enter school through a different door, or even to arrive in their own clothes, carrying their uniform and dressing in school later once they felt able to. The impact of this was that absence rates had significantly fallen and there were fewer issues at the school gates. This allowed class teachers to focus more on the classroom experience and teaching, rather than being pulled out to deal with issues arising if some children were struggling to come into school. Parents also reported that they had found this to be very supportive and helpful to their family.

One school stated that they had reoriented their school systems so that they could provide enhanced wellbeing support for pupils without the need for additional funding, as they noted that funding was limited for them due to their demographics. They opted to provide support for children as required, even before obtaining a diagnosis or targeted funding. They had found that by adjusting the general ethos and environment of the whole school community and with adjustments to staffing structures, they were able to provide this enhanced support for children's wellbeing in their school.

Ethos and Environment

This aspect was the most frequently mentioned, with many of the schools talking of being inclusive and focussing on wellbeing throughout the whole school community. This universal focus on wellbeing communicated awareness that every child had different needs and emotions and hence acceptance and support should be given to aid universal understanding of one another. Others spoke of a desire to provide broader opportunities and experiences, whereby the schools were intentionally seeking to provide opportunities which the children may otherwise not have such as trips to specific places or visitors into school to augment school life. Across the partnership of schools, there were group-wide opportunities for children with a clear remit that these events must accommodate the needs of children from their diverse schools, so that all children had equal chance to win and not be unfairly disadvantaged due to socio-economic context and access to chargeable activities. Many described an ethos of reinforcing positive aspects by modelling and embedding positive conversations to build the children's self esteem and resilience. Equally, open and sensitive communication was expressed as being key to ensuring that information about individual children's needs was conveyed as necessary. All of these efforts are potentially highly impactful but are low cost. They depend however on how the structures and mechanisms within schools are set up.

Case Study

One example of the schools working together was to organise a recipe competition. All of the schools in the collective invited the children to write up a recipe of their favourite meal and explain why they liked it. This was designed to supplement the inter-school sports competitions, which usually only included children who enjoyed partaking in sports. This different focus on recipes successfully involved different children. There were a few winners from each school, and all of the winners from each school were invited to a local restaurant to have lunch together during school one day. (The restaurant kindly donated the meal.) The children involved thoroughly enjoyed this and felt affirmed and valued for their different ideas and expression about food, rather than feeling excluded if they were not proficient at sport. Other similar and diverse opportunities are being explored across the collective.

Other strategies implemented by participant schools included evidence giving the children tools to manage their own feelings through vocabulary development. Others had introduced bespoke soothing spaces for focus children with significant anxieties to transition into school in the mornings. These spaces supported children to access school in a slightly different way than the majority of the cohort, resulting in them being more willing and happy to attend and inevitably being more ready and able to learn. Others in the project provided free clubs and activities at lunch time or after school as part of their wellbeing package. There was also evidence of approaches such as playtime buddies, buddy benches and a 'timeout' club where children could go at playtime if they wanted some quiet and calm space. These aspects of the ethos and environment required additional investment of time and funding but the schools who incorporated these details into their package found them to be beneficial.

Curriculum Teaching and Learning

Each of our participant schools included elements such as character development, self care, financial, physical and emotional wellbeing in their PSHE curriculum, in addition to science, literacy and maths. Participants emphasised that this embedding enabled holistic wellbeing to be fully integral to school life and hence beneficial to all children within the school. Many of the schools in our study expressed that wellbeing underpins learning, so that when children had a good sense of wellbeing, they would be more able to learn effectively, although conversely if they felt anxious, their learning would be negatively impacted. Such attitudes and ways of working had been incorporated into the behaviour policies of many participant schools, so that it had been amended to be more aligned to the schools revised understanding and approaches to wellbeing. As you consider your strategy for wellbeing, it is therefore key to consider broader aspects such as the behaviour policy must be amended, in addition to how your approaches can permeate throughout the whole curriculum.

Case Study

One school observed that Monday morning seemed a particularly difficult time for many children to transition into school. So they adjusted the daily timetable so that the first 20 minutes of Monday's classroom activity was a wellbeing activity, to give the children a more pleasant and gentle start to the day. They also ensured that staff finished teaching five minutes early at the end of each day and used that time to praise the children for specific tasks where they had shown resilience and determination during their learning that day. Both of these initiatives sought to set the ethos of the classroom to feel more affirming and supportive with the aim of ensuring that supporting a child's sense of wellbeing at the beginning of the week would aid their capacity to be ready to learn.

Enabling Student Voice to Influence Decisions

This was the principle with the least evidence exhibited in the research interviews, demonstrating limited activity across all of the school settings. Only one of the schools stated that their student council was active in decision making about pupil wellbeing policies and activities. This is a key area to focus efforts as you are formulating your strategy - to listen to the student voice and take note of what they express.

Staff Development

All of the participant schools were confident in identifying the staff training needs and many explained that they had actively promoted this amongst the staff team, encouraging them to raise training needs. All of the schools had provided some pastoral training to some staff, with some of these being school leaders and in some cases teaching assistants. Only one of the schools had intentionally invested significantly into training all of their staff in quality first teaching for children with SEND techniques. The impact of this was that every classroom was neurodiverse friendly and all children universally received early help, regardless of funding being obtained. Further to this, all of the schools explained that some of their staff members had received training in specific therapies or approaches, such as Lego therapy, art therapy, social thinking and the use of social stories. Whilst these training opportunities had incurred cost implications, the schools had all found that they had considerably strengthened their efforts and enabled specific and targeted support as needed in their particular context. So, consideration of how your strategy is dependent on or provides opportunities for specific training of staff is of critical importance.

Identifying Need and Monitoring Impact

All of the participant schools expressed an acute awareness of the individual child's needs by getting to know each child and finding out about their needs and any gaps or mismatches in their interests and opportunities. The schools also explained extensive systems and processes which had been devised to identify and report specific children's needs, with many emphasising the importance of early intervention. Building these processes and monitoring into your strategy is of paramount importance to ensure the effectiveness and wide adoption of approaches by school staff. Having a designated staff member to identify specific issues seems to work well. In our study this was most commonly the SENCO or Designated Safeguarding Lead and in one school there was a specialist pastoral worker who supplemented this team. Mental Health First Aiders were also mentioned. Other aspects which were only observed in some of the schools were continual awareness and review of the requirements of the school building to meet the needs of children's wellbeing, creativity and how to use opportunities in the timetable to best foster the wellbeing of children in the school.

Working With Parents and Carers

Providing information and gaining consent was universal across all settings, and understanding families' perspectives, collaboration and training with them was evident in all of the settings, although in some cases this was minimal. The schools communicated that this was challenging as they were aware that some parents did not have the capacity to find appropriate support for their child so required the school to facilitate this, whilst other parents may be pleased for the school to take responsibility in this area. Collaborating with parents/carers was evidenced through meet and greet at the school gates, continuous conversation with parents if needs arise and to discuss the school and family interpretations of a child's behaviour, and parental workshops run in school by external agencies. Staff found these activities effective in breaking down barriers and enabling more authentic dialogue and collaboration. The training provided for parents/carers was either in terms of signposting to local services, running online curriculum and library sessions, mental health support groups with parents, equipping parents/carers with skills and awareness about the impact of overuse of technology and SEND/pastoral coffee afternoon. This broad range of activities demonstrates to diverse opportunities available to work with parents and to partner with them in the quest to support their child's mental health and well-being.

Case Study

Working directly with families can have many positive outcomes. For example, in a bid to engage with families in the community to boost school attendance the school organised and designed parent workshops. This had manifold impact in addition to raising attendance in the short term, such as increasing positive social interaction for families who were isolated, increasing employability through building skills, building support networks between families and enhancing staff relationships with the community.

Targeted Support and Appropriate Referral

There was not much evidence provided in the staff interviews of activity towards this principle. Many participants attributed this to funding and resource limitations, which greatly frustrated the research participants. Three of the schools were making targeted use of external agencies within the school; mainly the mental health support team, whilst two were making targeted use of external agencies or professionals outside of the school premises, so that the children went offsite to visit these professionals or organisations. In addition to this, three of the schools had been trained or bought in resources to use targeted and specific tools such as self esteem and resilience training. Such training could be beneficial to roll out across a group of schools to gain maximum impact of individual training sessions.

7. STEPS FOR BUILDING YOUR OWN STRATEGY

Know your context. Time spent gathering information and having a secure understanding of the "here and now" in your school are crucial.

Have a clear idea of what needs improving and why. Use your knowledge of how things stand to see where you want your school to be and why this is important.

Get people onside. Taking people with you is key. It is great to have seen or read something that makes you excited or drives you, but you also need to get others excited about it too. Be aware of everyone's workload - change always comes with a price - so think about the price of everyone going on this journey with you, whether that be staff within the school, parents, governing bodies, trust boards, local schools or local community members.

Use your connections. Think about which successful schools you know and consider what makes them successful. What is it they do which makes a difference? Is there any way you can share best practice between your team or use knowledge exchange? Are there any resources you can share? It would also be a good idea to contact your local provider of teacher education as partnerships are very important to them and they have a ready and well motivated team of trainee teachers who are able to share their research and current skills through working on projects in schools.

Read widely. Whatever your target area is, take time to find out who the current thinkers are and sign up to their social media, subscribe to websites, read educational journals in the area as well as engaging in current national guidance.

Reflect and take time. Always take time to stop and think, question yourself and key people again. How are things progressing? Are there any unforeseen obstacles/ challenges that people have faced? Always think on what you have learnt, what you will take forward and why?

Celebrate your successes. Running any project or approach being aware of the outcome you need and then seeing them come to life is extremely rewarding. Make sure you celebrate them with staff, partnership (whether that is formally or informally) as widely across your stakeholder base as you can. Thank your staff and your leaders for the support they have given you.

Case Study: Forest School

Research, data and observations of children at play showed that children had little interaction with each other apart from school and nature and became uneasy and anxious when outdoors. This led to fractious relationships which often spilt over during lunchtimes and break times when there was no "Teacher supervision". After extensive research for an appropriate approach to follow including visiting local provision, Forest School was felt to be the most appropriate for both context and need. Key staff were trained to deliver sessions and coached other staff on elements of pedagogy on the completion of their training. Families were engaged through after school sessions delivered by support staff, where they were assured of their child's safety.

The approach built resilience, built children's engagement in learning and their families, offered a shared experience for the children as well as a real understanding of issues such as care for living things and sustainability.

8. CONCLUSIONS AND RECOMMENDATIONS

Schools have a constant balance between what they consider best for their children and outside pressures of accountability. This was again illuminated through our study, with schools seeing approaches to mental health and wellbeing as key to the future success for children, but also feeling that the time they spend in supporting the children in this way is not formally measured or documented. Consequently, these approaches often do not feel valued since they do not necessarily feed into school accountability measures. This accountability is largely measured by comparative national data in areas such as attainment in the core subjects and through monitoring of statutory bodies. These pressures play a huge role in how a school operates and the strategies and planning.

As seen in our study, schools saw the value of connecting ideas across the curriculum as crucial. Learning about wellbeing through teaching about money management, for example, is extremely worthwhile in the present financial climate and can be used to help families and the wider school community in a really proactive way, as well as teaching valuable mathematical skills in an authentic real life situation. This can further help dilute anxiety and build confidence in a small way, while teaching children valuable life skills. This also helps illustrate another key issue when considering your strategy for mental health and wellbeing in school - context is key. A good leader will have an acute awareness of local data, whether that be aspects of children's physical health, such as dental hygiene, or knowledge of vulnerable family units, since these aspects can impact negatively on a child's attendance and engagement in school (D'Alessandro et al., 2022). This then brings opportunities to create approaches to meet these precise needs and improve outcomes. Research is central to this. Being proactive and anticipating children's needs is much more valuable than firefighting, in terms of success and time spent on any particular challenge. This emphasises the importance of effective leadership as you devise these strategies.

Currently, schools are using many proven approaches based on strong research and pedagogy to support mental health and wellbeing. Some use these as interventions but all have been used successfully as whole school approaches. These include, Forest School, Nurture Bases, Zones of Regulation as well as more therapeutic methods such as Mindfulness, Peer Massage, Yoga, Lego and Art therapies. There are also other approaches such as Mental Health First AIders and Emotional Learning and Support Assistants (ELSAs). Crucially for schools, some carry a high cost implication, but there are many that can be provided on a small budget such as Mindfulness. Again the support of leadership is crucial to this and this is where research can drive change. If an approach has proven positive impact, it is much more likely any request for financial support will be met if it is possible to do so. And again, think about how these investments and cost implications could be spread across a group of schools.

We have mentioned leadership many times, but wellbeing is everyone's responsibility in schools. And staff have a responsibility to practise self-care too. Where there was evidence in our research of supporting staff wellbeing also, it was very much appreciated by staff. Designated roles, such as Safeguarding Lead, SENDCo and Family Liaison/Attendance Officer, all play a key part in supporting the wider school community in their mental health and wellbeing and maintaining sensitive data and that privacy and confidentiality is a focus at all times. Some families will unfortunately face very challenging times and sadly children living with trauma is not rare and levels of anxiety are rising in even our youngest children. It is leadership's responsibility to develop strategies to ensure that the right people are in the right role in order to deal with circumstances as they arise keeping in mind the school's values and policies as appropriate.

Ultimately, our research findings highlight the benefits of sharing resources across a group of schools, but also emphasise the need for each school to establish its own strategy, according to the needs and challenges identified in the school. Despite belonging to any form of collaborative working group, each school therefore needs to carefully consider how they can effectively develop their own individual approaches to support the wellbeing of children in their school.

Here are some recommendations:

Wellbeing and mental health should be central to all that schools do. The best schools are those who build this into the fabric of their culture and values and their related artefacts.

Schools who educate children in their younger years (for example, 3 to 11 years old) should continue to build their knowledge of contemporary research, and consider how these new insights can be incorporated into your school's ethos and way of working. This helps to enhance each child's holistic wellbeing and in turn boost their educational engagement and attainment, preparing them well for high school education.

Schools in similar socio-economic areas should actively seek opportunities to work collaboratively. Research projects are an excellent way to do this as they can help and support schools to achieve similar goals or outcomes, cut costs by sharing knowledge, experience and resources, build relationships,trust and cohesion across communities that can be challenging to reach, build a sense of place and achievement across the schools' communities.

Schools should be seen as individual, and in context and as valuable entities, rather than simply schools following a ready-made guide in order to comply. Approaches should always be selected to fit the individual school environment, children and families.

You could even try setting up your own research project in your school, to help you to view what is achieved over time.

REFERENCES

Cavioni, V., Grazzani, I. and Ornaghi, V., 2020. Mental health promotion in schools: A comprehensive theoretical framework.

D'Alessandro, A. M., Butterfield, K. M., Hanceroglu, L., & Roberts, K. P. (2022). Listen to the children: Elementary school students' perspectives on a mindfulness intervention. *Journal of Child and Family Studies*, 31(8), 2108–2120. DOI: 10.1007/s10826-022-02292-3 PMID: 35505672

Department for Education, 2019. ITT Core Content Framework. Crown copyright.

Dolton, A., Adams, S., & O'Reilly, M. (2020). In the child's voice: The experiences of primary school children with social, emotional and mental health difficulties. *Clinical Child Psychology and Psychiatry*, 25(2), 419–434. DOI: 10.1177/1359104519859923 PMID: 31257914

Holmes, S. (2019). Play-based interview techniques with young children. In *Using innovative methods in early years research* (pp. 92–108). Routledge. DOI: 10.4324/9780429423871-8

Holmes, S. E., & Sinclair, V. (2024). pending. What is working? A Qualitative Comparative Analysis of approaches to pupil well-being in a MAT in NorthWest England. *British Educational Research Journal*.

Huang, Y., Edwards, J., & Laurel-Wilson, M. (2020). The shadow of context: Neighborhood and school socioeconomic disadvantage, perceived social integration, and the mental and behavioral health of adolescents. *Health & Place*, 66, 102425. DOI: 10.1016/j.healthplace.2020.102425 PMID: 32911129

Lyon, A. R., & Bruns, E. J. (2019). From evidence to impact: Joining our best school mental health practices with our best implementation strategies. *School Mental Health*, 11(1), 106–114. DOI: 10.1007/s12310-018-09306-w PMID: 31709018

Public Health England, 2021

Richter, A., Sjunnestrand, M., Romare Strandh, M., & Hasson, H. (2022). Implementing school-based mental health services: A scoping review of the literature summarizing the factors that affect implementation. *International Journal of Environmental Research and Public Health*, 19(6), 3489. DOI: 10.3390/ijerph19063489 PMID: 35329175

Tomé, G., Almeida, A., Ramiro, L., & Gaspar, T. (2021). Intervention in schools promoting mental health and well-being: A systematic. *Global J Comm Psychol Pract*, 34, 3–23.

Verhoog, S., Eijgermans, D. G. M., Fang, Y., Bramer, W. M., Raat, H., & Jansen, W. (2022). Contextual determinants associated with children's and adolescents' mental health care utilization: A systematic review. *European Child & Adolescent Psychiatry*, 1–15. PMID: 36129544

Chapter 3

Strengthening Socio-Emotional Skills For Students at Risk for Mental Health Issues Within School-Wide Positive Behavioral Interventions and Supports

Lefki Kourea
https://orcid.org/0000-0003-4572-6377
University of Nicosia, Cyprus

Fotini Lytra
University of Nicosia, Cyprus

ABSTRACT

Student mental health has received increased attention over the last years, with researchers and governments trying to identify the best ways to support students and adolescents (e.g., Johns Hopkins Bloomberg School of Public Health & United Nations Children's Fund, 2022). Efforts have concentrated on initiating mental health services and increasing school-and program-based mental health supports to address student needs at individual and school levels. Recently, some researchers have suggested teaching social-emotional skills within a prevention-focused school-

DOI: 10.4018/979-8-3693-5325-7.ch003

wide tiered model because simply adopting a socio-emotional curriculum does not lead to adequate implementation or improved student outcomes (Greenberg et al., 2017). This chapter describes the mental health challenges at-risk students face and suggests strengthening their socio-emotional skills within the tiered continuum of supports of the School-wide Positive Behavioral Interventions and Supports framework.

INTRODUCTION

Schools are among the most important social contexts where students blossom academically, socially, and emotionally (e.g., Greenberg et al., 2017). However, for many students, the pressure to excel and navigate the complexities of adolescence can create significant mental health challenges. Recognizing the importance of promoting mental health in schools is critical for fostering resilient and academically successful students and nurturing a generation of well-rounded, balanced individuals.

The prevalence of mental health issues among students is a growing global health problem. According to the State of the World's Children 2021 report (United Nations, 2021), an estimated 86 million adolescents 15-19 years old and 80 million 10-14 years old live with a mental disorder (e.g., depression, anxiety, bipolar, eating disorder, autism, schizophrenia, attention-deficit/hyperactivity disorder [ADHD], etc). Adolescent boys are more likely to experience mental disorders than girls in both age groups. However, girls are more likely to experience mental health issues (e.g., distress, a lack of life satisfaction, a lack of sense of flourishing and happiness) (Johns Hopkins Bloomberg School of Public Health & United Nations Children's Fund, 2022). What is alarming is that researchers from the United States (U.S.) National Institute of Health found that rates of preteen suicide (ages 8-12) have been increasing by approximately 8% annually since 2008. The increases are most evident among female preteens and some ethnic minority preteens (e.g., Hispanic, American Native) (e.g., Ruch et al., 2024).

In an international study about the prevalence rates of mental disorders in youngsters aged 5–17 years, Erskine et al. (2017) found that the mean percentage rates were Conduct Disorder: 5.0%, ADHD: 5.5%, Autism Spectrum Disorder: 16.1%, Eating Disorders: 4.4%, Depression: 6.2%, Anxiety: 3.2%. Previously, Erskine and colleagues (2015) concluded that mental and substance use disorders constitute the leading cause of disability in students and adolescents globally.

Mental Health and Student Academic
and Socio-Emotional Outcomes

Mental health issues impact students' academic and social lives. First, the relationship between *mental health and academic achievement* is well-established (e.g., Firose et al., 2023). Students struggling with mental health challenges often experience difficulties with concentration, motivation, and emotional regulation. This can manifest as decreased engagement in class, lower academic performance, and increased absenteeism. For instance, Fernandez-Castillo & Rojas (2009) found that depression scores of Spanish students aged 12 to 16 were inversely correlated with lower grades in nearly every subject area, but anxiety scores were not. Similarly, Burnett-Zeigler et al. (2012) targeted a sample of American adolescents aged 12 to 18 years old and showed that lower grades predicted the presence of mental health problems, namely anxiety, and depression, after controlling for gender, age, ethnicity, and drug and alcohol use.

The above findings lend support to McLeod et al.'s study (2012), which concluded that the negative social consequences of mental health problems are not solely due to an individual's impaired functional ability; instead, the consequences reflect the negative impact of the social environment. Specifically, McLeod and colleagues investigated the relationship between mental health, behavior problems, and academic achievement among adolescents. Even after controlling for aptitude, attention problems, delinquency, and substance use remained significant predictors of low academic achievement.

Recently, Dunkan and colleagues (2021) aimed to investigate the association between *mental health factors with academic achievement and problem behaviors* (e.g., truancy, incomplete homework, and days missed due to health issues) in Canadian secondary school students. Results showed that lower depression and higher psychosocial well-being were consistently associated with better academic performance and reduced problem behaviors. Furthermore, problem behaviors were associated with low academic performance, such that students who had more frequent absences, skipped classes, and had incomplete homework tended to show lower grades. Several studies have also shown a correlation between mental health and school absenteeism. For instance, Kearney and Graczyk (2020) concluded that school absenteeism is a key indicator of maladaptive functioning in students, whereas regular school attendance is critical for adaptive functioning. Recently, Sharpe et al. (2023) further examined the predictive relationship between mental health difficulties and school absenteeism among 9-year-old students and concluded with four distinct mental health student categories: (1) students at high risk for both emotional and behavioral difficulties; (2) students at high risk primarily for emotional difficulties; (3) students at high risk for behavioral challenges; and (4) students at low risk for emotional and behavioral difficulties. Sharpe and colleagues found that students in the high-risk group had significantly higher odds of absenteeism compared to the low-risk group. Additionally, the high-risk groups were more likely to experience multiple family, school, and demographic risk factors. In sum, the relationship between mental health and school absenteeism in students should not be ignored when developing school-based mental health interventions.

Contributing Factors to Student Mental Health

Primary and secondary school students face unique challenges that can contribute to the development of mental health issues. To this end, family (e.g., parent relationships) and school (e.g., peer pressure, school climate, academic performance) factors play a key role in students' mental health. Specifically, *family relations* can affect a child's mental health condition. Damsgaard et al. (2014) investigated the parent-child relationship with respect to trusted communication and the frequency of emotional symptoms in students. Additionally, they explored whether the family's socio-economic status influenced this relationship. Results showed that students that had not experienced trusted communication with parents had a higher odds ratio for daily emotional symptoms than those who had experienced trusted communication. Interestingly, this association remained unaffected by the family's socio-economic status.

Several studies have verified the important role *supportive relationships* play in mitigating poor mental health. Butler et al. (2022) aimed to investigate the relative impact of three types of supportive relationships (school, family, peer) on mental health with 2,074 students aged 8–15 years in the United Kingdom. Results showed that all three sources of support were independently associated with mental well-being. Moreover, students with multiple sources of support were more protected and exhibited higher levels of well-being than the ones with fewer levels of support. Nonetheless, students with lower levels of family support still benefited from school sources of support. Peer support emerged as particularly crucial. Students with high peer support (even if they had low family and school support) had similar levels of mental well-being as those with high family and school support (but low peer support). Finally, high peer support was determined as equal to having two other protective factors.

Buli and colleagues (2024), utilizing student data from repeated cross-sectional surveys between 2004 and 2020, aimed to investigate whether certain *school-related factors* (i.e., school liking, school-related parental support, teacher support, and the school physical environment) influence trends in mental health problems (i.e., psychosomatic symptoms [PSS], depressive symptoms [DS], suicidal ideations [SI], and suicide attempts [SA]) among 15-year-old students having low or high socio-economic status (SES). Research findings suggested a general improvement in all school factors over the years in both SES groups. School physical environment was associated with decreases in mental health issues, such as PSS and DS in both SES groups. Over time, mental health problems increased among adolescents with low SES and decreased among those in the high SES group. Similarly, Skoric and colleagues (2023) investigated the association between school factors and life satisfaction, symptoms of depression, and psychosomatic health complaints. To this end, researchers obtained data from the 2018 Health Behavior in School-aged Students (HBSC) survey. The main findings showed that schoolwork pressure and bullying experiences were positively associated with depression symptoms. However, teacher and peer support were negatively related to depression symptoms. Regarding the association between psychosomatic complaints and school factors, Skoric et al. found that schoolwork pressure and being bullied at school were positively correlated to psychosomatic symptoms, but teacher and peer support, as well as satisfaction with school, were negatively correlated.

In conclusion, schools are an essential context where mental health and resilience can be cultivated for all students, regardless of their family background. They also play a critical role in fostering positive peer relationships and supportive teacher-student relationships. By recognizing the various factors that impact student mental health and implementing strategies to promote emotional well-being, we can better support the development of happy and healthy young people.

Students at Risk and Mental Health Challenges

Students face significant pressure and challenges that put their mental health at risk. While they may not express themselves in the same way as adults, the foundation for emotional well-being is laid in the early years. Identifying risk factors contributing to mental health issues and promoting positive mental health practices is crucial for fostering a generation of resilient and thriving individuals.

When trying to identify students who are at risk of developing mental health issues, there is a range of aspects that one must take into consideration. First, *family income and living conditions* play a significant role in a child's or an adolescent's mental and psychological state. Coley et al. (2018) studied the associations between family income and youth mental and behavioral health by examining economic risks derived from family, neighborhood, and school contexts. The study targeted a nationally representative sample of high school students with an average age of 16 years old. Concerning school contexts, the results showed that adolescents who studied in schools with more affluent schoolmates were at risk of using drugs, being intoxicated, or committing property crimes. However, youth at poorer schools reported different risks related to mental health issues, such as greater depressive and anxiety symptoms and engagement in violence and intoxication, especially for male adolescents. In relation to family income and neighborhood, they were far less predictive of adolescent mental and behavioral health outcomes.

When considering students at risk, it is crucial to investigate *the role of ethnicity and discrimination*. A study conducted in the Netherlands (Andriaanse et al., 2014) investigated the relationship between ethnicity, social disadvantage, and mental health outcomes in school-aged students. The sample consisted of Dutch, Moroccan, and Turkish students. Key findings showed that ethnic minorities exhibited more externalizing problems and fewer internalizing ones than the majority youth. Moreover, what's interesting is that perceived discrimination and living in an unstable social environment were associated with mental health issues, regardless of ethnicity. Finally, social disadvantage was strongly correlated with mental health issues and was more common in ethnic minority youth.

Furthermore, students who face *academic difficulties* are at risk for mental health issues. In their meta-analysis, Nelson and Harwood (2011) showed that more depressive and anxious symptoms were found in students with reading difficulties compared to the general population. Similarly, Ihbour et al. (2023) aimed to examine the associations between reading difficulties, anxiety, depressive symptoms, self-esteem status, and academic achievement among students aged 9 to 16 years old. Findings showed that weak readers and intermediate-level readers exhibited more frequent emotional disturbances compared to good readers. These emotional disturbances included symptoms of anxiety and depression. In addition, academic achievement and reading level were negatively correlated with anxious-depressive symptoms and positively correlated with self-esteem.

Similar findings came from a recent systematic review (Vieira et al., 2024), which examined the association between learning difficulties (e.g., math, reading difficulties, unspecified learning difficulties) and emotional problems (e.g., anxiety, depression, physical complaints, and social withdrawal). Researchers also looked at factors that might influence the severity of these emotional problems. Overall, individuals with learning difficulties were more likely to experience internalizing problems compared to those without any learning difficulties. Interestingly, the effect size was moderate, indicating a moderate association between learning difficulties and emotional problems. The study also explored moderators (e.g., age, specific types of internalizing problems, and anxiety types). Unfortunately, the study didn't reveal clear patterns for how these moderators influenced the results. In conclusion, this research suggests a connection between learning difficulties and internalizing problems, but the strength of that connection may vary depending on individual circumstances.

To sum up, mental health concerns are a significant issue for primary and secondary school students. By recognizing the risk factors, school staff and families can collaborate to create a nurturing environment that prioritizes up and foremost, emotional well-being. To achieve this, research has already documented school-wide approaches to achieve this. The section below describes the School-Wide Positive Behavioral Interventions and Supports framework and its empirical evidence on strengthening student socio-emotional skills.

School-Wide Positive Behavioral Interventions and Supports

School-Wide Positive Behavioral Interventions and Supports is an empirically validated organizational framework (Center for PBIS, 2023, 2024; Sugai & Horner, 2020) (for further analysis, readers may check the chapter *"Whole-School Approaches and Their Impact on School Climate and Student Psycho-Emotional Being: The Example of School-Wide Positive Behavioral Interventions and Supports (SWPBIS) Framework"*). Its principles are based on public health and prevention science (see Simeonsson, 1994), applied behavior analysis (Horner & Sugai, 2015; Horner & Kittleman, 2021; Simonsen & Sugai, 2019), and implementation science (e.g., Fixen et al., 2005). SWPBIS is not a curriculum or an intervention program but an approach that aims to improve student academic performance and social competence by establishing a continuum of tiered instructional supports and systems in and outside of classrooms. Its overall aim is to strengthen teacher and administrator efforts to build safe, supportive, and positive learning environments for all students (e.g., Sugai & Lewis, 1999). Stated differently, SWPBIS seeks to alter the school's organizational context and work with adults to implement with fidelity evidence-based practices and make data-based decisions related to student academic and social behaviors.

SWPBIS follows the three-tiered public health prevention logic (Walker et al., 1996), which entails the provision of behavioral and academic supports across a continuum. Some students, due to environmental and personal risk factors, need targeted support either at small group or individualized level. To this end, a school should be reorganized so that three tiers of supports are available to students.

Figure 1. Three-tiered School-wide Positive Behavioral Interventions and Supports Framework

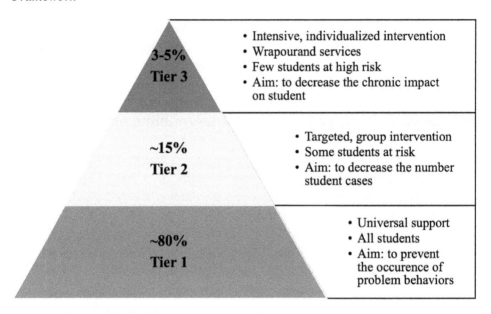

Tier 1: Universal Prevention

As Figure 1 shows, Tier 1 or universal/primary prevention is designed to be implemented across all school settings in a consistent, proactive, and instructional manner. It consists of systems and practices supporting teacher efforts to improve student social skills. When a school decides to implement the first tier of prevention, a school leadership team is established, composed of one teacher per grade level, a member from the administration team (school principal or assistant school principal), a special education teacher, and/or a school counselor. Additionally, a parent representative and a student representative may also be included in the team. The leadership team is trained by external coaches from ministry/school district or university staff, and its main role is to lead the development, implementation, and evaluation of Tier 1 core elements for students and teachers, as shown in Figure 2 (Missouri School-wide Positive Behavior Support, 2019; Simonsen et al., 2008).

Figure 2. SWPBIS Tier 1 Core Elements

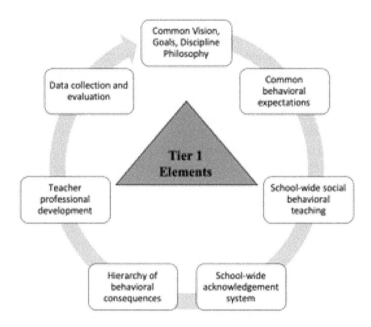

A school vision and a discipline philosophy are developed that emphasize pre-vention, relationship building, and collaboration. Three to five schoolwide behav-ioral expectations are defined (e.g., be respectful, be cooperative, be safe) in each school setting, representing student and community cultural values. Each behavioral expectation is defined in an observable and measurable way in every setting so that all teaching staff develops a clear understanding of the instructional objectives (e.g., in class: "be respectful means wait for your turn to talk", in hallways: "be respect-ful means keep your voice level to 1", etc.). Teachers are committed to improving student social behaviors by teaching those explicitly and systematically, providing frequent positive reinforcement for expected behaviors, and addressing inappropriate behaviors consistently in an instructional and respectful manner.

A continuum of strategies is developed and implemented to provide specific positive feedback to student behaviors. Teachers aim at delivering behavior-specific praise (e.g., Ennis et al., 2020; Royer et al., 2019) and individual and/or group rewards contingent upon the occurrence of expected behaviors (e.g., Tyre et al., 2023). The goal is for adults to increase their attention and thus, their behavior-specific praise to students' appropriate behaviors at higher rates than they address inappropriate behaviors (e.g., Caldarella et al., 2020; Miller et al., 2023). As students become fluent in demonstrating behavioral expectations, teachers fade out tangible rewards and shift to natural reinforcers (e.g., verbal praise, public recognition).

For managing student problem behaviors, the leadership team develops and implements a schoolwide continuum of practices and strategies that determine which behaviors are staff-managed or office-managed so that problem behaviors are handled predictably and consistently. Teachers manage problem behaviors the same way as academic problems. First, they interpret problem behaviors as social errors, meaning students have not learned adequately and have not become fluent in the expected behavioral steps. Second, teachers correct social errors following the same feedback approach as the one for academic errors. For this reason, a range of direct and indirect evidence-based practices are implemented to discourage inappropriate behavior and elicit the expected behavior in a respectful and non-confrontational way. Practice opportunities for the expected behaviors are essential when correcting student social errors (Scott, 2017).

Finally, the last two Tier 1 components pertain to developing a system for supporting teacher efforts in implementing universal practices with fidelity and a system for progress monitoring Tier 1 implementation and student response. For the first system, school staff receives frequent short professional development training on Tier 1 practices (e.g., Palmer & Noltemeyer, 2019) and coaching support to enhance the quality and, thus, sustainability of teacher implementation (e.g., Bethun, 2017; Freeman et al., 2017; Hershfeld et al., 2012; Kraft et al., 2018). Coaching is provided internally as well as externally. Internal coaches are assigned school staff responsible for training and strengthening teacher practices. External coaches are district or university staff that assist SWPBIS leadership teams in designing and implementing Tier 1 elements and assisting with problem-solving issues. In a survey study examining the perceptions of SWPBIS Tier 1 leadership team members regarding the amount and importance of coaching activities received, the 264 teachers with at least three years of Tier 1 implementation experience perceived the external coach's assistance with action planning, data collection, and sharing SWPBIS knowledge as the most important activities for school team members (Bastable et al., 2020).

Furthermore, ongoing monitoring of the fidelity implementation and student response to Tier 1 practices requires developing a data collection and analysis system where teaching staff is informed about the quality of implementation and student responsiveness across tiers. Schools collect student behavioral data (e.g., discipline referrals, rule violations, problem behavior incidences, attendance) and analyze them to determine students' responsiveness to Tier 1 practices. Non-respondents to universal prevention will receive additional support at Tiers 2 and 3. Additionally, school teams assess, with the assistance of an external coach, the fidelity of Tier 1 implementation to determine the degree to which systems and practices are implemented as intended. The fidelity assessment is a critical component of the data collection system because empirical evidence has documented the positive association between implementation and student outcomes (e.g., Childs, Kincaid, George, & Gage, 2016; Flannery, Fenning, Kato, & McIntosh, 2014). In a recent study, Elrod and colleagues (2022) investigated relationships between SWPBIS fidelity, school climate, and office discipline referrals with a student sample of 204,701 students in 288 middle and high schools. Their main results showed that additional years of SWPBIS implementation were related to greater fidelity, stronger school climate, and fewer ODRs.

Tier 1 is the stepping stone for a successful implementation of Tier 2. Hence, universal systems and practices must be implemented with fidelity so that at-risk students are identified correctly and receive additional support (Van Camp et al., 2021). It is evident that identifying students at risk in a classroom and school context, whereby primary prevention practices are implemented with low quality, leads to increased numbers of students needing targeted interventions. Stated differently, implementing Tier 1 as intended and with high fidelity is cost-effective and minimizes school resources.

Tier 2: Secondary Prevention

Tier 2 prevention is designed to provide early behavioral and/or academic support to students (approximately 10-15%) at risk for school failure due to certain risk factors (e.g., low academic skills, limited family support, low social skills). Specifically, Tier 2 interventions purport to decrease the development of any unexpected new behavior, to prevent the existing problem behaviors from worsening and intensifying, to identify environmental triggers that maintain problem behavior and eliminate those, and to teach and strengthen a replacement behavior. Targeted interventions are delivered in small groups or individualized in the classroom, and they address student skill deficits related to acquisition or performance (e.g., Anderson & Borgmeier, 2010; Mitchell et al., 2011).

For students who need to develop social or academic skills, they participate in targeted academic interventions, small group social skills, anger management programs, character education programs, etc. (e.g., Missouri School-wide Positive Behavior Support, 2019). For students who can perform the target skill but need to become fluent in it, they would benefit from added structure and increased adult feedback so that they can maintain and generalize the expected behavior over time and across settings. Examples of such interventions include self-monitoring systems (e.g., Van Camp et al., 2021), Check-in Check-out program (e.g., Drevon et al., 2019; Todd et al., 2008;), and Check & Connect (e.g., Maynard et al., 2014; Powers et al., 2017). When Tier 2 systems and practices are implemented with fidelity, it is expected that 10%-15% of students will have their behavioral needs met (McDaniel et al., 2015).

According to Mitchell and her colleagues (2015), secondary prevention presents some key features (see Figure 3). Tier 2 supports should be *continuously available* so that students at risk can be included at any time. This means that interventions should be organized well and can be implemented quickly. Tier 2 supports must *be easily accessible* and can be delivered within 72 hours from student identification. Any environmental change added in the classroom context should require *low teacher effort*. Otherwise, it will not be sustained over time. Given how busy places classrooms are, changes to methods and strategies should be kept to a minimum so that teachers can devote a few more minutes only (Bruhn et al., 2021). Another critical element of Tier 2 is the *consistent alignment of behavioral expectations across tiers*. Whatever expected behaviors will be introduced to students at Tier 2 these should have already been in place and have been taught at Tier 1. Maintaining the same schoolwide expectations across tiers allows for greater consistency in implementation and helps at-risk students experience a safe and predictable learning environment. Tier 2 systems and practices are described clearly to the staff so everyone understands the rationale and purpose. Assigned staff members should be trained in interventions and implement those with fidelity. It is important that targeted interventions may require some modifications depending on student needs (e.g., McDaniel et al., 2017). Thus, *staff flexibility* is requested to tailor intervention components to student needs. Any intervention selected should serve the function of the student's behavioral needs (e.g., Lindsey & White, 2009). Administrators are instrumental in providing necessary support and schedule adjustments to ease staff efforts in Tier 2 implementation. Finally, *ongoing monitoring* of student responsiveness and intervention fidelity is imperative to ensure that targeted supports meet student needs.

Figure 3. SWPBIS Tier 2 Core Elements

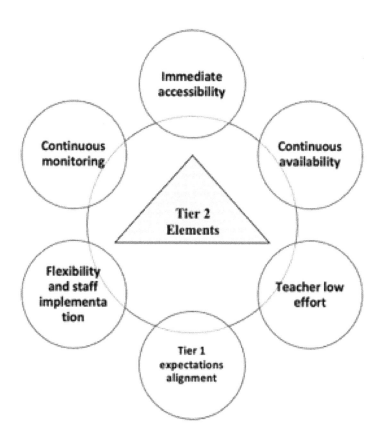

With the rising research interest in understanding Tier 2 systems and practices in depth and supporting school staff to implement them efficiently and effectively (Bruhn et al., 2021), empirical evidence has yielded positive effects on student academic, social, and behavioral outcomes (e.g., Cho Blair et al., 2021; Drevon et al., 2019; Kern et al., 2020; Lane et al., 2012). For instance, in an experimental single-case multiple-baseline-across-subjects-design study, Hawken and Horner (2003) collaborated with a local middle school with 487 students to provide targeted intervention to those who had received at least five office discipline referrals and had not been receiving any other individualized behavior support. Four male students were identified between 12 and 13 years old and were introduced to the Behavior Education Program, which included five components (Hawken et al., 2020). First, students were paired with an adult who served as a mentor. Students had to check in with the adult at the beginning of the school day to receive the daily progress report card and be reminded of the behavioral expectations. Second, participants took the card in the classroom and handed it to their teacher. At the end of each instructional period, classroom teachers provided specific behavior feedback on student behavior by recording points on the card and verbally. Third, students met with their mentor at the end of the school day to review their card progress and calculate the points earned. If their daily behavioral goal were met, students would receive their reinforcer. If they did not reach their target goal, the mentor would provide information as to what to work on the next day. Fourth, students took the card home so that parents would sign it. Last, participants would return the signed card to their mentor the following day. Research results showed a modest functional relationship between intervention and reduction of problem behaviors, indicating the positive impact of this simple, cost-effective, and teacher-friendly program. Similar replicated studies demonstrate the effectiveness of the Check In Check Out (a.k.a. Behavior Education Program) intervention (see Drevon et al., 2019; Todd et al., 2008).

There are instances in which students do not respond satisfactorily to Tier 2 interventions, and schools should consider providing individualized intervention supports (e.g., Missouri School-wide Positive Behavior Support, 2019).

Tier 3: Tertiary Prevention

As shown in Figure 1, the last tier of the pyramid is focused on students with chronic behavioral and academic complex needs who benefit from individualized intensive support (e.g., Walker et al., 2022). Tertiary prevention is initiated when universal and secondary prevention have not been successful for certain students. In most cases, these students present extended academic and behavioral difficulties for a prolonged time, and schools can only support them and their teachers when another layer of prevention is added to the continuum of support. It is estimated that up to 5% of the student population would require Tier 3 support (e.g., Kurth et al., 2016).

According to Figure 4, Tier 3 presents certain core features to be in place, which enable a comprehensive and efficient approach to students with extensive support needs. First, the center of the planning process is the target student, who decides his planning support team. *Person-centered planning* gives a voice to students so that adults can understand their needs and interests. Second, Tier 3 teams prioritize certain *quality-of-life* dimensions that should be incorporated into their intervention planning. Such dimensions include social inclusion, physical well-being, emotional well-being, interpersonal relationships, etc. (Carr, 1999). School staff should spend considerable time discussing with the student and his family those dimensions and/ or identifying others so that any school intervention attempts must capture a good quality of life for this particular student. Third, a critical survival skill to be introduced and taught to students with extensive needs is *self-determination*. This is a functional skill in which the person acts independently, realizes, and regulates his actions. Tier 3 support team discusses with the student what behavioral aspects are important for successful independent living and incorporates processes and practices where the student can demonstrate autonomous thinking and decision making. At Tier 3, school teams focus on developing and implementing *function-based interventions* to minimize disruptive behaviors and teach students replacement behaviors that serve the same function (e.g., Strickland-Cohen et al., 2019). Goh and Bambara (2012) conducted a meta-analysis of 83 studies representing 145 participants with extensive needs and found functional behavioral assessments and function-based interventions are effective in reducing problem behaviors and increasing appropriate skills. A fifth critical feature in Tier 3 support is the *ongoing monitoring* of student responsiveness to intensive interventions and fidelity of implementation (e.g., Freeman et al., 2024). According to Cumming and colleagues (2019), a data-based individualization process is initiated to make decisions about how and when to intensify intervention support for meeting student academic and behavioral needs. It is important to note that students in Tier 3 should be assessed more frequently than those in Tier 1 and 2 so that the intervention components match their individualized needs. Lastly, *multidisciplinary teaming* allows school members to collect input from internal and external professionals and develop a comprehensive behavior support plan that would support students over time (Nese et al., 2021)

Figure 4. SWPBIS Tier 3 Core Elements

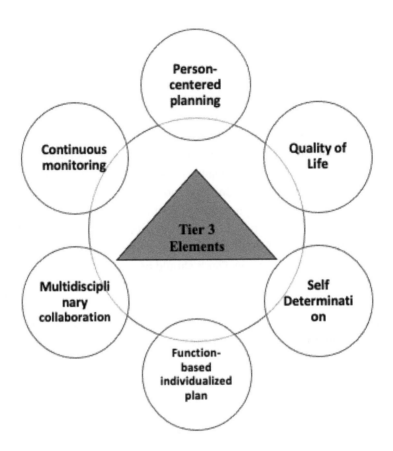

SWPBIS is an applied example of inclusion for all students. The provision and implementation of tiered support for students with extensive behavioral needs is challenging because it demands school resources (e.g., time and money) that are often times limited. To this end, school teams need to re-think how they allocate and manage their time efficiently, and administrators should consider allocating financial resources cost-effectively to maximize student inclusion. Interestingly, in a recent survey research measuring teachers' perceptions of the educational involvement of students with complex support needs in schools, Zagona and her colleagues (2024) found that teachers responded differently about student educational placement, and their response differences were statistically significant. Specifically, teachers working in schools where students with complex support needs were included in general education classrooms had positive perceptions about teaching schoolwide expectations to all simultaneously and managing problem behaviors the same way for all students. However, teachers working in segregated settings (separate classrooms, special schools) were less likely to agree with teaching students school-wide expectations as they considered those not to be appropriate for students with complex behavioral needs. Such finding reflects the self-fulfilling prophecy.

School-Wide Positive Behavioral Interventions and Socio-Emotional Learning

As described above, SWPBIS is a schoolwide application of behavioral systems and practices to change student and staff behavior in schools. It provides a safe and positive learning environment for students at risk for mental health issues through the continuum of tiered support and consistent implementation. However, SWPBIS focuses mainly on social behaviors and less on emotions and cognitions. Unlike SWPBIS, the Collaborative for Academic, Social, and Emotional Learning has introduced the Socio-Emotional Learning (SEL) framework (e.g., Weissberg et al., 2017) consisting of five interconnected domains of cognitive, affective, and behavioral competencies: self-awareness, self-management, social awareness, relationship skills, and responsible decision making, which are taught in a systemic schoolwide approach targeting students, families, and communities.

Some authorities argue integrating SEL and SWPBIS in a unified approach as they are not antithetical (e.g., Bradshaw et al., 2014; Eber et al., 2019). Barrett and colleagues (2018) proposed teaching SEL skills within SWPBIS systems and practices as described in the previous section. Specifically, a school team leads the efforts to communicate among staff the SEL emphasis and collects data that indicate a behavioral pattern for SEL challenges. Then, school teams prioritize specific SEL skills to be taught across the SWPBIS continuum. SEL skills are integrated within the SWPBIS universal language, and teachers model, teach, and provide lots of practice opportunities with specific positive feedback. Promoting teacher wellness through a nurturing and supportive school environment with coaching and professional development training increases the possibility of staff becoming engaged in the schoolwide unified approach. Interestingly, Cook and colleagues (2015) conducted a matched quasi-randomized control design to examine the independent and combined effects of SWPBIS Tier 1 and SEL at the fourth and fifth-grade classroom level across two large elementary schools (n=8 classrooms). Two classrooms were assigned to each of the four experimental conditions: business-as-usual control, SWPBIS Tier 1 only, SEL curriculum only, and SWPBIS-SEL condition. Some of the main dependent measures included teacher measures on student internalizing and externalizing behavior. Results yielded significantly greater improvements in mental health and externalizing behaviors under the SWPBIS-SEL condition than the other three conditions. Positive gains were noted under the SWPBIS and SEL only conditions.

School efforts to support student mental health and strengthen SEL skills can be enhanced within the SWPBIS structures. According to Eber and colleagues (2019), SWPBIS school teams at Tier 1 should expand their composition to include students, families, and clinical experts in mental health. All team members engaged in a shared decision-making process where everybody benefits. For instance, clinicians are removed from their traditional consultant role, and now they engage and interact with school staff, students, and families. Teachers come to appreciate how interventions related to depression and anxiety can be supported at the classroom level and progress monitored. Integrating mental health within the SWPBIS logic maximizes prevention efforts in identifying and addressing student mental health issues openly and as early as possible.

Bradshaw and her colleagues (2014) have proposed an 11-step process for integrating SWPBIS and SEL based on empirical work conducted through the John Hopkins Center for Prevention and Early Intervention. The step-by-step approach includes the following: (1) School leadership commits to a unified approach of SWPBIS and SEL. This means that school stakeholders have read and understood the research supporting both frameworks and have realized the importance of coordinated efforts to bring the unified approach to fruition. (2) School leadership must secure staff buy-in by asking teachers to vote formally or informally. Like in SWPBIS, the expected staff buy-in rate should be at least 80%. (3) School leadership invites staff to form a leadership committee with key players, including students, families, paraprofessionals, community members, clinicians, and grade-level teachers. Given the large number of persons attending, a smaller committee is formed (aka steering committee) that is authorized to make decisions about planning and implementation. (4) School team develops a shared vision based on the SEL domains and it is presented to staff for buy-in and adoption. (5) School team should identify their school improvement goals by conducting a schoolwide strengths, weaknesses, opportunities, and threats analysis (SWOT). Such an assessment enhances the team's efforts to work smart and effectively and align the unified approach demands with other intended school initiatives. (6) School team defines the content of each tier and makes decisions about student referral. It is important to note that school teams should carefully select intensive programs and services offered by community agencies, especially for students with the greatest needs. The emphasis is to build a strong Tier 1 foundation. (7) School team develops an action plan with the goals, actions, timeline, and expected outcomes. (8) School team ensures that ongoing professional development and coaching are provided to staff throughout the year. Emphasis is placed to help teachers realize the importance of the unified approach and maximize implementation fidelity. (9) School team is instrumental in launching the integrated approach according to the four-step implementation logic: exploration, installation, initial implementation, full implementation, and continuous revisit. (10) The district or ministry ensures that ongoing coaching support is provided to the school team in each implementation phase. (11) Finally, the school team ensures ongoing evaluation throughout the year to assess fidelity implementation and student responsiveness from the unified approach.

In a nutshell, strengthening student socio-emotional skills requires selecting and implementing evidence-based practices incorporated in an organizational theoretically-driven framework. Thus, SWPBIS systems and practices, as analyzed earlier, can be unified with the SEL logic, and careful attention should be given to designing and delivering implementation drivers within and outside of school to maximize student outcomes and fidelity of implementation.

Implications for Practice

Improving student mental health is a shared responsibility among schools, families, and communities. Family active involvement in the three-tiered continuum is necessary to develop a common socio-emotional and behavioral language between home and school settings. School members should keep parents/guardians in close collaboration throughout the build-up of prevention logic and ensure that family cultural perspectives are incorporated in identifying school vision, behavioral expectations, and SEL domains. Family input can be sought through participation in the school leadership team, interviews, or survey questionnaires at every implementation stage. Family involvement becomes critical in secondary and tertiary prevention because parents/guardians should provide their consent for their child's participation in academic or behavioral intervention. Open communication between home and school from the beginning of the year helps solve implementation issues or prevent possible parental resistance.

The SWPBIS prevention logic requires staff to work in teams and develop a shared approach in instructional practices. This is difficult to achieve because teachers are not trained to work collectively. Thus, targeted ongoing professional development trainings accompanied by internal and or external coaching support ensures that SWPBIS practices are implemented with fidelity. Professional development seminars should be kept short and concise and provide staff with many opportunities to practice. Coaching entails frequent interaction with classroom teachers and opportunities to build trust. An effective coach must use many skills, such as active listening, reflection, and collaborative problem solving to promote teacher change. Teachers who are overwhelmed with challenging behaviors are in need of a coach willing to listen and support. Sharing real-life classroom solutions grounded in educational principles gains teacher trust.

Finally, community stakeholders are key players in generalizing the prevention tiered logic in community neighborhoods. To achieve this, school leadership should invite community stakeholders early on in the SWPBIS leadership team and become involved in building behavioral expectations and rules within and outside of school. Community agencies play an instrumental role in providing mental health services to students with the greatest needs. Thus, agency members should communicate openly with the SWPBIS leadership team from the beginning of the school year.

CONCLUSION

Strengthening the socio-emotional and behavioral skills of all students, particularly those at risk for mental health issues, requires a multidisciplinary and integrated approach. SWPBIS provides the empirical foundation for integrating other frameworks, such as CASEL's SEL domains, across the three tiers of prevention. By incorporating empirical evidence and knowledge from implementation science, school stakeholders can make a positive change in the lives of at-risk students for mental health.

REFERENCES

Adriaanse, M., Veling, W., Doreleijers, T., & van Domburgh, L. (2014). The link between ethnicity, social disadvantage and mental health problems in a school-based multiethnic sample of children in The Netherlands. *European Child & Adolescent Psychiatry*, 23(11), 1103–1113. DOI: 10.1007/s00787-014-0564-5 PMID: 24927803

Anderson, C. M., & Borgmeier, C. (2010). Tier II interventions within the framework of School-Wide Positive Behavior Support: Essential features for design, implementation, and maintenance. *Behavior Analysis in Practice*, 3(1), 33–45. DOI: 10.1007/BF03391756 PMID: 22479670

Barrett, S., Eber, L., McIntosh, K., Perales, K., & Romer, N. (2018). *Teaching social-emotional competencies within a PBIS framework*. OSEP Technical Assistance Center on Positive Behavioral Interventions and Supports.

Bastable, E., Massar, M. M., & McIntosh, K. (2020). A survey of team members' perceptions of coaching activities related to tier 1 SWPBIS implementation. *Journal of Positive Behavior Interventions*, 22(1), 51–61. DOI: 10.1177/1098300719861566

Behavioral Interventions and Supports and Social Emotional Learning Weist, M. D., Lever, N. A., Bradshaw, C. P., & Owens, J. S. (Eds.), *Handbook of school mental health: Research, training, practice, and policy* (pp. 101–118). Springer.

Bethune, K. S. (2017). Effects of coaching on teachers' implementation of Tier 1 School-Wide Positive Behavioral Interventions and Support strategies. *Journal of Positive Behavior Interventions*, 19(3), 131–142. DOI: 10.1177/1098300716680095

Bradshaw, C.P., Bottiani, J. K., Osher, D., & Sugai, G. (2014). The integration of Positive

Bruhn, A. L., & McDaniel, S. C. (2021). Tier 2: Critical issues in systems, practices, and data. *Journal of Emotional and Behavioral Disorders*, 29(1), 34–43. DOI: 10.1177/1063426620949859

Buli, B. G., Larm, P., Nilsson, K. W., Hellstrom-Olsson, C., & Giannotta, F. (2024). Trends in mental health problems among Swedish adolescents: Do school-related factors play a role? *PLoS One*, 19(3), e0300294. DOI: 10.1371/journal.pone.0300294 PMID: 38457463

Burnett-Zeigler, I., Walton, M. A., Ilgen, M., Barry, K. L., Chermack, S. T., Zucker, R. A., Zimmerman, M. A., Booth, B. M., & Blow, F. C. (2012). Prevalence and correlates of mental health problems and treatment among adolescents seen in primary care. *The Journal of Adolescent Health*, 50(6), 559–564. DOI: 10.1016/j.jadohealth.2011.10.005 PMID: 22626481

Butler, N., Quigg, Z., Bates, R., Jones, L., Ashworth, E., Gowland, S., & Jove, M. (2022). The contributing role of family, school, and peer supportive relationships in protecting the mental well-being of children and adolescents. *School Mental Health*, 14(3), 776–788. DOI: 10.1007/s12310-022-09502-9 PMID: 35154501

Caldarella, P., Larsen, R. A. A., Williams, L., Downs, K. R., Wills, H. P., & Wehby, J. H. (2020). Effects of teachers' praise-to-reprimand ratios on elementary students' on-task behaviour. *Educational Psychology*, 40(10), 1306–1322. DOI: 10.1080/01443410.2020.1711872

Carr, E. G. (1999). *Positive behavior support for people with developmental disabilities: A research synthesis*. AAMR.

Center on PBIS. (2023). *PBIS: An evidence-based framework for making schools safe, positive, predictable, and equitable*. Center on PBIS, University of Oregon. www.pbis.org

Center on PBIS. (2024). *PBIS improves student & adult mental health and wellbeing*. Center on PBIS, University of Oregon. www.pbis.org

Childs, K. E., Kincaid, D., George, H. P., & Gage, N. A. (2016). The relationship between school-wide implementation of Positive Behavior Intervention and Supports and student discipline outcomes. *Journal of Positive Behavior Interventions*, 18(2), 89–99. DOI: 10.1177/1098300715590398

Cho Blair, K. S., Park, E. Y., & Kim, W. H. (2021). A meta-analysis of Tier 2 interventions implemented within School-Wide Positive Behavioral Interventions and Supports. *Psychology in the Schools*, 58(1), 141–161. DOI: 10.1002/pits.22443

Coley, R. L., Sims, J., Dearing, E., & Spielvogel, B. (2018). Locating economic risks for adolescent mental and behavioral health: Poverty and affluence in families, neighborhoods, and schools. *Child Development*, 89(2), 360–369. DOI: 10.1111/cdev.12771 PMID: 28245340

Colomeischi, A. A., Duca, D. S., Bujor, L., Rusu, P. P., Grazzani, I., & Cavioni, V. (2022). Impact of a school mental health program on children's and adolescents' socio-emotional skills and psychosocial difficulties. *Children (Basel, Switzerland)*, 9(11), 1661. DOI: 10.3390/children9111661 PMID: 36360389

Cook, C. R., Frye, M., Slemrod, T., Lyon, A. R., Renshaw, T. L., & Zhang, Y. (2015). An integrated approach to universal prevention: Independent and combined effects of PBIS and SEL on youths' mental health. *School Psychology Quarterly*, 30(2), 166–183. DOI: 10.1037/spq0000102 PMID: 25602629

Cumming, T. M., & O'Neill, S. C. (2019). Using data-based individualization to intensify behavioral interventions. *Intervention in School and Clinic*, 54(5), 280–285. DOI: 10.1177/1053451218819203

Damsgaard, M. T., Holstein, B. E., Koushede, V., Madsen, K. R., Meilstrup, C., Nelausen, M. K., Nielsen, L., & Rayce, S. B. (2014). Close relations to parents and emotional symptoms among adolescents: Beyond socio-economic impact? *International Journal of Public Health*, 59(5), 721–726. DOI: 10.1007/s00038-014-0600-8 PMID: 25178736

Drevon, D. D., Hixson, M. D., Wyse, R. D., & Rigney, A. M. (2019). A meta-analytic review of the evidence for check-in check-out. *Psychology in the Schools*, 56(3), 393–412. DOI: 10.1002/pits.22195

Duncan, M. J., Patte, K. A., & Leatherdale, S. T. (2021). Mental health associations with academic performance and education behaviors in Canadian secondary school students. *Canadian Journal of School Psychology*, 36(4), 335–357. DOI: 10.1177/0829573521997311

Eber, L., Barrett, S., Perales, K., Jeffrey-Pearsall, J., Pohlman, K., Putnam, R., Splett, J., & Weist, M. D. (2019). Advancing Education Effectiveness: Interconnecting School Mental Health and School-Wide PBIS, Volume 2: An Implementation Guide. Center for Positive Behavior Interventions and Supports. University of Oregon Press.

Elrod, B. G., Rice, K. G., & Meyers, J. (2022). PBIS fidelity, school climate, and student discipline: A longitudinal study of secondary schools. *Psychology in the Schools*, 59(2), 376–397. DOI: 10.1002/pits.22614

Ennis, R. P., Royer, D. J., Lane, K. L., & Dunlap, K. D. (2020). Behavior-specific praise in pre-K–12 settings: Mapping the 50-year knowledge base. *Behavioral Disorders*, 45(3), 131–147. DOI: 10.1177/0198742919843075

Erskine, H. E., Baxter, A., Patton, G. C., Moffitt, T. E., Patel, V., Whiteford, H., & Scott, J. F. (2017). The global coverage of prevalence data for mental disorders in children and adolescents. *Epidemiology and Psychiatric Sciences*, 26(4), 395–402. DOI: 10.1017/S2045796015001158 PMID: 26786507

Erskine, H. E., Moffitt, T. E., Copeland, W. E., Costello, E. J., Ferrari, A. J., Patton, G., Degenhardt, L., Vos, T., Whiteford, H. A., & Scott, J. G. (2015). A heavy burden on young minds: The global burden of mental health and substance use disorders in children and youth. *Psychological Medicine*, 45(7), 1551–1563. DOI: 10.1017/S0033291714002888 PMID: 25534496

Fernandez-Castillo, A., & Rojas, M. E. G. (2009). Atencion selectiva, ansiedad, sintomatologia depressive y rendimiento academico en adolescentes. *Electronic Journal of Research in Educational Psychology*, 7(1), 49–76.

Firose, M., Musthafa, M.M., Marikar, & F.M.M.T. (2023). Mental health and self-esteem correlated with the academic achievements of youths from Sri Lankan schools. *Psihiatru.ro, 73(2)*, 27-32.

Fixsen, D. L., Naoom, S. F., Blase, K. A., Friedman, R. M., & Wallace, F. (2005). *Implementation research: A synthesis of the literature* (FMHI Publication No. 231). University of South Florida, Louis de la Parte Florida Mental Health Institute, National Implementation Research Network.

Flannery, K. B., Fenning, P., Kato, M. M., & McIntosh, K. (2014). Effects of school-wide positive behavioral interventions and supports and fidelity of implementation on problem behavior in high schools. *School Psychology Quarterly*, 29(2), 111–124. DOI: 10.1037/spq0000039 PMID: 24188290

Freeman, J., Sugai, G., Simonsen, B., & Everett, S. (2017). MTSS coaching: Bridging knowing to doing. *Theory into Practice*, 56(1), 29–37. DOI: 10.1080/00405841.2016.1241946

Freeman, R., Simacek, J., Jeffrey-Pearsall, J., Lee, S., Khalif, M., & Oteman, Q. (2024). Development of the tiered onsite evaluation tool for organization-wide person-centered Positive Behavior Support. *Journal of Positive Behavior Interventions*, 26(3), 131–141. DOI: 10.1177/10983007231200540

Goh, A. E., & Bambara, L. M. (2012). Individualized positive behavior support in school settings: A meta-analysis. *Remedial and Special Education*, 33(5), 271–286. DOI: 10.1177/0741932510383990

Greenberg, M., Domitrovich, C., Weissberg, R., & Durlak, J. (2017). Social and emotional learning as a public health approach to education. *The Future of Children*, 27(1), 13–32. DOI: 10.1353/foc.2017.0001

Hawken, L. S., Crone, D. A., Bundock, K., & Horner, R. H. (2020). *Responding to problem behavior in schools*. Guilford Publications.

Hawken, L. S., & Horner, R. H. (2003). Evaluation of a targeted intervention within a schoolwide system of behavior support. *Journal of Behavioral Education*, 12(3), 225–240. DOI: 10.1023/A:1025512411930

Hershfeldt, P. A., Pell, K., Sechrest, R., Pas, E. T., & Bradshaw, C. P. (2012). Lessons learned coaching teachers in behavior management: The PBIS*plus* Coaching Model. *Journal of Educational & Psychological Consultation*, 22(4), 280–299. DOI: 10.1080/10474412.2012.731293 PMID: 23599661

Horner, R. H., & Kittelman, A. (2021). Advancing the large-scale implementation of Applied Behavior Analysis. *Behavior and Social Issues*, 30(1), 94–105. DOI: 10.1007/s42822-021-00049-z

Horner, R. H., & Sugai, G. (2015). School-wide PBIS: An example of Applied Behavior Analysis implemented at a scale of social importance. *Behavior Analysis in Practice*, 8(1), 80–85. DOI: 10.1007/s40617-015-0045-4 PMID: 27703887

Ihbour, S., Essaidi, O., Laaroussi, M., Najimi, M., & Chigr, F. (2023). Links between reading acquisition level, emotional difficulties, and academic performance in school-aged children. *The Journal of Mental Health Training, Education and Practice*, 18(2), 135–145. DOI: 10.1108/JMHTEP-05-2021-0040

Johns Hopkins Bloomberg School of Public Health & United Nations Children's Fund. (2022). *On My Mind: How adolescents experience and perceive mental health around the world*. JHU and UNICEF.

Kearney, C. A., & Graczyk, P. A. (2014). A response to intervention model to promote school attendance and decrease school absenteeism. *Child and Youth Care Forum*, 43(1), 1–25. DOI: 10.1007/s10566-013-9222-1

Kearney, C. A., & Graczyk, P. A. (2020). A multidimensional, multitiered system of supports model to promote school attendance and address school absenteeism. *Clinical Child and Family Psychology Review*, 23(3), 316–337. DOI: 10.1007/s10567-020-00317-1 PMID: 32274598

Kern, L., Gaier, K., Kelly, S., Nielsen, C. M., Commisso, C. E., & Wehby, J. H. (2020). An evaluation of adaptations made to Tier 2 social skill training programs. *Journal of Applied School Psychology*, 36(2), 155–172. DOI: 10.1080/15377903.2020.1714858

Kraft, M. A., Blazar, D., & Hogan, D. (2018). The effect of teacher coaching on instruction and achievement: A meta-analysis of the causal evidence. *Review of Educational Research*, 88(4), 547–588. DOI: 10.3102/0034654318759268

Kurth, J. A., & Enyart, M. (2016). Schoolwide positive behavior supports and students with significant disabilities: Where are we? *Research and Practice for Persons with Severe Disabilities : the Journal of TASH*, 41(3), 216–222. DOI: 10.1177/1540796916633083

Lane, K. L., Capizzi, A. M., Fisher, M. H., & Ennis, R. P. (2012). Secondary prevention efforts at the middle school level: An application of the behavior education program. *Education & Treatment of Children*, 35(1), 51–90. DOI: 10.1353/etc.2012.0002

Lindsey, B., & White, M. (2009). Tier 2 behavioral interventions for at-risk students. *School social work: Practice, policy, and research*, 665-673.

Maynard, B. R., Kjellstrand, E. K., & Thompson, A. M. (2014). Effects of check and connect on attendance, behavior, and academics: A randomized effectiveness trial. *Research on Social Work Practice*, 24(3), 296–309. DOI: 10.1177/1049731513497804

McDaniel, S. C., Bruhn, A. L., & Mitchell, B. (2015). A Tier 2 framework for identification and intervention. *Beyond Behavior*, 24(1), 10–17. DOI: 10.1177/107429561502400103

McDaniel, S. C., Bruhn, A. L., & Troughton, L. (2017). A brief social skills intervention to reduce challenging classroom behavior. *Journal of Behavioral Education*, 26(1), 53–74. DOI: 10.1007/s10864-016-9259-y

McLeod, J. D., Uemura, R., & Rohrman, S. (2012). Adolescent mental health, behavio problems, and academic achievement. *Journal of Health and Social Behavior*, 53(4), 482–497. DOI: 10.1177/0022146512462888 PMID: 23197485

Miller, F. G., Swenson Wagner, N., & Robers, A. C. (2023). Examining behavior specific praise as an individual behavior management strategy in a high-need educational setting. *Preventing School Failure*, 1–11. DOI: 10.1080/1045988X.2023.2269891

Missouri School-wide Positive Behavior Support. (2019). *Missouri Schoolwide Positive Behavior handbook*. MO SWPBS.

Mitchell, B. S., Bruhn, A. L., & Lewis, T. J. (2015). Essential features of Tier 2 & 3 school-wide positive behavioral supports. In Jimerson, S. R., Burns, M. K., & VanDerHeyden, A. M. (Eds.), *Handbook of response to intervention: The science and practice of assessment and intervention* (2nd ed., pp. 539–562). Springer.

Mitchell, B. S., Stormont, M., & Gage, N. A. (2011). Tier two interventions implemented within the context of a tiered prevention framework. *Behavioral Disorders*, 36(4), 241–261. DOI: 10.1177/019874291103600404

Nelson, J. M., & Harwood, H. (2011). Learning disabilities and anxiety: A meta-analysis. *Journal of Learning Disabilities*, 44(1), 3–17. DOI: 10.1177/0022219409359939 PMID: 20375288

Nese, R. N. T., Kittelman, A., Strickland-Cohen, M. K., & McIntosh, K. (2023). Examining teaming and Tier 2 and 3 practices within a PBIS Framework. *Journal of Positive Behavior Interventions*, 25(1), 16–27. DOI: 10.1177/10983007211051090

Palmer, K., & Noltemeyer, A. (2019). Professional development in schools: Predictors of effectiveness and implications for statewide PBIS trainings. *Teacher Development*, 23(5), 511–528. DOI: 10.1080/13664530.2019.1660211

Powers, K., Hagans, K., & Linn, M. (2017). A mixed-method efficacy and fidelity study of Check and Connect. *Psychology in the Schools*, 54(9), 1019–1033. DOI: 10.1002/pits.22038

Royer, D. J., Lane, K. L., Dunlap, K. D., & Ennis, R. P. (2019). A systematic review of teacher-delivered behavior-specific praise on K–12 student performance. *Remedial and Special Education*, 40(2), 112–128. DOI: 10.1177/0741932517751054

Ruch, D. A., Horowitz, L. M., Hughes, J. L., Sarkisian, K., Luby, J. L., Fontanella, C. A., & Bridge, J. A. (2024). Suicide in US preteens aged 8 to 12 years, 2001-2022. *JAMA Network Open*, 7(7), e2424664. DOI: 10.1001/jamanetworkopen.2024.24664 PMID: 39078634

Scott, T. (2017). *Teaching behavior*. Corwin., DOI: 10.4135/9781506337883

Sharpe, J., Bunting, B., & Heary, C. (2023). A latent class analysis of mental health symptoms in primary school children: Exploring associations with school attendance problems. *School Mental Health*, 15(4), 1128–1144. DOI: 10.1007/s12310-023-09610-0

Simeonsson, R. J. (Ed.). (1994). *Risk, resilience & prevention: Promoting the well-being of all children*. Paul H. Brookes Publishing Co.

Simonsen, B., & Sugai, G. (2019). School-wide positive behavioral interventions and supports: A systems-level application of behavioral principles. In Little, S. G., & Akin-Little, A. (Eds.), *Behavioral interventions in schools: Evidence-based positive strategies* (2nd ed., pp. 35–60). American Psychological Association., DOI: 10.1037/0000126-003

Simonsen, B., Sugai, G., & Negron, M. (2008). Schoolwide Positive Behavior Supports: Primary systems and practices. *Teaching Exceptional Children*, 40(6), 32–40. DOI: 10.1177/004005990804000604

Skoric, D., Rakic, J. G., Jovanovic, V., Backovic, D., Soldatovic, I., & Zivojinovic, J. I. (2023). Psychosocial school factors and mental health of first-grade secondary school students—Results of the health behavior in school-aged children survey in Serbia. *PLoS One*, 18(11), e0293179. DOI: 10.1371/journal.pone.0293179 PMID: 37943735

Strickland-Cohen, M. K., Pinkelman, S. E., Jimerson, J. B., Berg, T. A., Pinkney, C. J., & McIntosh, K. (2018). Sustaining effective individualized behavior support: Barriers and enablers. *Preventing School Failure*, 63(1), 1–11. DOI: 10.1080/1045988X.2018.1456399

Sugai, G., & Horner, R. H. (2020). Sustaining and scaling positive behavioral interventions and supports: Implementation drivers, outcomes, and considerations. *Exceptional Children*, 86(2), 120–136. DOI: 10.1177/0014402919855331

Sugai, G., & Lewis, T. J. (1999). Developing positive behavioral support systems. In Sugai, G., & Lewis, T. J. (Eds.), *Developing positive behavioral support for students with challenging behavior* (pp. 15–23). Council for Children with Behavioral Disorders.

Todd, A. W., Campbell, A. L., Meyer, G. G., & Horner, R. H. (2008). The effects of a targeted intervention to reduce problem behaviors: Elementary school implementation of check in—check out. *Journal of Positive Behavior Interventions*, 10(1), 46–55. DOI: 10.1177/1098300707311369

Tyre, A., Begay, K. K., Beaudoin, K., & Feuerborn, L. (2023). Understanding middle and high school student preferences for acknowledgements in the context of schoolwide PBIS. *Preventing School Failure*, 68(2), 139–148. DOI: 10.1080/1045988X.2023.2186339

United Nations Children's Fund. (2021). [*On my mind. Promoting, protecting and caring for children's mental health.* UNICEF Office of Global Insight and Policy.]. *The State of the World's Children*, 2021.

Van Camp, A. M., Wehby, J. H., Copeland, B. A., & Bruhn, A. L. (2021). Building from the bottom up: The importance of Tier 1 supports in the context of Tier 2 interventions. *Journal of Positive Behavior Interventions*, 23(1), 53–64. DOI: 10.1177/1098300720916716

Vieira, A. P. A., Peng, P., Antoniuk, A., DeVries, J., Rothou, K., Parrila, R., & Georgiou, G. (2024). Internalizing problems in individuals with reading, mathematics and unspecified learning difficulties: A systematic review and meta-analysis. *Annals of Dyslexia*, 74(1), 4–26. DOI: 10.1007/s11881-023-00294-4 PMID: 38135829

Walker, H. M., Horner, R. H., Sugai, G., Bullis, M., Sprague, J. R., Bricker, D., & Kaufman, M. J. (1996). Integrated approaches to preventing antisocial behavior patterns among school-age children and youth. *Journal of Emotional and Behavioral Disorders*, 4(4), 194–209.

Walker, V. L., & Loman, S. L. (2022). Strategies for including students with extensive support needs in SWPBIS. *In Practice*, 1(1), 23–32.

Walker, H. M., Horner, R. H., Sugai, G., Bullis, M., Sprague, J. R., Bricker, D., & Kaufman, M.

Weissberg, R. P., Durlak, J. A., Domitrovich, C. E., & Gulotta, T. P. (2017). Social emotional learning: Past, present, and future. In Durlak, J. A., Domitrovich, C. E., Weissberg, R. P., & Gullotta, T. P. (Eds.), *Handbook of Social and Emotional Learning: Research and Practice* (pp. 3–19). The Guildford Press.

Zagona, A. L., Hara, M., Loman, S., Kurth, J. A., & Walker, V. L. (2024). Educators' perceptions on the involvement of students with complex support needs in PBIS: The role of educational placement. *Research and Practice for Persons with Severe Disabilities : the Journal of TASH*, •••, 15407969241263515. DOI: 10.1177/15407969241263515

Chapter 4
Behavior Problems in the School Community:
Prevention and Intervention Strategies

Efi Glymitsa
http://orcid.org/0009-0001-5315-7904
National and Kapodistrian University of Athens, Greece

Eleni Zafiriadou
http://orcid.org/0009-0002-1265-4653
National and Kapodistrian University of Athens, Greece

Maria Zafiropoulou
http://orcid.org/0009-0009-3930-999X
Thessaly University, Greece

Evangelia Galanaki
http://orcid.org/0000-0002-7519-6146
National and Kapodistrian University of Athens, Greece

ABSTRACT

This chapter presents strategies that teachers can use for preventing and dealing with students' behavior problems in the school community. These strategies are based on behavioral, cognitive behavioral, ecosystemic, and humanistic approaches. The basic premise of this chapter is that the effectiveness of prevention and intervention is enhanced when strategies from all these approaches are used by educators. The basic principles of behavioral, cognitive behavioral, ecosystemic, and humanistic models are briefly presented based on which, management strategies are described that teachers can implement to prevent and deal with children's behaviour problems

DOI: 10.4018/979-8-3693-5325-7.ch004

as well as to increase desirable behaviours. These prevention and intervention programs are delivered at the individual, classroom, whole school, and family levels. Specific examples are given for all these strategies. Finally, two case studies or scenarios are presented with the aim of illuminating the effective use of these strategies in real situations within the school community.

INTRODUCTION

This chapter focuses on prevention and intervention strategies regarding children's behavior problems in school. First, behavior and behavior problems are defined, as well as their types and consequences, and then basic theoretical models of human behavior are briefly presented, namely the behavioral, cognitive behavioral, ecosystemic, and humanistic models. Based on these models, we describe behavior management techniques that the teacher can use to reduce children's behavior problems and increase desirable behaviors. The techniques presented are indicative and by no means exhaustive. Finally, two case studies or scenarios are presented with the aim of illustrating the use of these techniques in the educational practice.

Behavior and Behavior Problems

Definitions and Determining Factors

Behavior is defined as "the set of characteristic actions of a person or animal, the specific way of reacting to external or internal stimuli" (Cambridge University Press, n.d.). The term *behavior problems* is used to refer to children's inappropriate, ineffective, or unsuccessful attempts to adapt to the demands of their environment (Galanaki, 2011).

Factors determining or contributing to the onset of behavior problems may be intrinsic and/or extrinsic ones (Carr, 2016). Negative internal and/or external factors acting gradually and cumulatively can cause emotional or behavioral dysfunction (Sameroff, 2000). Examples of intrinsic factors are the individual's temperament, genetic, and physical factors (American Psychiatric Association [APA], 2013; Bromley et al., 2006; Gardner & Shaw, 2008). Examples of extrinsic factors are parenting practices, school context, social environment, and the culture (APA, 2013; Gardner & Shaw, 2008). The emergence of undesirable behaviors may be the result of personal predisposing factors, environmental and social contextual predisposing factors, personal and environmental factors that maintain problem behavior, and catalytic factors (e.g., adolescence, loss, victimization, etc.) (Carr, 2016). Research evidence (for a meta-analysis see Carneiro et al., 2016) indicates that common risk factors for children's behavior problems are environmental risk factors (i.e., demographic factors, socio-economic status, parental education, and age), parental mental health factors and parenting factors (i.e., parents' substance abuse and mental health), disciplinary practices, parental interaction, expectations and concerns for the child, and child risk factors (i.e., gender and temperament).

Types of Behavior Problems and Their Consequences

Achenbach (1966) proposed a taxonomy of behavior problems by distinguishing between *externalizing problems* and *internalizing problems*. This taxonomy is included in contemporary dimensional systems of psychopathology and has proved useful in clinical and school practice, as well as in research. According to Achenbach and Rescorla (2001), externalizing problems take the form of aggressive, rule-breaking, and delinquent behavior, whereas internalizing problems include withdrawal, anxiety/depression, and physical complaints. Internalizing problems are not easily recognized, although they entail subjective distress, whereas externalizing problems are easily recognizable because they involve behavior directed towards others (Abry et al., 2017; Achenbach & Rescorla, 2019; Kalantzi-Azizi & Zafiropoulou, 2004).

Students with behavior problems exhibit deficits in social, emotional, and academic skills. This means that they experience problems regarding psychosocial adjustment and adaptation to the demands of school life (Austin & Sciarra, 2016; Kourkoutas, 2011; Kourkoutas et al., 2018; Steele & Steele, 2014). Therefore, effective management of behavior problems is essential in the school community (Sciarra et al., 2022).

Models of Human Behavior

The Behavioral Model

The principles of behaviorism have been extensively applied in educational settings. The first model of behaviorism is *classical conditioning*, as formulated by Ivan P. Pavlov (1927) and John B. Watson (1914) through their experimental work with animals. According to this model, an initially neutral stimulus can elicit, by itself, a specific response in the individual if this stimulus has been previously associated with another stimulus that produces this response, which is often a reflex (Zafiropoulou, 2000; see Figure 1).

Figure 1. **Classical conditioning**

stimulus ⟶ response

A step further was taken by Edward Thorndike (1898) who, after experiments on how cats behave when placed in a puzzle box, introduced the law of effect, in other words the effect of consequences. When behavior has a pleasant consequence, it is more likely to be repeated, whereas a behavior followed by an unpleasant event tends to be discontinued. In addition to classical conditioning, this model introduced the concept of consequences and the involvement of the individual's will. Thus, behaviors are not simply reflexive, but involve their effects, which are the critical element for their repetition. Building on Thorndike's model, B. F. Skinner (1966) introduced operant conditioning, which emphasizes the role of positive and negative reinforcement in acquiring and strengthening desired behaviors and the role of punishment in reducing or eliminating undesired ones (see Figure 2). Radical behaviorism (both classical and operant conditioning) claims that behavior science is a branch of natural science. Within this viewpoint, individuals' thoughts, feelings, and behaviors are the products of their environments and experiences and do not exist on their own (Baum, 2011).

Figure 2. **Operant conditioning**

stimulus ⟶ response ⟷ consequences

The Cognitive Behavioral Model

While the involvement of cognitive and social factors in the manifestation of behavior was ignored by radical behaviorism (classical and operant conditioning), the cognitive revolution, which emerged in the 1970s (Dember, 1974; Miller, 2003), addressed the shortcomings of behaviorism. This new approach complemented behaviorism, by combining the influence of external/environmental factors on behavior with the internal, non-obvious processes that take place within the individual. These processes intervene between stimuli and response and are related to the perception and interpretation of the situation from which the behavior arises (Muhajirah, 2020).

In this way, a new view of behavior emerged (see Figure 3), in which the individual is not a passive receptor of external stimuli, but an *active agent*.

Figure 3. **The cognitive behavioral model**

stimulus ⟶ individual (cognitive, emotional processes) ⟶ response

Within the cognitive behavioral model, the *reciprocal determinism model* (Bandura, 1977, 1978; see Figure 4) emphasizes the interdependence among the environment, the individuals' behavior and their characteristics and processes (Little, 2018). More specifically, *observational learning*, that is, learning by observing a model and imitating his/her behavior, has been suggested by Bandura (1986) in the framework of his social learning theory. Four processes need to take place for the student to successfully imitate a desirable behavior: attention, retention, motor production, and motivation.

Figure 4. **The reciprocal determinism model**

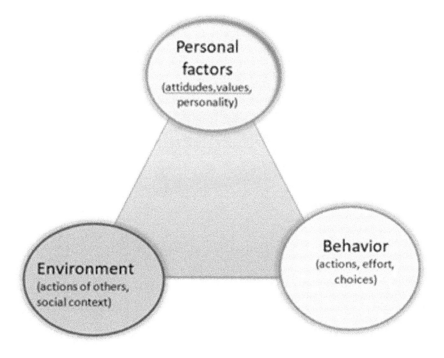

Conscious and unconscious factors such as thoughts have the power to modify behavior as behavioral reinforcers (Homme, 1965). In the 1960s and 1970s, studies by Ellis (1962) and later by Beck (1976) supported the idea that pathological behavior, in both its internalized and externalized forms (Achenbach & Rescorla, 2019), is due to dysfunctional cognitive processes. This approach can be summarized as follows: thoughts elicit emotions and the latter lead to behaviors which, in turn, reinforce the thoughts; this process continues in a cyclical form (see Figure 5).

Figure 5. **Associations between inner processes, behavior, and reality**

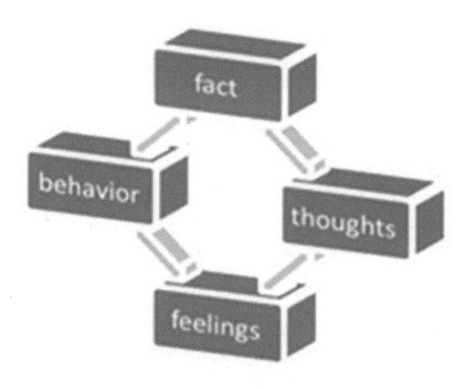

The Ecosystemic Model

According to the *general systems theory* introduced by von Bertalanffy (1968/2013) and to the *ecological model* introduced by Bronfenbrenner (1979), every individual is a member of social systems, such as microsystems, mesosystems, exosystems, and macrosystems. Each behavior is a part of these systems, influences the other parts, and is influenced by them. A *system* is an organized set of interrelated elements, which function to achieve specific goals, and strives to maintain its homeostasis. The microsystem consists of significant others, such as family, peers, school environment, friends. The relationships between microsystems form the mesosystem. Other domains, such as extended family, work, and health services among others, form the exosystem, which is included in the macrosystem. The macrosystem is the wider society, with its laws, cultural values, customs, and traditions. All these contexts and systems affect the developing individuals, who are embedded in the microsystem, and are affected by them. They are in constant interaction, and each is open to the influences of the environment and other exogenous factors (see Figure 6). If the interactions are positive, then the individual's development is positive and the microsystem is characterized as facilitative of the individual's development (Bronfenbrenner, 1979; Galanaki, 2000a, 2000b; Pianta, 1999; Shelton, 2018; von Bertalanffy, 1968/2013).

Figure 6. **The ecosystemic model**

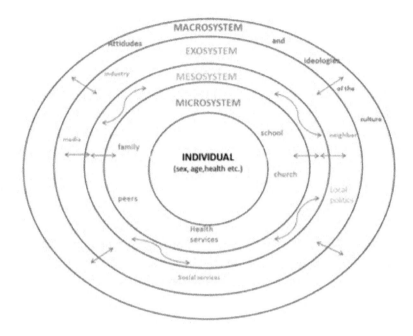

Within the ecosystemic model, behaviors are not conceptualized in a linear way (i.e., as cause and effect), but in a holistic way, based upon the principle of *circular causality*, according to which every behavior is both cause and effect, action and reaction. This model also considers multiple interacting factors that lead to the manifestation of behavior and treats each relationship created in a microsystem as dependent on the other relationships created within it and outside of it, open to causing and receiving constant change (Bronfenbrenner, 1979; Pianta, 1999; Shelton, 2018; von Bertalanffy, 1968/2013; Watzlawick, 1981).

The Humanistic Model

The humanistic model, which appeared in the 1970s, has as its basic principle the involvement of the *whole person*, as a unique personality consisting of emotions, cognitions, and behavior. According to the *hierarchy of needs* introduced by Abraham Maslow (1968, 1987), the aim of education is the *self-actualization* of the student, which is attained when all the other human needs are satisfied (see Figure 7).

Figure 7. **Maslow's hierarchy of needs**

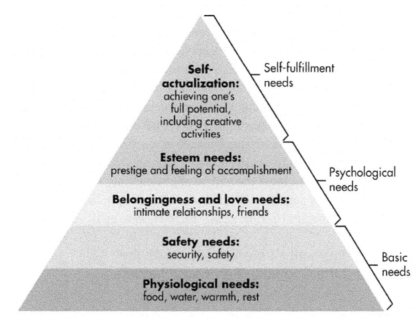

Source: https://www.simplypsychology.org/maslow.htm

According to this model, teachers should facilitate the satisfaction of their students' needs for safety, love, effective social skills, and self-esteem. Education should aim not only to cognitive but also to emotional learning. The implementation of *social and emotional learning* (SEL) programs is, therefore, considered essential for the promotion of children's wellbeing (for meta-analyses see Durlak et al., 2022; Grand et al., 2023; Green et al., 2021; Sutherland et al., 2018).

Emotional learning should not be separated from the rest of the school curriculum (Brown, 1987). The teacher sends verbal and non-verbal messages to his/her students with the aim of making them feel responsible, competent, and valued. Teachers create a warm emotional climate and enable students develop *positive self-concept* and a *sense of self-worth* (Purkey, 1970, 1978, 1991). Collaborative learning, the use of "I-messaging" (i.e., the use of the first-person singular in conversation; e.g., "I see how... I feel... I believe...", etc.), active listening, enhancement of empathy, and the promotion of values are the core principles of the humanistic model.

Behavior Management Strategies

Based on the aforementioned models, below we present a series of behavior management strategies. In addition, we suggest teacher practices that can be applied on the individual and on the class and school level, as well as in the relationship between family and school. A large body of research supports the effectiveness of these strategies and practices in preventing and dealing with students' behavior problems, in developing their social skills, enhancing their resilience, improving student-teacher relationships, engaging students in the educational process, etc. (for meta-analyses see Chafee et al., 2017; Kincade et al., 2020; Sheridan et al., 2019; Sutherland et al., 2018). Additionally, research indicates that programs integrating ideas and methods from multiple theoretical approaches are significantly more effective. This integration amplifies the strengths of each approach while mitigating their respective weaknesses (Cooper et al., 2020; Heward et al., 2016).

Behavior Management Strategies Based on the Behavioral and the Cognitive Behavioral Models

A) Behavior management in the classroom is largely based on techniques derived from behavioral theories. The basic premise of these approaches is that to change undesirable behaviors, we must target the *context* within which these behaviors appear.

Below we describe in detail the main behavioral strategies used for effective classroom management.

1. Promoting desirable behaviors through reinforcement

Reinforcement can be either positive or negative (Skinner, 1966). *Positive* reinforcement refers to something that the individual desires and receives; in other words, the individual's behavior is followed by a pleasant consequence, which increases the likelihood that this behavior will appear in the future. In everyday school life, an example of positive reinforcer is the teacher's phrase *"Well done!!!"*, as a response to a student's desirable behavior. *Negative* reinforcement means that an unpleasant or aversive stimulus is removed, thus, again, the likelihood that the desirable behavior will appear is increased. Negative reinforcement can be characterized as relieving the student from a difficult task when he/she behaves in the desired manner. Negative reinforcement may then be followed by positive one, as a result of the student's desirable behavior.

In an educational setting, reinforcers may be given whenever the desired behavior occurs either at specific intervals (reinforcement by fixed or variable intervals), or according to the number of positive behaviors exhibited (ratio-based reinforcement).

In the first case, a continuous aid program is applied, while in the second case, a periodic aid program is applied. Continuous reinforcement of a student is appropriate when trying to establish a new behavior, because the student must realize as soon as possible that the manifestation of the desired behavior will be followed by something positive. However, continuous reinforcement programs are not suitable for maintaining new behaviors, because continuous reinforcement can lead to saturation (Angeli & Vlachou, 2004). In practice, the use of periodic reinforcement programs seems to be more effective. This is because the individual continues to manifest the desired behavior as he/she does not know when the reinforcement will be applied (Hulac & Briesch, 2017). Positive reinforcement motivates students to exhibit the desired behavior more often and fosters a strong relationship between educators and students (Nisar et al., 2022). To be effective, positive reinforcement needs to be specific, which means that the teacher identifies the target –a student or a group–, describes the behavior, and aligns the intervention with the school-wide expectations (Missouri Department of Elementary and Secondary Education, 2018).

2. Reducing undesirable behaviors through extinction

Extinction results when a behavior that was reinforced in the past is reinforced no more. If all children who used to laugh when their classmate was joking stop doing so, then it is expected that this student will gradually stop joking. However, in such situations, initially the *extinction burst effect* is observed: an increase in the intensity, duration, and frequency of the undesirable behavior occurs, before it is eventually eliminated (Whittingham & Coyne, 2019; Hulac & Briesch, 2017).

3. Reducing undesirable behaviors through punishment

Punishment is defined as stimuli that reduce the likelihood that a child's undesirable behavior will occur (Alberto & Troutman, 2013). Punishment can be either positive or negative (Hulac & Briesch, 2017; Zafiropoulou, 2000). *Positive* punishment means that an aversive stimulus is presented to suppress the undesirable behavior. For example, when the student has incomplete home assignments, the teacher gives him a low grade. In *negative* punishment, something desirable is taken away after the negative behavior occurs, such as not allowing the student to play his/her favorite game at recess. It is important to note that misinterpretation of strict, punitive, dismissive, and rigid discipline standards may have questionable or often harmful effects on students (Missouri Department of Elementary and Secondary Education, 2018; see meta-analysis by Noltemeyer et al., 2015). Although punishment may temporarily suppress behavior problems, these problems tend to reappear or even become aggravated. This occurs because punitive approaches focus on undesirable behaviors, inadvertently rewarding and reinforcing them (Burt et al., 2021). Another negative effect of the punitive approaches is that they harm teacher-student relationships and weaken students' connection to the school (Bear, 2020; Pyne, 2019).

4. Reducing undesirable behaviors through time out

Time out means that the student is removed from a reinforcing environment (i.e., time-in environment) and placed in a non-reinforcing one. Depending on the age of the child and the circumstances, the removal may be (a) from an activity, inside the classroom in a specially designed area so that the child can attend but not participate in the activities or (b) outside the classroom. In the latter case, which is not appropriate except in rare circumstances, the presence of an adult near the child must be ensured, as much as the fact that no reinforcement is provided to the child there.

5. Reducing undesirable behaviors through the path of least resistance

It is common for the teacher to give in to the child's demands. When giving in to the child's disobedience is reduced, it is expected that the child's undesirable behavior will also be reduced.

6. Behavior management through functional behavior analysis

Functional behavior analysis is based on the principles of agentic learning and aims at managing students' behavior in the classroom (Zafiropoulou, 2004). In the framework of this analysis, the teacher produces a clear and precise description of the environmental conditions within which the behavior problem occurs and of the factors that trigger and maintain this problem (Ferster, 1965). The process of functional behavioral assessment involves the following: (a) defining the behavior problem in a positive, observable, and measurable way; (b) gathering information about the context, timing, and circumstances in which the behavior problem occurs and does not occur, including what happens before and after the behavior; and (c) developing hypotheses about the purpose of the behavior problem, so as to understand its possible associations with the context in which it occurs (Neitzel & Bogin, 2008; O'Neill et al., 2015). This process, also known as the *ABC of behavior*, involves the following three elements: the *antecedents* of the behavior (A), the *behavior* itself (B), and its *consequences* (C) (Landrum & Kauffman, 2006; Morgan & Jenson, 1988; Zirpoli, 2005).

The antecedents are all those circumstances that preceded the specific behavior, such as the people involved, the place, the time of day, etc. Identifying the circumstances usually reveals what triggers a dysfunctional behavior and is a very useful tool for preventing it. The consequences of the behavior are also very likely to influence whether it will re-emerge or not. Identifying the consequences allows us to reveal evidence about the feasibility of the behavior in order to reduce it or reinforce an alternative, positive behavior with similar feasibility (Morgan & Jenson, 1988). A thorough examination of the dysfunctional behavior through the ABC process will provide us with the necessary information to design the behavior modification (Crone et al., 2015).

7. Implementing token economy

Reinforcers may take various forms such as points, stickers, etc. and can be exchanged with various rewards, thus acting as a kind of classroom "currency" or token economy. Rewards may be edible (e.g., candy), material (e.g., small gifts), activity (e.g., five minutes more recess), or social (praise from the school principal). It is better to implement token economy at the classroom level than at the student level, because it is easier for the teacher to manage it, while avoiding discrimination among students (Filcheck et al., 2004).

8. Implementing the self-instructional method

The self-instructional method (Meichenbaum, 1977) is one of the first behavioral techniques influenced by Bandura's (1977) theory of modeling. According to this method, the individual is trained to find desired solutions through an internal dialogue that includes self-instructions and self-directions. Thus, perception, attention, judgment, behavioral modification, and search for alternatives are positively influenced (Koliadis, 2010). This method is effective in reducing hyperactivity, aggression, anxiety, and learning difficulties (Karmba & Zafiropoulou, 1997, 2002; Ronen, 2003). A self-instructional program for students consists of the following five steps:

Step 1: The teacher acts as a role model (cognitive modeling).
Step 2: The student performs the same activity under the guidance of the teacher (overt external guidance).
Step 3: The student guides himself/herself by expressing out loud his/her thoughts and actions (overt self-guidance).
Step 4: The student guides himself/herself whispering as he/she performs the activity (faded self-guidance).

Step 5: The student performs the activity while mentally repeating the instructions to himself/herself (covert self-guidance).

9. Implementing self-management

Self-management or self-monitoring is a technique used when students are trained to take a more active role in modifying their behavior (Briesch & Briesch, 2016). For example, the teacher asks the student to record every time he/she breaks a rule (e.g., speaking without raising his/her hand). To ensure the effectiveness of this method, the teacher needs to check the reliability of the child's recordings, use reinforcers and/or token economy, and monitor the child's performance over time. The discussion of the results of the student's recording leads to evaluation and reinforcement, first by the teacher and later by the student in the form of *self-evaluation* and *self-reinforcement*.

B) According to the cognitive behavioral theory (Ellis, 1962), a triggering event (Activity-A) activates the individual's rational or irrational beliefs (Beliefs Rational or Irrational-B), which in turn lead to corresponding emotional reactions (Consequent Affect or Emotion-C). If the person adopts irrational thoughts, he/she receives help to challenge them and replace them with alternative, rational thoughts (Dispute-D). Challenging and modifying irrational thoughts leads to different results on both emotional and behavioral levels (Effect-E). Following are some examples of students' irrational thoughts: "I still have a problem to solve. I'll never get it done"; "Nobody loves me. I'll never have friends at school!"; "Why should I study if I always fail?", etc. (Manning & Payne, 1996). The teacher, according to the *ABCDE model*, is asked to help the student to *name his/her thoughts and feelings* and then with appropriate questions the teacher leads the student to *question and reformulate his/her thoughts*.

A similar method is *problem solving* (Braswell & Kendall, 1988; D'Zurilla & Goldfried, 1971). This method aims at facilitating students to cope with problems and improve their socio-emotional state. It consists of the following five steps: (1) identification of the problem ("What is the problem?"; "What am I thinking?"; "What am I feeling?"; "What do I do when...?"); (2) setting specific, measurable, and realistic goals, with timeframes for their achievement; (3) generating alternative solutions through brainstorming ("What else could I do?"); (4) making a decision after evaluating the consequences of each idea ("If... then" for each idea); and (5) implementing the solution and evaluating it.

Behavior Management Strategies based on the Ecosystemic Model

According to the ecosystemic model (Bronfenbrenner, 1979; von Bertalanffy, 1968/2013), a child's behavior problem is the result of the processes taking place within the systems in which the child lives, and it helps maintain the balance or homeostasis of these systems. In this sense, the problem behavior serves a specific function, for example, to ensure that the systems keep their coherence. Because the school is conceptualized as a system, behavior management strategies should be implemented not only at the individual level but also at the interface between the micro-systems within the school as well as between family and school. Consequently, the reduction of behavior problems is likely to occur if the whole microsystem and its relationships with other microsystems are involved. In other words, a child's behavior is improved if there is a change in the teacher's and/or the peers' behavior towards the child, in addition to any interventions implemented at the individual level (Galanaki, 2000b; Molnar & Lindquist, 2009).

Following are a series of strategies inspired by the ecosystemic model (Molnar & Lindquist, 2009).

1. *Reframing*

Reframing is defined as an alternative, usually positive, interpretation of problem behavior and a change of perspective. Reframing modifies the structure and the processes of the ecosystem and leads to a new, improved homeostasis. It resembles the ripple effect caused when we throw a stone into the water (Galanaki, 1997). This strategy involves the following elements: (a) awareness of the problem behavior; (b) formulation of an alternative, usually positive, interpretation of that behavior; (c) verbal expression of the new interpretation of the problem behavior; and (d) specific actions that confirm this interpretation. In short, with this strategy the teacher can find a new context for the problem behavior that is functional and entails a different way of reacting to it.

2. *Identifying positive motives and functions*

With this strategy, we identify positive motives and functions of the problem behavior that facilitate the modification of it. The basic elements of this strategy are the following: (a) identifying reasons why the child is exhibiting such behavior; (b) focusing on the positive motives and functions of this behavior; (c) selecting a positive aspect of this behavior; (d) verbally expressing the positive aspect; and (e) acting in a way that recognizes the positive motives and functions. Being able to identify positive aspects of an undesirable behavior requires observation and reflection.

3. *Influencing the problem indirectly*

With this strategy, the teacher selects a positive aspect of the child's behavior and makes positive comments about it in the appropriate time and space. It is also called the *storming-the-back-door technique.*

4. *Encouraging problem behavior to continue in different ways and at different times*

When the direct attempts to reduce the problem behavior have failed, we may focus on how this challenging behavior may continue, but in different ways and in different times. It is a paradoxical technique, also called the *symptom prescription technique*, because the teacher urges the student to continue manifesting symptoms – differently.

5. Focusing on what is not a problem

With this strategy, the teacher identifies exceptions, that is, strengths, within the student and uses them to improve his/her behavior. The focus is on the "background" (i.e., the non-problem behavior) and not on the "form" (i.e., the problem behavior). The teacher (a) identifies instances where the challenging behavior does not occur; (b) reflects on the reasons why this happens; (c) selects a non-problem behavior; and (d) reinforces it.

Intervention in the School Settings

Below we briefly present a series of strategies for managing students' behavior which are considered effective for both the classroom and the whole school setting and lead to changes not only in the students' behavior but also in the relationships between all people involved in the educational process (for a meta-analysis see Chafee et al., 2017; Goldberg et al., 2019; Kincade et al., 2020). These interventions are based on the Positive Behavioral Interventions and Supports (PBIS) or Positive Behavior Support (PBS) approaches. These approaches are inspired by operant learning (Skinner, 1966), observational learning (Bandura, 1986), and positive psychology (Mendes de Oliveira et al., 2022). Positive psychology does not focus on what is "pathological" but on positive subjective experience and the positive characteristics of individuals and institutions. It places emphasis on the individuals' strengths (rather than on their weaknesses) and on their willingness to work with the aim of developing their potential and using their talents. This perspective aims at improving the quality of life so that individuals, communities and societies prosper (Selligman

& Csikszentmihalyi, 2000). PBS is an evidence-based framework of prevention and intervention strategies designed to improve the school climate, supports the entire student population on behavioral, social, emotional, and academic levels, and has a strong preventive orientation (Barker et al., 2022; OSEP, 2019; Sugai & Horner, 2002; Sugai & Simonsen, 2012). Interventions are developed on three interrelated levels of intensity (Horner & Monzalve, 2018). The first level includes preventive interventions that target the entire student population and all areas of the school with the aim of creating a predictable, stable, and safe school climate and improving interpersonal relationships among all members of the school community (Horner et al., 2009). At the second level, additional, targeted interventions are developed to support small groups of students who cannot benefit from universal services. Their main characteristics are their differentiated structure and greater family involvement (Horner & Sugai, 2015). Finally, the third level involves the design of intensive individualized interventions for students who cannot benefit from the first and the second level interventions (Bradshaw et al., 2008). School-based positive behavior interventions have been shown to contribute to improved social and emotional skills (Bradshaw et al., 2012; Cook et al., 2015), increases in positive behavior (Lee & Gage, 2020; Park et al., 2019), and decreases in behavior problems (Bradshaw et al., 2012; Flannery et al., 2014; Lee & Gage, 2020; Noltemeyer et al., 2019).

Strategies for Managing Students' Behavior

1. Establishing school-level expectations for student behavior and communicating them to students and parents.
2. Facilitating students to comply with school rules and regulations.
3. Enabling students to take responsibilities within the school context, under the guidance of teachers.
4. Promoting strategies and procedures for early identification, referral, and intervention regarding behavior problems.
5. Implementing regular meetings with both students and parents to ensure consistency of expectations and goals between family and school.
6. Promoting communication among all teachers of the student who exhibits problem behavior. Recording incidents and finding time to discuss these incidents.
7. Providing opportunities and finding alternative activities for the student who exhibits undesirable behavior.
8. Ensuring adequate training for all teachers in the use of collaborative methods and appropriate strategies to manage behavior problems.
9. Enhancing consistent behavior of all teaching staff regarding management strategies and consequences for both negative and positive student behaviors.

Intervention at the Classroom Level

Creating positive climate in classrooms (Wang et al., 2020) plays an important role not only in promoting children's academic and socioemotional wellbeing and resilience, but also in preventing and addressing behavioral problems (Allen et al., 2018; Doll et al., 2014; Vogiatzoglou & Galanaki, 2011). The positive classroom climate is facilitated by the following practices: (a) improving relationships among classroom members; (b) setting clear boundaries; (c) enhancing social skills; (d) providing nurturing; (e) having high expectations and expressing them; (f) providing opportunities for all members of the school community to actively participate in school life and learning (Henderson & Milstein, 2003); and (g) implementing social and emotional learning (SEL) programs (Collaborative for Academic, Social and Emotional Learning [CASEL], n.d.; Social and Emotional Aspects of Learning [SEAL]; for a meta-analysis see Durlak et al., 2022).

Creating a Positive Classroom Climate

Classroom structure and organization reduces students' stress and tension, improves their behavior, and increases their school performance and achievements (Bapst et al., 2023). A flexible classroom, in which the level of noise and movement of students is tolerated, the interactions among all members are promoted, the teacher has clear expectations, and all objects (e.g., desks, materials, bags, etc.) are ergonomically arranged, provides children with a sense of happiness, security, and freedom to explore. The organization of the classroom environment is a key factor in promoting desirable behaviors. A beautifully decorated space, with all necessary materials being well organized and accessible, strengthens the positive mood among class members. Therefore, it is important that students contribute to the decoration of their classroom with their own works.

Regarding the arrangement of desks, teachers should be sensitive to the dynamics of their group (Doll et al, 2014; Henderson & Milstein, 2003). To achieve an appropriate arrangement, the teacher reflects on the following issues: (a) how does he/she want the students to interact; (b) which students will interact most often; (c) how easy will it be for him/her to reach each child; (d) whether there are children with attention or distraction issues; and (e) the type of teaching that will take place (student-centered, group-cooperative, teacher-centered). The traditional arrangement is in rows (see Figure 8). The row arrangement enhances focus on the learning task over other arrangements (Wannarka & Ruhl, 2008). Frontal arrangement in rows encourages individual work and the monitoring of teacher presentations by the teacher. In the "Π" shaped arrangement (see Figure 9), students face each other, and the teacher has easy access to all students. The group arrangement (see Figure

10) favors cooperation among students and promotes discussion and collaboration among them but is likely to reinforce disruptive behaviors.

Figure 8. **Arrangement of desks in rows**

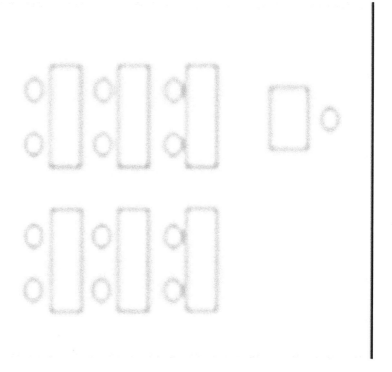

Figure 9. **Arrangement of desks in "П" shape**

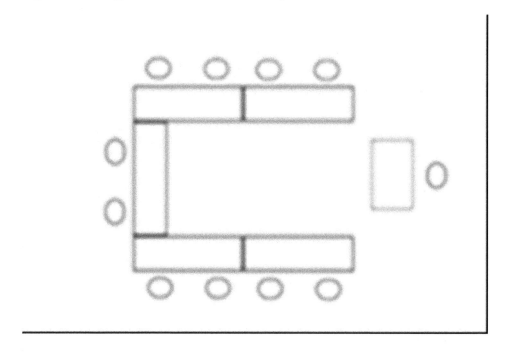

Figure 10. **Arrangement of desks in groups**

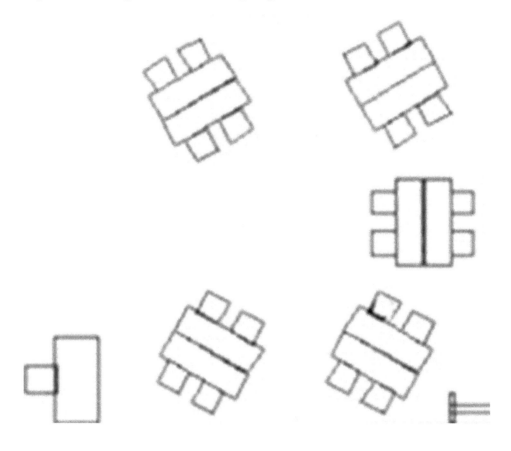

Teaching Rules and Expected Behavioral Routines

Students themselves tend to associate behavior management efficacy mainly with rules and class organization as well as with teacher proximity (Bapst et al., 2023). Knowing in advance what is expected of the student and what he/she is or is not allowed to do in the classroom should not be taken for granted. It is necessary at the beginning of each school year to clearly set out expectations and rules and to allow sufficient time for teaching them. Classroom rules should be co-decided by plenary discussion, be few, that is, four to six (Gable et al., 2009), positively worded (e.g., "I speak in a low voice and do not shout"), age-appropriate, realistic, and understandable. They should also be detailed and consistent. Children's compliance with them should be monitored and noted. Children with behavior problems are likely to disregard the rules; therefore, it is advisable that teachers inform their students that they are going to monitor and record their behavior.

The classroom rules should address the following issues: (a) how I move around the classroom; (b) when and how I speak; (c) how I work and what I do after I have finished my work; and (d) what I should do if a classmate misbehaves or says something that I find inappropriate. In addition, some flexibility in the rules is necessary. Strict and absolute rules will hardly be followed by children with behavior problems. The consequences of the rules must also be important and *meaningful* to the children. A positive consequence of obedience and a negative consequence of disobedience are necessary as long as they are *reasonable* and *proportionate* to the situation. Finally, consequences must be applied *consistently*. It is common for adults to express threats of punishment that are not realized. The teachers should avoid taking decisions in the heat of the moment, in times of tension, because when they calm down, they may change their mind and not implement them.

In addition to rules, it is necessary for students to have specific *routines* in the classroom (Greenberg et al., 2014; Rubie-Davies, 2007). These routines involve procedures to follow during daily activities, that is, how to collect and hand in assignments, how to move from one lesson to another, how to enter and leave the classroom, how to get help, how to discuss in groups, etc. It is adamant that routines and rules are taught step-by-step and are enriched with examples, counterexamples, and continuous reinforcement. As in teaching any new skill, we follow a process that involves presentation, demonstration, and continued application before we reach generalization. More specifically:

1. the teacher, after presenting the routine, starts implementing it while saying out loud what he/she is doing;
2. the teacher describes what needs to be done step-by-step with the use of the first person (I, we);
3. the students follow the procedure while describing it aloud;
4. the students follow the procedure while describing it from memory;
5. examples and counterexamples are presented by the teacher and/or students and the class decide on the "right" and the "wrong".

It is noteworthy that, at each stage, the necessary feedback and reinforcement are provided. Even the way students are greeted and welcomed into the classroom reduces challenging behaviors and improves students' engagement in the educational process (Darling & Cook, 2018; Shields-Lysiak et al., 2020). Consequently, welcoming activities that have become "rituals" make group members feel special, loved, and accepted, promote social and emotional development, enhance group bonding, and improve classroom climate. For example, the adoption of ritualistic complimenting, namely, the Positive Peer Reporting (PPR), has been shown to enhance social interactions and peer acceptance (Moroz & Jones, 2002).

Using Effective Teaching Practices

Certain appropriate teaching practices that promote students' functional behavior are presented below (Alberta Learning, 2000; Barkley & Benton, 2013; Hulac & Briesch, 2017).

1. *Active listening*: it reflects genuine interest in what is being said, so that the student feels important and validated. In active listening:
   - open questions are used that allow the interlocutor to speak by answering beyond "yes" or "no" (e.g., "How about...?"; "How come ...?"; "What options do you have...?", etc.);
   - the idea or thought of the interlocutor is repeated or paraphrased (e.g., "Oh, you're telling me that ...", etc.);
   - the interlocutor reflects on feelings (e.g., "You look... what happened?"; "That would make you proud, huh?", etc.);
   - a summary of what is said is given (e.g., "So what happened is that...", etc.);
   - reframing offers alternative perspectives on what is said (e.g., "Have you thought that maybe...?", etc.);
   - it is preferable to use messages in the first person (e.g., "When..., I feel... and think that... I would like...").
2. *Effective communication of instructions*:
   - An effective way to improve attention is to make eye contact with the student. If the child looks away, the teacher needs to help the child so that his/her gaze returns to him/her. It may even be necessary for the teacher to come down to the child's height so that eye contact is possible.
   - We avoid lengthy instructions. Usually, children can follow one instruction at a time; therefore, when the teacher wants the child to perform a more complex task, it is better to break the task into smaller steps.
   - We ask for measurable things, for example, "Look at the first act"; "Try harder to get your letters on the line".
   - We check the implementation of the instruction.
   - When we give instructions, we avoid threats. Threats are fear-based techniques, whereas instructions simply express what behavior we expect.
   - We really mean what we ask from the child.

- We do not present the instruction as a wish or a question. We express it in a simple, clear, and unambiguous way, so that it can be fully understood by the child.
- It is necessary for the child to know when to follow an instruction, whether it is something that must be done immediately or whether it has a certain time limit.
- When we give an instruction, we should reduce disruptive factors as much as possible. When something else attracts the child's interest while we give an instruction, then it is very likely that the child will not be able to pay attention to the instruction, not understand it, and therefore not follow it.
- When we think that the student has not shown the required attention or when his/her attention span is short, we must repeat the instruction to make sure that it will be carried out.
- We should reward immediately the child's compliance with the instruction.

3. *Precise requests*:

The teacher calls the child's name and makes the request in a firm voice, looking the child in the eyes. The teacher waits for about five minutes and then, if the student responds, he/she praises him/her. If not, he/she uses more imperative tone and repeats the instruction saying: "It is necessary to...". Depending on the student's attitude, the teacher either gives praise or reminds him/her of the rule and the agreed-upon consequence which will be applied.

Cooperation Among Students in the Classroom

It is important to encourage students to participate in school activities and to have an active role in classroom life in the following ways: (a) taking initiatives and acknowledging their responsibilities regarding, for example, their work or the classroom tidiness and cleanliness; (b) cooperating with each other; (c) accepting and respecting all their classmates; (d) helping their classmates deal with challenging behaviors and learning difficulties through the peer teaching method; and (e) rewarding positive behaviors of any of their classmates (Alberta Learning, 2000; Doll et al., 2014; Henderson & Milstein, 2003). A sense of care and support from peers (Hamm & Faircloth, 2005) and a sense of belonging (Allen et al., 2018) contribute to children's social adjustment and academic progress. In general, it is advisable for the teacher to act according to the following principle: "Avoid doing in the school setting what children can do themselves".

Individual Intervention

We have designed and implemented an individual intervention program, which can be applied especially when the usual strategies and behavioral instructions in the classroom are not effective (Glymitsa, 2019; Zafiriadou, 2019; Zafiropoulou, 2019). The purpose of this individual intervention program is to reduce undesirable behaviors, facilitate the emergence of functional behavioral patterns, and increase academic progress. To achieve the overall purpose of the intervention, individual goals need to be small and specific. They also need to be set gradually, with increasing difficulty, so that after mastering one goal students can smoothly move on to the next.

In the framework of this intervention, a variety of strategies, based on social and emotional learning programs, are used:

1. techniques for recognizing the physical symptoms of emotions such as anger and anxiety, for example, an increase in the heart rate;
2. relaxation techniques, such as mindful breathing exercises (Kuyken, 2013), for the effective management of difficult emotions;
3. self-monitoring and self-observation techniques;
4. social skills acquisition techniques;
5. problem solving techniques.

In general, the teacher should bear in mind that challenging behaviors are likely to reoccur. These relapses are common and should be treated as such. In addition, for the effective reduction of a problem behavior, the following must have been achieved: (a) the child's behavior must have improved and (b) the way in which a problem behavior is interpreted by other members of the school system, especially the child's teacher(s) and other educational staff, must have changed (Molnar & Lindquist, 2009).

School-family Cooperation

Considering that school-family cooperation has a direct impact on students' development and progress (Dearing et al., 2006; Pianta, 1999; Shelton, 2018; Sheridan et al., 2019; Smith et al., 2019), it is necessary to briefly mention ways that teachers can suggest to parents for managing their children's behavior problems. Research evidence indicates that parents' involvement plays a crucial role in the effectiveness of interventions (for a meta-analysis see Epstein et al., 2015; for a meta-analysis regarding externalizing problems see Mingebach et al., 2018). Some ways of supporting parents are as follows (Alberta Learning, 2000):

1. Encouraging frequent meetings with parents so that (a) parents understand the teachers' interest and awareness of their child's difficulties, individual needs, family and cultural values, and the school's respect for them; (b) parents understand the school's objectives regarding the child's behavior, the consequences of their own behavior, and the school's expectations of them.
2. Keeping a communication diary between the school and the family, in which both sides will record what is considered important regarding the child's behavior and will be carried daily from school to home and vice versa.
3. Encouraging parents to create a motivational program at home with clear goals and benefits for the child and in direct concordance with the child's behavior program at school.
4. Assisting parents in creating a structured, stable, predictable, rule-based home environment. Such an environment reinforces positive behaviors and reduces the occurrence of behavior problems.
5. Encouraging parents to become active listeners, to observe and record target behaviors, so that they can adequately communicate information to specialists and to the school.
6. Encouraging parents to discover their child's interests and organize activities that they can enjoy together.
7. Supporting parents to ensure that they are adequately informed about their child's behavior problem and referring them to specialists (psychologists, special educators, social workers, etc.) when necessary.
8. Informing parents of the goals and objectives teachers have set for their child's behavior. The goals should be small and achievable to increase the likelihood that they will be attained. It is also a good idea to identify their child's strengths and weaknesses and focus on the positive aspects of the child's behavior.

In general, the aim of interventions for parents is to change the behavior of the parents themselves, not just that of their child's (Kalantzi-Azizi & Galanaki, 2001). The emergence of behavior problems in children is often the result of parents' laissez-faire practices, miscommunication between the parental couple, lack of boundaries or even a negative attitude towards boundaries, among others.

Practical Applications

Case Study 1: Panagiotis

Panagiotis is a sixth-grade student. His physical development makes him look older than his age. Intellectually, he performs better than the average student in the class and this seems to give him an advantage over his classmates. He often corrects them or makes derogatory comments after hearing an incorrect answer. The teacher, in vain, tries to explain to him that this is not right and that he must stop judging or mocking others for their efforts. Panagiotis loses control when he does not get one of the best marks in the class on a written test. For example, in a recent math test, surprisingly, he did not do as well as usual; actually, he got one of the worst marks in the class. As soon as he saw his grade, he started yelling at the teacher: "You take that back! Do you hear me?". At recess, he was so angry about a classmate of his who laughed at his failure, that he threw him up against the railing of the school and hit him hard. His parents, after being called to the school, claimed that he was right, that he was provoked and that he had to react that way; so do those who can. The other teachers at the school wished Panagiotis' teacher "good luck" in dealing with him!

Designing the Intervention

The first step when dealing with a behavior problem is the functional analysis of it. Therefore, we suggest applying *functional analysis* on Panagiotis' behavior, focusing on his behavior towards his classmates (irony, aggression) and his teacher. Subsequently, we suggest recording the teacher's emotions, thoughts, and interpretations of the student's behavior. In addition, the use of a *sociogram* will map the dynamics of the classroom and indicate Panagiotis' status among his classmates. Because Panagiotis' family seems to consider aggression as a normative behavior, the school should provide guidelines to help this student modify his values and improve his social behavior and social status. The intervention objectives are presented in Table 1.

Table 1. The intervention objectives

Long-term objectives	Short-term objectives
The student accepts that he will not always be the first one.	When something displeases or frustrates the student, he expresses it and asks for help.

continued on following page

Table 1. Continued

Long-term objectives	Short-term objectives
The student speaks politely, even if something bothers him.	When others make mistakes, no negative comments on the part of the student are accepted.
His parents understand that violence is not a functional way of responding.	His parents accept the school's view of their child's behavior at school.

Intervention at the Individual Level

At the onset of Panagiotis' undesirable behavior, the teacher is advised to adopt a consistent attitude which is briefly discussed below.

A. For Panagiotis' dismissive and rude attitude towards the teacher, the teacher

1. keeps his temper;
2. looks at the student with a serious, steady gaze; and
3. talks to him using the first person. For example, "Panagiotis, *I understand* it's disappointing that your performance is different from what you expected. But *when you* react like this, *I feel* insulted. *I would like you* to express your opinion in a polite way. Now, you need to calm down. Go get some water. Then, during the break, we'll discuss any questions you have. Remember, in our classroom we speak politely".

Subsequently, in the *discussion* with the student, when the student is calm and able to listen, the teacher guides the student in identifying his thoughts, feelings, and behavior as well as its consequences, with the aim of achieving *cognitive restructuring*. Panagiotis should be informed that such behaviors are not acceptable, and that there will be consequences if he engages in them.

Finally, the teacher asks Panagiotis to agree on a *mutual contract* that includes how he should behave when (a) he gets angry and (b) his classmates make mistakes. At this point, it is suggested that the student create a self-direction card using an acronym that he will carry with him (see Figure 11). Moreover, the adoption of "*secret signals*" (e.g., a gesture or a wink) in the teacher-child communication is likely to enable the child to control his/her behavior.

Figure 11. **Visualization of a self-management strategy**

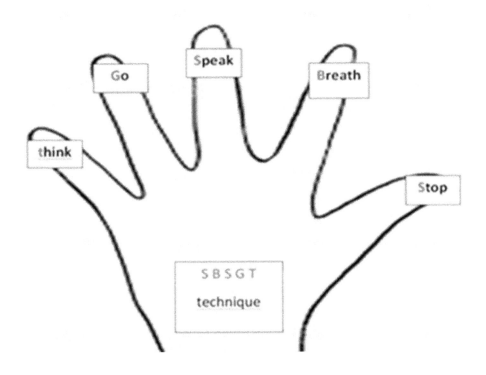

B. For Panagiotis' dismissive and rude attitude towards his peers:
1. We discuss with the student the ways he can help and guide his classmates in group activities without criticizing them. For this purpose, an *empathy game*, such as "The Other Person's Chair", can be played first with the teacher and then with the whole class. In this game, two chairs are placed opposite to each other: one for the "criticizer" and one for the "criticized". The student first sits in the "criticizer" position and asks the teacher sitting in the "criticized" position to express his *thoughts* (e.g., "He/she is rude. I am incompetent") and *feelings* (e.g., anger, frustration, sadness, guilt). Then, the roles are reversed. This exercise facilitates the discussion which leads to *cognitive restructuring*, that is, the identification of the dysfunctional thoughts and their replacement by alternative, more functional thoughts.
2. The ecosystemic technique of *reframing* can be used, according to which the teacher gives an alternative explanation of the student's behavior. For example, the teacher recognizes that the student's intention is to establish his position within the peer group and to impose his values.

3. By *encouraging the problem behavior to continue in different ways and at different times*, Panagiotis' cognitive abilities and physique can be used to the benefit of his class. For example, Panagiotis can act as a helper when other students in the class have cognitive difficulties and/or his physical superiority can be used, for example, when they need to arrange the high shelves of the library.
4. Using *the-storming-the-back-door technique*, the teacher can recognize the positive aspects of Panagiotis' behavior and capitalize on them to achieve change. For example, the teacher may focus on the student's high learning motivation.
5. A multidisciplinary and holistic approach to the problem is also considered necessary, with the involvement of the school psychologist, the social worker and/or the teacher of the school's integration department. This approach is expected to be effective, especially because the class teacher does not always have the necessary time to intervene drastically at the individual level.

Intervention at the Classroom Level

Intervention at the classroom level can easily and effectively be implemented by the teacher and will benefit both the student who exhibits the problem behavior and the group which he belongs to (for a meta-analysis see Chafee et al., 2017). This type of intervention is considered as a prerequisite to the promotion of a positive classroom climate, to the use of effective strategies, and to the implementation of social and emotional learning programs aiming at identifying, expressing, and managing emotions and dealing with conflict.

Below we suggest a series of interventions at the classroom level.

1. *Implementing an anger management program in the classroom.* The components of such a program are presented in Table 2.

Table 2. Components of an anger management program

Axes	Instruments
Recognition of anger in the body: warning signs	Reading and processing of relevant scenarios
Identifying the causes	Role-playing games
Examples of effective and ineffective management by identifying the consequences	Worksheets, artistic creations

2. *Redefining the classroom rules and the consequences of breaking them.* A democratic process of formulating classroom rules is suggested, in which everyone has both *rights* (safety, learning opportunities, dignity, etc.) and *obligations,* and in which the violation of each other's rights is not tolerated.
3. *Learning ways of self-management of behavior.* "What I do when I (feel)... and when someone...".
4. *Applying collaborative learning techniques and providing opportunities for group collaborative activities.*
5. *Using token economy and response cost.* For example, in the game "Cost of Actions" (Hulac & Briesch, 2017), the name of each child or group is written on a board and below it numbers are written from 25 back to 1. When the student or group breaks a rule, the highest number is deleted. At the end of the day, the student or team gets as many points as the highest number left (e.g., 25, 24, 23, 22, 21, 20, 19, 18, 17, 16, ... 1; if the numbers from 25 to 22 are crossed out, the student or team gets 21 points). The winner(s) of the week win whatever they draw from the reward jar. This can be reduced homework, free time, or whatever the class agrees upon as a reward.
6. *Setting a time for the whole class to discuss issues of concern.* Papers (either anonymous or not) with the issues each student wants to discuss with the class group are put in a box and some of the issues are randomly selected for discussion.
7. *Implementing a compliment game.* For example, in the "Giant and Dwarf" game, a secret draw takes place, and each child receives a card with the name of his "dwarf", that is, his protégé. At the same time, each child will be the "dwarf" of another child. The obligation of each child is to leave a little note every day (for the five days of the given week) with compliments, something nice for his/her "dwarf" that will make him/her feel good. The "giant-dwarf" pairing will be secret and will be revealed on a designated day, at which time there will be a class discussion on whether it was carried out correctly, how the children felt as dwarves and giants, and what the class got out of it. At this point, praise/rewards are given by the teacher to the giants who have successfully completed the task.

Intervention at the School Level

Intervention at the school level is necessary, as mentioned above, to achieve a change in Panagiotis' behavior. Initially, after discussing the student's behavior problems with all the teachers and the rest of the school staff, a common response pattern should be adopted by all. Therefore, all staff should:

1. pay increased attention to Panagiotis' behavior during the break;
2. consistently apply the rules of the school;
3. use "the same language" about the limits of the student's behavior;
4. remind Panagiotis the alternative ways of anger relief already agreed upon;
5. inform the principal, all other school staff, and Panagiotis' parents when necessary;
6. record serious incidents in the school life book.

Intervention at the Family Level

Families, as another key factor in children's education, should not be left out of every effort to support children. The cooperation of the two systems, that is, family and school, is necessary. Otherwise, the child finds himself/herself between the two systems, with his/her challenging behavior reflecting the conflict between the two; this causes great confusion and distress (Galanaki, 2000b). Therefore, Panagiotis' parents need to be invited to a meeting during which they are informed about the problem and the deep concern of the teachers about their child's adjustment difficulties. The parents also need to have an appointment with the school psychologist and the social worker. Finally, the school needs to state explicitly which behaviors are permissible and which are not, within its operating framework, and to maintain a firmness in the application of the consequences rules entail, especially when the parents' attitudes and values set obstacles to their child's adjustment in school.

Case Study 2: Anna

Anna, a first-grade student, is an only child. She always comes to school very well-groomed. Her clothes, shoes and possessions are always of the latest fashion. On the cognitive level, she already knows how to read and write as well as the basic concepts in mathematics. In class she finishes her tasks very quickly and gets up saying, "I'm done" and "I'm bored". She often complains about being annoyed by her classmates who are untidy, do not understand the lessons quickly, sit on the floor and play silly games. She finds no interest in her peers and, as a result, she often mocks or ignores them, saying she has nothing to talk about with them because "they act like babies". She always prefers to stay next to her teacher and chat with her during the break time; she does the same with teachers while they supervise students at break time. Besides, her speech, interests, and general knowledge are very well developed for her age. Her teacher's colleagues consider her very lucky to have a child like Anna in her class. The teacher herself, however, finds it difficult to cope with this situation. She worries about Anna and is tired of Anna's overall behavior. On the contrary, her parents are proud of their daughter and don't seem to worry about anything.

Designing the Intervention

Detailed observation and clear recording of the student's behavior is the first step of behavior modification. Therefore, Anna's challenging behavior is described as follows: (a) Anna goes to the teacher at times when she should be with other children or working; and (b) Anna adopts a judgmental attitude, both verbally and non-verbally, towards her classmates.

Subsequently, for each of the above "problems", functional behavior analysis is applied, and the frequency of these behaviors is recorded over a one-week period (see Table 3, where, for the sake of brevity, only one of the five observation days are presented).

Table 3. Diary of the frequency of behavior

	Monday	Tuesday	Wednesday	Thursday	Friday
1st hour	**II**				
2nd hour	III				
1st break	I				
3rd hour	IIII				
	Monday	Tuesday	Wednesday	Thursday	Friday
4th hour	II				
2nd break	II				
5th hour	IIII				
3rd break	II				
6th hour	IIIII				
Total	25				
Average per hour	4.2				

This process ensures an objective approach to the "problem", which enables us to formulate clear and measurable intervention objectives (see Table 4).

Table 4. The intervention objectives

Long-term objectives	Short-term objectives
The student interacts with same-age children.	The student has reduced her approach to the teacher to twice a day.
The student talks to other children without judgment.	The student has reduced dismissive attitudes towards peers to two points each day.
	The student talks to a classmate at recess for at least five minutes.
	When she finishes a task, the student can keep herself busy, either independently or with her classmates who have also finished their task, in the corner of the classroom and with an alternative activity (e.g., reading literature books, playing board games, etc.).

Intervention at the Individual Level

In Anna's case study, it is clear that her teacher experiences unpleasant feelings regarding Anna's behavior. The application of *reframing* will help the teacher view the situation from a different perspective by focusing on the positive aspects of it. In other words, she may realize that Anna is a child with cognitive abilities who can be her "assistant" and provide help and support to her classmates, if needed. Furthermore, Anna is a keen learner and loves to explore and discover new things. Therefore, the teacher can protect her from experiencing boredom by assigning to her interesting and challenging new tasks. What is more, Anna likes order and cleanliness, which is what all teachers want from their students.

Another intervention is to focus on the *positive motives* of Anna's behavior, such as her desire for attention and for showing her potential and high cognitive level. With this perspective, an improvement in the bond between Anna and her teacher is expected to occur. Moreover, looking for positive motives in Anna's rejection of her classmates, her teacher could be able to reason that Anna's desire for order and organization makes it difficult for her to accept others' impulsive behaviors. Probably because of her lack of ability to clearly express her annoyance, Anna seems to adopt an arrogant attitude towards her peers. Teaching functional ways of expressing dissatisfaction could possibly help Anna change her behavior. By acting as a role model, the teacher can show the student what to do when she is annoyed.

This is an example of such a conversation: "Look, Anna, like you do, I also find some things non pleasant, for example, I'm annoyed by the mess in the teachers' office. It makes it difficult for me to concentrate and prepare my lesson. How would you think the teachers would feel if I yelled at them or said they were acting like babies? What would happen next? What could I do to let them know that the mess was bothering me? Have you ever felt that way? When? What did you do? What happened next? What else could you do to make them listen to you? So, what will you choose to do when you see some kids doing things you don't like?".

In addition, by applying the *storming-the-back-door technique*, the teacher can get to know the student's particular interests and inclinations (this should be done gradually with all students) and use some of her findings as reinforcers or "tools" to guide the child towards the desired goal, that is, the development of social skills. A useful practice for selecting reinforcers and getting to know each other more deeply is to use a questionnaire or drawing that explores what gives students joy and what does not in different contexts, such as home or school (e.g., favorite food, toy, hero, what would you do if you had a magic wand, etc.).

Because the aim is for the student to interact more with her peers and seek less interaction with adults, it seems appropriate for teachers to set clear boundaries. When the student approaches the teacher, the teacher could say in a firm tone: "Anna, I'm glad to see you, but now I have to do something else. Why don't you..." (suggest alternative). When the student criticizes her classmates or says that she is "bored", a good response would be: "I'm sorry you feel.... I'm sure you have lots of ideas about what you can do about it. Tell me some of them. If you do this... then what happens? So, what do you choose?".

An *individual contract* can also be used to increase Anna's proper social interaction and to reduce judgmental comments. Combined with the use of direct positive reinforcement and rewards in exchange for tokens collected, this strategy motivates the child to participate and interact with her peers without negative comments. For example, Anna could collect tokens when she "spots" a classmate doing something positive and then she could praise him/her or make kind remarks or positive comments about it. Then, she could earn a red marble on her individual report card for each detection and a yellow marble for each kind remark or positive comment. Then, she may be asked to use red and yellow to color a beautiful snail as quickly as possible (see Figure 12). The colorful snail provides the student with the necessary visual feedback about her performance and enhances her motivation to improve her behavior.

Figure 12. **The colorful snail**

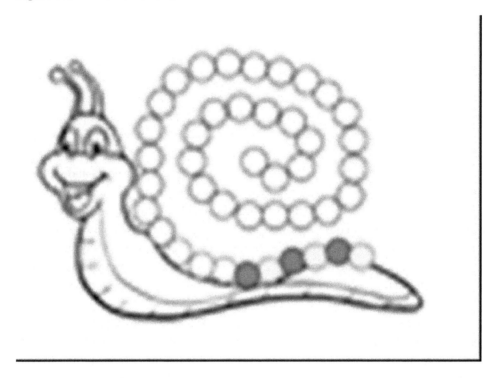

Intervention at the Classroom Level

Intervention at the classroom level is crucial in promoting Anna's social skills and reducing her isolation. Once teachers agree not to let Anna stay and chat with them often, she will be faced with isolation. It is at this point that the teaching of alternative forms of behavior with her peers' involvement becomes necessary. Special attention needs to be paid to the implementation of techniques from social and emotional programs with objectives such as the following:

1. Team bonding and trust in the team
2. Development of empathy
3. Cultivation of self-perception
4. Acceptance of diversity
5. Recognition, expression, and management of emotions, especially the "difficult" ones (e.g., anger, frustration, fear, sadness, boredom) in a way that shows respect for the other person.

In addition, the classroom needs to be designed to provide *places for those who finish their work*. For example, the *"anti-boredom corner"* can be created, where activities such as puzzles, mazes, books, educational games, etc., can be provided.

To enhance the *sense of belonging* in class, assignments of responsibilities could be given to all students, including mutual adoption of routines, rules, and fixed consequences. Increasing cooperative versus individual activities may seem difficult to implement at first; however, if adopted consistently, this attitude will benefit the whole group, as it is one of the principal ways to improve students' social skills.

It is also suggested to read *books* or invent a *narrative* or *story* (preferably with animals for these young children) related to the dilemma "being alone without concessions *vs* being with company with some concessions". Reading and narratives can be accompanied by role-playing and related experiential activities.

Furthermore, *a complimentary game* can be presented and played in the classroom. For example, in the game "Make My Day", one student at a time –after a draw– becomes "the person of the day". On that day, he receives a compliment from each of his/her classmates. First, the teacher explains the procedure. Then, the children follow it by applying the four steps that are presented in Table 5.

Table 5. The "Make My Day" game

How do I make a compliment?	
I think of something good about the child (what he/she has-characteristics, what he/she did, what he/she said)	
I look *into the eyes* of the child.	
I'm smiling.	
I make a positive comment (e.g., "He is a good and helpful friend")	

Finally, during the break, *group activities* and *games* can be organized to ensure Anna's participation in them. For example, Anna can bring a rope and during the break she can play with her classmates and the teacher. Gradually, the teacher withdraws, and the duration of her withdrawal will increase depending on the amount of Anna's participation in the group.

Intervention at the School Level

As mentioned in the previous case study, the involvement of the whole system (the school) is necessary for a successful intervention to a problematic situation. Anna's difficulties, once discussed by the school staff, should be addressed by the adoption of a common attitude towards her behavior by all teachers. Thus, it is advisable that all teachers:

1. reduce the amount of time Anna spends talking to them;
2. give her positive reinforcement when she interacts with other children;
3. use "the same language" about setting boundaries and providing alternatives (e.g., "I have to watch the kids in the yard, why don't you talk about your favorite game with...");
4. suggesting games with other children (e.g., picking up leaves in the yard).

Intervention at the Family Level

To increase the effectiveness of the intervention, we need to involve the family system as well. When discussing with parents, the teacher needs to:

1. describe Anna's behaviors which cause serious concern to her teachers and explain why;
2. agree on common school-family goals;
3. inform parents about the school's actions for the management of Anna's behavior;
4. ask the family to encourage and support their child's socialization and participation in structured and non-structured group activities.

CONCLUSION

Behavioral, cognitive behavioral, ecosystemic, and humanistic models have the potential to provide educators with very useful strategies for managing children's behavior problems at school. Combining strategies from all the above perspectives (Chafee et al., 2017) and working within a whole-school approach (Goldberg et al., 2019) are expected to increase teachers' effectiveness in prevention and intervention. Finally, it should be noted that, as existing research indicates (Lei et al., 2016), the implementation of these strategies presupposes a general teacher attitude which is characterized by affection, care, and trust, as well as by the setting of firm and clear boundaries.

References

Abry, T., Bryce, C. I., Swanson, J., Bradley, R. H., Fabes, R. A., & Corwyn, R. F. (2017). Classroom-level adversity: Associations with children's internalizing and externalizing behaviors across elementary school. *Developmental Psychology*, 53(3), 497–510. DOI: 10.1037/dev0000268 PMID: 28045283

Achenbach, T., & Rescorla, L. (2019). *Handbook for the SAEBA school-age questionnaires and profiles*. EHRC. https://archive.org/details/manualforasebasc0000ache

Achenbach, T. M. (1966). The classification of children's psychiatric symptoms: A factor-analytic study. *Psychological Monographs*, 80(7), 1–37. DOI: 10.1037/h0093906 PMID: 5968338

Achenbach, T. M., & Rescorla, L. A. (2001). *Manual for the ASEBA School-Age Forms and Profiles*. University of Vermont Research Center for Children, Youth, & Families.

Aggeli, K., & Vlachou, M. (2004). Problem-solving techniques and methods in the classroom. In Kalantzi-Azizi, A., & Zafiropoulou, M. (Eds.), *School adjustment: Prevention and intervention* (pp. 26–50). Ellinika Grammata. (in Greek)

Alberta Learning. (2000). *Teaching students with emotional disorders and/or mental illnesses*. Alberta Learning, Special Programs Branch.

Alberto, P. A., & Troutman, A. C. (2013). *Applied behavior analysis for teachers* (9th ed.). Pearson.

Allen, K., Kern, M. L., Vella-Brodrick, D., Hattie, J., & Waters, L. (2018). What schools need to know about fostering school belonging: A meta-analysis. *Educational Psychology Review*, 30(1), 1–34. DOI: 10.1007/s10648-016-9389-8

American Psychiatric Association. (2013). *Diagnostic and statistical manual of mental disorders* (5th ed.)., DOI: 10.1176/appi.books.9780890425596

Austin, V., & Sciarra, D. (2016). *Difficult students and disruptive behavior in the classroom: Teacher responses that work*. W. W. Norton & Company.

Bandura, A. (1977). *Social learning theory*. Prentice Hall.

Bandura, A. (1978). The self-system in reciprocal determinism. *The American Psychologist*, 33(4), 344–358. DOI: 10.1037/0003-066X.33.4.344

Bandura, A. (1986). *Social foundations of thought and action: A social cognitive theory*. Prentice-Hall.

Bapst, M. S., Genoud, P. A., & Hascoët, M. (2023). Taking a step towards understanding interactions between teacher efficacy in behavior management and the social learning environment: A two-level multilevel analysis. *European Journal of Psychology of Education*, 38(3), 1129–1144. DOI: 10.1007/s10212-022-00647-4

Barker, K., Poed, S., & Whitefield, P. (Eds.). (2022). *School-Wide Positive Behavior Support: The Australian handbook*. Routledge. DOI: 10.4324/9781003186236

Barkley, R., & Benton, C. (2013). *Your defiant child: 8 steps to better behavior* (2nd ed.). The Guilford Press.

Baum, W. M. (2011). What is radical behaviorism? A review of Jay Moore's conceptual foundations of radical behaviorism. *Journal of the Experimental Analysis of Behavior*, 95(1), 119–126. DOI: 10.1901/jeab.2011.95-119

Bear, G. G. (2020). *Improving school climate: Practical strategies to reduce behavior problems and promote social and emotional learning*. Routledge. DOI: 10.4324/9781351170482

Beck, A. T. (1976). *Cognitive therapy and emotional disorders*. International Universities Press.

Bradshaw, C. P., Waasdorp, T. E., & Leaf, P. J. (2012). Effects of school-wide positive behavioral interventions and supports on child behavior problems. *Pediatrics*, 130(5), 1136–1145. DOI: 10.1542/peds.2012-0243 PMID: 23071207

Braswell, L., & Kendall, P. C. (1988). Cognitive-behavioral methods with children. In Dobson, K. S. (Ed.), *Handbook of cognitive-behavioral therapies* (pp. 167–213). The Guilford Press.

Briesch, A. M., & Briesch, J. M. (2016). Meta-analysis of behavioral self-management interventions in single-case research. *School Psychology Review*, 45(1), 3–18. DOI: 10.17105/SPR45-1.3-18

Bromley, E., Johnson, J. G., & Cohen, P. (2006). Personality strengths in adolescence and decreased risk of developing mental health problems in early adulthood. *Comprehensive Psychiatry*, 47(4), 315–324. DOI: 10.1016/j.comppsych.2005.11.003 PMID: 16769307

Bronfenbrenner, U. (1979). *The ecology of human development experiments*. Harvard University Press. DOI: 10.4159/9780674028845

Brown, G. I. (1971). *Human teaching for human learning. An introduction to confluent education*. Viking Press.

Burns, M. K., & Ysseldyke, J. E. (2009). Reported prevalence of evidence-based instructional practices in special education. *The Journal of Special Education*, 43(1), 3–11. DOI: 10.1177/0022466908315563

Burt, S. A., Clark, D. A., Gershoff, E. T., Klump, K. L., & Hyde, L. W. (2021). Twin differences in harsh parenting predict youth's antisocial behavior. *Psychological Science*, 32(3), 395–409. DOI: 10.1177/0956797620968532 PMID: 33577745

Cambridge University Press. (n.d.). Behavior. In *Cambridge Dictionaries Online*. https://dictionary.cambridge.org/dictionary/english/abortion

Carneiro, A., Dias, P., & Soares, I. (2016). Risk factors for internalizing and externalizing problems in the preschool years: Systematic literature review based on the child behavior checklist 11/2-5. *Journal of Child and Family Studies*, 25, 2941–2953. DOI: 10.1007/s10826-016-0456-z

Carr, A. (2016). *The handbook of child and adolescent clinical psychology: A contextual approach* (3rd ed.). Routledge.

Chaffee, R. K., Johnson, A. H., & Volpe, R. J. (2017). A meta-analysis of class-wide interventions for supporting student behavior. *School Psychology Review*, 46(2), 149–164. DOI: 10.17105/SPR-2017-0015.V46-2

Collaborative for Academic. Social and Emotional Learning (CASEL). (n.d.). *Program guide*. https://pg.casel.org/

Cook, C. R., Fiat, A., Larson, M., Daikos, C., Slemrod, T., Holland, E. A., Thayer, A. J., & Renshaw, T. (2018). Positive greetings at the door: Evaluation of a low-cost, high-yield proactive classroom management strategy. *Journal of Positive Behavior Interventions*, 20(3), 149–159. DOI: 10.1177/1098300717753831

Cook, C. R., Frye, M., Slemrod, T., Lyon, A. R., Renshaw, T. L., & Zhang, Y. (2015). An integrated approach to universal prevention: Independent and combined effects of PBIS and SEL on youths' mental health. *School Psychology Quarterly*, 30(2), 166–183. DOI: 10.1037/spq0000102 PMID: 25602629

Cooper, J., Heron, T., & Heward, W. (2020). *Applied behavior analysis* (3rd ed.). Pearson Education.

Crone, D., Hawken, L., & Horner, R. (2015). *Building positive behavior support systems in schools: Functional behavioral assessment* (2nd ed.). The Guilford Press.

D'Zurilla, T. J., & Goldfried, M. R. (1971). Problem solving and behavior modification. *Journal of Abnormal Psychology*, 78(1), 107–126. DOI: 10.1037/h0031360 PMID: 4938262

Darling-Hammond, L., & Cook-Harvey, C. M. (2018). *Educating the Whole Child: Improving School Climate to Support Student Success*. Learning Policy Institute. DOI: 10.54300/145.655

Dearing, E., Kreider, H., Simpkins, S., & Weiss, H. B. (2006). Family involvement in school and low-income children's literacy performance: Longitudinal associations between and within families. *Journal of Educational Psychology*, 98(4), 653–664. DOI: 10.1037/0022-0663.98.4.653

Dember, W. N. (1974). Motivation and the cognitive revolution. *American Psychologist, 29*(3), 161–168. [REMOVED HYPERLINK FIELD]DOI: 10.1037/h0035907

Doll, B., Zucker, St., & Brehm, K. (2014). *Resilient classrooms: Creating healthy environments for learning*. The Guilford Press.

Durlak, J. A., Mahoney, J. L., & Boyle, A. E. (2022). What we know, and what we need to find out about universal, school-based social and emotional learning programs for children and adolescents: A review of meta-analyses and directions for future research. *Psychological Bulletin*, 148(11-12), 765–782. DOI: 10.1037/bul0000383

Ellis, A. (1962). *Reason and emotion in psychotherapy*. Lyle Stuart.

Epstein, R. A., Fonnesbeck, C., Potter, S., Rizzone, K. H., & McPheeters, M. (2015). Psychosocial interventions for child disruptive behaviors: A meta-analysis. *Pediatrics*, 136(5), 947–960. DOI: 10.1542/peds.2015-2577 PMID: 26482672

Filcheck, H. A., McNeil, C. B., Greco, L. A., & Bernard, R. S. (2004). Using a whole-class token economy and coaching of teacher skills in a preschool classroom to manage disruptive behavior. *Psychology in the Schools*, 41(3), 351–361. DOI: 10.1002/pits.10168

Flannery, K. B., Fenning, P., Kato, M. M., & McIntosh, K. (2014). Effects of school-wide positive behavioral interventions and supports and fidelity of implementation on problem behavior in high schools. *School Psychology Quarterly*, 29(2), 111–124. https://psycnet.apa.org/doi/10.1037/spq0000039. DOI: 10.1037/spq0000039 PMID: 24188290

Gable, R. A., Hester, P. H., Rock, M. L., & Hughes, K. G. (2009). Rules, praise, ignoring, and reprimands revisited. *Intervention in School and Clinic*, 44(4), 195–254. DOI: 10.1177/1053451208328831

Galanaki, E. (1997). Applications of systems theory in school: The reframing technique. [in Greek]. *Tetradia Psychiatrikis*, 59, 67–79.

Galanaki, E. (2000a). Systemic approach of the school. In Kalantzi-Azizi, A., & Besevegis, E. G. (Eds.), *Training/awareness-raising issues for child and adolescent mental health professionals* (pp. 215–220). Ellinika Grammata. (in Greek)

Galanaki, E. (2000b). Systems theory as a framework for dealing with the child's behavior problems at school. [in Greek]. *Educational Review*, 30, 7–25.

Galanaki, E. (2011). Adjustment difficulties of children and adolescents: Definition, specificities, distinction from normal behavior. In Kalantzi-Azizi, A., & Zafiropoulou, M. (Eds.), *School adjustment: Prevention and intervention* (2nd ed., pp. 163–180). Pedio. (in Greek)

Gardner, F., & Shaw, D. S. (2008). Behavioral problems of infancy and preschool children. In M. Rutter, D. Bishop, D. Pine, S. Scott, J. Stevenson, E. Taylor, & A. Thapar (Eds.), *Rutter's child and adolescent psychiatry* (5th ed., pp. 882–894). Wiley-Blackwell. DOI: 10.1002/9781444300895.ch53

Glymitsa, E. (2019). Andreas doesn't want to wear his shoes. In Zafiropoulou, M. (Ed.), *The "difficult" child at home and at school* (pp. 108–123). Pedio. (in Greek)

Goldberg, J. M., Sklad, M., Elfrink, T. R., Schreurs, K. M., Bohlmeijer, E. T., & Clarke, A. M. (2019). Effectiveness of interventions adopting a whole school approach to enhancing social and emotional development: A meta-analysis. *European Journal of Psychology of Education*, 34(4), 755–782. DOI: 10.1007/s10212-018-0406-9

Grant, N., Meyer, J. L., & Strambler, M. J. (2023). Measuring social and emotional learning implementation in a research-practice partnership. *Frontiers in Psychology*, 14, 1052877. DOI: 10.3389/fpsyg.2023.1052877 PMID: 37564314

Green, A. L., Ferrande, S., Boaz, T. L., Kutash, K., & Wheeldon-Reese, B. (2021). Social and emotional learning during early adolescence: Effectiveness of a classroom-based SEL program for middle school students. *Psychology in the Schools*, 58(6), 1056–1069. DOI: 10.1002/pits.22487

Greenberg, J., Putman, H., & Walsh, K. (2014). Training our future teachers: Classroom management. https://files.eric.ed.gov/fulltext/ED556312.pdf

Henderson, N., & Milstein, M. M. (2003). *Resiliency in schools: Making it happen for students and educators* (updated ed.). Corwin Press.

Heward, W. L., Alber-Morgan, S. R., & Konrad, M. (2016). *Exceptional children: An introduction to special education* (11th ed.). Pearson.

Homme, L. E. (1965). Perspectives in psychology: XXIV Control of coverants, the operants of the mind. *The Psychological Record*, 15(4), 501–511. DOI: 10.1007/BF03393622

Horner, R., Sugai, G., Smolkowski, K., Eber, L., Nakasato, J., Todd, A. W., & Esperanza, J. (2009). A randomized, waitlist-controlled effectiveness trial assessing school-wide positive behavior support in elementary schools. *Journal of Positive Behavior Interventions*, 11(3), 133–144. DOI: 10.1177/1098300709332067

Horner, R. H., & Monzalve, M. M. (2018). A framework for building safe and effective school environments: Positive behavioral interventions and supports. *Pedagogická Orientace*, 28(4), 663–685. DOI: 10.5817/PedOr2018-4-663

Horner, R. H., & Sugai, G. (2015). School-wide PBIS: An example of applied behavior analysis implemented at a scale of social importance. *Behavior Analysis in Practice*, 8(1), 80–85. DOI: 10.1007/s40617-015-0045-4 PMID: 27703887

Hulac, D. M., & Briesch, A. M. (2017). *Evidence-based strategies for effective classroom management*. The Guilford Press.

Kalantzi-Azizi A., & Galanaki, E. (2001). Psychotherapy as a system and the need for "openings": Examples of the systemic perspective of the cognitive behavioral psychotherapy. *Psychology: The Journal of the Hellenic Psychological Society, 8*(2), 153–172. (in Greek). https://doi.org/DOI: 10.12681/psy_hps.24111

Karmba, C., & Zafiropoulou, M. (2002). Cognitive behavior modification and learning disabilities. In Scrimali, T., & Grimaldi, L. (Eds.), *Cognitive psychotherapy toward a new millennium: Scientific foundations and clinical practice* (pp. 219–222). Kluwer Academic/Plenum Publishers.

Kincade, L., Cook, C., & Goerdt, A. (2020). Meta-analysis and common practice elements of universal approaches to improving student-teacher relationships. *Review of Educational Research*, 90(5), 710–748. DOI: 10.3102/0034654320946836

Koliadis, E. A. (2010). Cognitive-behavioral/cognitive techniques. In Koliadis, E. A. (Ed.), *Behavior at school: We explore possibilities - We cope with problems* (pp. 184–208). Grigoris. (in Greek)

Kourkoutas, E., Stavrou, P. D., & Plexousakis, S. (2018). Teachers' emotional and educational reactions toward children with behavioral problems: Implication for school-based counseling work with teachers. *Journal of Psychology and Behavioural Science*, 6(2), 17–34. DOI: 10.15640/jpbs.v6n2a3

Kourkoutas, H. (2011). *Behavioral problems in children: Interventions in the context of the family and the school*. Topos. (in Greek)

Kuyken, W., Weare, K., Ukoumunne, O. C., Vicary, R., Motton, N., Burnett, R., Cullen, C., Hennelly, S., & Huppert, F. (2013). Effectiveness of the mindfulness in schools programme: Non-randomised controlled feasibility study. *The British Journal of Psychiatry*, 203(2), 126–131. DOI: 10.1192/bjp.bp.113.126649 PMID: 23787061

Landrum, T. J., & Kauffman, J. M. (2006). Behavioral approaches to classroom management. In Evertson, C. M., & Weinstein, C. S. (Eds.), *Handbook of classroom management: Research, practice, and contemporary issues* (pp. 47–71). Erlbaum.

Lee, A., & Gage, N. (2020). Updating and expanding systematic reviews and meta-analyses on the effects of school-wide positive behavior interventions and supports. *Psychology in the Schools*, 57(5), 783–804. DOI: 10.1002/pits.22336

Lei, H., Cui, Y., & Chiu, M. M. (2016). Affective teacher-student relationships and students' externalizing behavior problems: A meta-analysis. *Frontiers in Psychology*, 1311, 7. DOI: 10.3389/fpsyg.2016.01311 PMID: 27625624

Little, B. (2018). Reciprocal determinism. In Zeigler-Hill, V., & Shackelford, T. (Eds.), *Encyclopedia of personality and individual differences*. Springer., DOI: 10.1007/978-3-319-28099-8_1807-1

Maslow, A. H. (1968). Toward a psychology of being (2nd ed.). D. Van Nostrand.

Maslow, A. H. (1987). *Motivation and personality* (3rd ed.). Addison-Wesley.

Meichenbaum, D. (1977). Cognitive behavior modification. *Scandinavian Journal of Behaviour Therapy*, 6(4), 185–192. DOI: 10.1080/16506073.1977.9626708

Mendes de Oliveira, C., Santos Almeida, C. R., & Hofheinz Giacomoni, C. (2022). School-based positive psychology interventions that promote well-being in children: A systematic review. *Child Indicators Research*, 15(5), 1583–1600. DOI: 10.1007/s12187-022-09935-3

Miller, G. A. (2003). The cognitive revolution: A historical perspective. *Trends in Cognitive Sciences*, 7(3), 141–144. DOI: 10.1016/S1364-6613(03)00029-9 PMID: 12639696

Mingebach, T., Kamp-Becker, I., Christiansen, H., & Weber, L. (2018). Meta-meta-analysis on the effectiveness of parent-based interventions for the treatment of child externalizing behavior problems. *PLoS One*, 13(9), e0202855. DOI: 10.1371/journal.pone.0202855 PMID: 30256794

Missouri Department of Elementary and Secondary Education. (2018). *Missouri Schoolwide Positive Behavior Support, Tier 1 Team Workbook 2018-2019*. https://pbismissouri.org/wpcontent/uploads/2018/05/MO-SW-PBS-Tier-1-2018.pdf

Molnar, A., & Lindquist, B. (2009). *Changing problem behavior in schools*. Information Age Publishing.

Morgan, D. P., & Jenson, W. R. (1988). *Teaching behaviorally disordered students: Preferred practices*. Prentice Hall.

Moroz, K. B., & Jones, K. M. (2002). The effects of positive peer reporting on children's social involvement. *School Psychology Review*, 31(2), 235–245. DOI: 10.1080/02796015.2002.12086153

Muhajirah, M. (2020). Basic of learning theory: Behaviorism, cognitivism, constructivism, and humanism. *International Journal of Asian Education*, 1(1), 37–42. DOI: 10.46966/ijae.v1i1.23

Neitzel, J., & Bogin, J. (2008). *Steps for implementation: Functional behavior assessment*. The National Professional Development Center on Autism Spectrum Disorders, Frank Porter Graham Child Development Institute, The University of North Carolina.

Nisar, H., Elgin, D., Bradshaw, C., Dolan, V., Frey, A., Horner, R., Owens, J., Perales, K., & Sutherland, K. (2022). *Promoting social and behavioral success for learning in elementary schools: Practice recommendations for elementary school educators, school and district administrators, and parents*. 2M Research Services. Contract No. 92990019F0319.

Noltemeyer, A., Palmer, K., James, A., & Petrasek, M. (2019). Disciplinary and achievement outcomes associated with school-wide positive behavioral interventions and supports implementation level. *School Psychology Review*, 48(1), 81–87. DOI: 10.17105/SPR-2017-0131.V48-1

Noltemeyer, A., Ward, R., & Mcloughlin, C. (2015). Relationship between school suspension and student outcomes: A meta-analysis. *School Psychology Review*, 44(2), 224–240. DOI: 10.17105/spr-14-0008.1

O'Neill, R. E., Allbin, R. W., Storey, K., Horner, R. H., & Sprague, J. R. (2015). *Functional assessment and program development for problem behavior*. Cengage Learning.

Office of Special Education Programs (OSEP) Technical Assistance Center on Positive Behavioral Interventions and Supports. (2019). *Positive Behavioral Interventions & Supports*. U.S. Department of Education, Office of Special Education www.pbis.org

Park, J., Lee, H. J., & Kim, Y. (2019). School-wide positive behavior support in six special schools of South Korea: Processes and outcomes across years. *International Journal of Developmental Disabilities*, 65(5), 337–346. DOI: 10.1080/20473869.2019.1647729 PMID: 34141357

Parsonson, B. S. (2012). Evidence-based classroom behaviour management strategies. *Kairanga, 13*(1), 16–23. https://api.semanticscholar.org/CorpusID:17274857

Pavlov, I. P. (1927). *Conditioned reflexes: An investigation of the physiological activity of the cerebral cortex*. Oxford University Press.

Pianta, R. C. (1999). How the parts affect the whole: Systems theory in classroom relationships. In Pianta, R. C. (Ed.), *Enhancing relationships between children and teachers* (pp. 23–43). American Psychological Association., DOI: 10.1037/10314-002

Purkey, W. W. (1970). *Self-concept and school achievement*. Prentice-Hall.

Purkey, W. W. (1978). *Inviting school success: A self-concept approach to teaching and learning*. Wadsworth Publishing Company.

Purkey, W. W. (1991). *Invitational teaching, learning, and living. Analysis and action series* (ED340689). https://files.eric.ed.gov/fulltext/ED340689.pdf

Pyne, J. (2019). Suspended attitudes: Exclusion and emotional disengagement from school. *Sociology of Education*, 92(1), 59–82. DOI: 10.1177/0038040718816684

Ronen, T. (2003). *Cognitive constructivist psychotherapy with children and adolescents*. Kluwer Academic/Plenum Publishers. DOI: 10.1007/978-1-4419-9284-0

Rubie-Davies, C. M. (2007). Classroom interactions: Exploring the practices of high and low expectation teachers. *The British Journal of Educational Psychology*, 77(2), 289–306. DOI: 10.1348/000709906X101601 PMID: 17504548

Sameroff, A. J. (2000). Dialectical processes in developmental psychopathology. In A. J. Sameroff, M. Lewis, & S. M. Miller (Eds.), *Handbook of developmental psychopathology*. Springer. https://doi.org/DOI: 10.1007/978-1-4615-4163-9_2

Sciarra, D. S., Austin, V. L., & Bienia, E. J. (2022). *Working with students with emotional and behavioral disorders: A guide for K-12 teachers and service providers*. Vernon Press.

Seligman, M. E. P., & Csikszentmihalyi, M. (2000). Positive psychology: An introduction. *The American Psychologist*, 55(1), 5–14. DOI: 10.1037/0003-066X.55.1.5 PMID: 11392865

Shelton, L. (2018). *The Bronfenbrenner primer: A guide to develecology*. Routledge. DOI: 10.4324/9781315136066

Sheridan, S. M., Smith, T. E., Kim, E. M., Beretvas, S. N., & Park, S. (2019). A meta-analysis of family-school interventions and children's social-emotional functioning: Moderators and components of efficacy. *Review of Educational Research*, 89(2), 296–332. DOI: 10.3102/0034654318825437

Shields-Lysiak, L., Boyd, M. P., Iorio Jr, J., & Vasquez, C. R. (2020). Classroom greetings: More than a simple hello. *Iranian Journal of Language Teaching Research,* 8(3 (Special Issue), 41–56. DOI: 10.30466/ijltr.2020.120933

Skinner, B. F. (1966). Contingencies of reinforcement in the design of a culture. *Behavioral Science*, 11(3), 159–166. DOI: 10.1002/bs.3830110302 PMID: 5935977

Sklad, M., Diekstra, R., Ritter, M., Ben, J., & Gravesteijn, C. (2012). Effectiveness of school-based universal social, emotional and behavioral programs: Do they enhance students' development in the area of skill, behavior and adjustment? *Psychology in the Schools*, 49(9), 892–909. DOI: 10.1002/pits.21641

Smith, T. E., Sheridan, S. M., Kim, E. M., Park, S., & Beretvas, S. N. (2019). The effects of family-school partnership interventions on academic and social-emotional functioning: A meta-analysis exploring what works for whom. *Educational Psychology Review*, 32(2), 511–544. DOI: 10.1007/s10648-019-09509-w

Social and Emotional Aspects of Learning (SEAL). https://sealcommunity.org/

Steele, H., & Steele, M. (2014). Attachment disorders: Theory, research, and treatment considerations. In M. Lewis & K. D. Rudolph (Eds.), *Handbook of developmental psychopathology* (3rd ed., pp. 357–370). Springer.

Sugai, G., & Horner, R. H. (2002). Introduction to the special series on positive behavior support in schools. *Journal of Emotional and Behavioral Disorders*, 10(3), 130–135. DOI: 10.1177/10634266020100030101

Sugai, G., & Simonsen, B. (2012). *Positive behavioral interventions and supports: History, defining features, and misconceptions.* Center for PBIS & Center for Positive Behavioral Interventions and Supports, University of Connecticut. www.PBIS.org

Sutherland, K. S., Conroy, M. A., McLeod, B. D., Kunemund, R., & McKnight, K. (2018). Common practice elements for improving social, emotional, and behavioral outcomes of young elementary school students. *Journal of Emotional and Behavioral Disorders*, 27(2), 76–85. DOI: 10.1177/1063426618784009

Thorndike, E. L. (1898). Animal Intelligence: An experimental study of associative processes in animals. *Psychological Monographs*, 2(4), i–109. DOI: 10.1037/h0092987

Vogiatzoglou, P., & Galanaki, E. (2011). Classroom life of children with behavioral problems. *Proceedings of the 2nd Panhellenic Conference of Special Education: "Special Education as a starting point for developments in science and practice".* Greek Society of Special Education - University of Athens. (in Greek)

von Bertalanffy, L. (2013). *General system theory: Foundations, development, applications* (rev. ed.). Braziller. (Original work published 1968)

Wang, M.-T., Degol, J. L., Amemiya, J., Parr, A., & Guo, J. (2020). Classroom climate and children's academic and psychological wellbeing: A systematic review and meta-analysis. *Developmental Review*, 57, 100912. DOI: 10.1016/j.dr.2020.100912

Wannarka, R., & Ruhl, K. (2008). Seating arrangements that promote positive academic and behavioural outcomes: A review of empirical research. *Support for Learning*, 23(2), 89–93. DOI: 10.1111/j.1467-9604.2008.00375.x

Watson, J. B. (1914). *Behavior: An introduction to comparative psychology*. Henry Holtand., DOI: 10.1037/10868-000

Watzlawick, P. (1981). *The language of change: Elements of therapeutic communication*. Basic Books.

Whittingham, K., & Coyne, L. W. (2019). Values and proto-values. In Whittingham, K., & Coyne, L. W. (Eds.), *Acceptance and commitment therapy: The clinician's guide for supporting parents* (pp. 153–186). Academic Press. DOI: 10.1016/B978-0-12-814669-9.00007-2

Zafiriadou, E. (2019). The tender and sensitive Mimis who has become completely unpredictable. In Zafiropoulou, M. (Ed.), *The "difficult" child at home and at school* (pp. 17–42). Pedio. (in Greek)

Zafiropoulou, M. (2000). *Understanding our behavior: The role of learning in the acquisition and development of behavior*. Kastaniotis. (in Greek)

Zafiropoulou, M. (2004). Cognitive-behavioral interventions at school. In Kalantzi-Azizi, A., & Zafiropoulou, M. (Eds.), *Adaptation to school prevention and coping with difficulties* (pp. 26–50). Ellinika Grammata. (in Greek)

Zafiropoulou, M. (2019). *The "difficult" child at home and at school*. Pedio. (in Greek)

Chapter 5
Overcome Mental Health Challenges in Educational Settings:
An In-Depth Guide on Effective Interventions and Practices

Maria Efstratopoulou
http://orcid.org/0000-0002-5162-2104
United Arab Emirates University, UAE

Hawraa Habeeb
http://orcid.org/0000-0002-1437-8544
United Arab Emirates University, UAE

Jehan Osama Abdulla
United Arab Emirates University, UAE

Dingfei Shen
United Arab Emirates University, UAE

ABSTRACT

This chapter will not only delve into the rising interest in mental health among children and adolescents but also provide a comprehensive examination of school-based mental health programs and interventions, providing practical guidance for stakeholders. The aim is to assess their effectiveness in supporting students facing mental health challenges. Importantly, this chapter will offer practical strategies and evidence-based solutions that are readily applicable in helping school districts implement effective mental health interventions tailored to the diverse needs of

DOI: 10.4018/979-8-3693-5325-7.ch005

students. By targeting prevalent challenges such as anxiety, depression, ADHD, trauma, and others, school communities can advocate for the well-being and safety of their students. Educators, mental health practitioners, and policymakers can benefit from understanding the most effective programs and areas for improvement in current interventions. Ultimately, this discussion will contribute to enhancing the efficacy and future implementation of school-based mental health interventions

There has been a consistent increase in the occurrence of mental health conditions among children and adolescents. Nevertheless, there is a dearth of information addressing the implementation procedures of mental health interventions and techniques in schools. This chapter suggests a thorough investigation of school-based mental health programs and interventions, acknowledging the significant influence of mental health on academic success and general well-being.

Psychological well-being is an essential aspect of general health, particularly for students in their educational environments. Schools are recognized as playing a crucial role in promoting and enabling the mental well-being of pupils (Madireddy & Madireddy, 2020). They have the ability to use a variety of strategies to meet the mental health requirements of pupils. Accordingly, this chapter provides a comprehensive analysis of literature reviews (Chiumento et al., 2022; Eschenbeck et al., 2019; Richter et al., 2022), systematic reviews (Fenwick-Smith et al., 2018; Martínez-García, 2022), and meta-analyses (Murano et al., 2020; Yang et al., 2019; Zhang et al., 2022), in order to identify the most effective evidence-based interventions (EBIs). The comprehensive literature search and evaluation revealed the 15 most advantageous mental health interventions used in schools.

This chapter serves as a comprehensive guide to effective mental health promotion interventions in schools, detailing their theoretical underpinnings, implementation strategies, and tangible outcomes. Each section also offers practical insights and implications for future application, empowering educators to effectively enhance their students' well-being. By prioritizing these programs, educators and policymakers can transform schools into nurturing environments that foster the holistic development of every student. This research lays the groundwork for a healthier and more empathetic society that values and supports mental health.

SCHOOLS' MENTAL HEALTH EBIS PROGRAMS

Positive Behaviour Interventions and Supports

Positive behaviour interventions and supports (PBIS) have gained popularity in schools because they improve student behavior and reduce special education needs (Taylor et al., 2023). PBIS uses multitiered EBIs to enhance educational environments and behavior (Corcoran & Edward Thomas, 2021) by building components that are classified into three categories: Tier I (universal support), Tier II (targeted support), and Tier III (custom support).

Schools used the three-tier framework to explore bullying and juvenile violence prevention with a preventative and integration method. Intervention schools received teaching, support, and the necessary instruments to conduct a consistent and long-term preventive plan. The first two years of implementation focused on establishing the core components and systems needed for three-tier implementation.

Kelm et al. (2014) completed a meta-analysis of 2007–2009 Canadian grade 4 and 7 instructor data. After partially implementing the intervention in the first year and entirely in the second, suspensions decreased, and academic achievement, conduct, and school safety improved. Classrooms created rules to avoid penalties and utilized informal evaluation to evaluate rule understanding.

Social Emotional Learning

Social emotional learning (SEL) is a new concept in education that strengthens our emotional intelligence (EI) abilities. It is well-documented that SEL skills can significantly support educators and students in improving self-management, relationship management, and task-management abilities. Research suggests that teacher-led programs have a more substantial effect than those led by school psychologists (Cefai, 2020). In 2020, Cyprus implemented a SEL program, which enhanced teachers' personal and professional development by fostering 12 distinct interpersonal and intrapersonal values (Cefai, 2020). The Health Education courses were divided into organized subcourses with lesson plans, modules, and practical activities. This program positively impacted teachers and helped reduce children's anxiety, aggressiveness, nervousness, competitiveness, indifference, and negativity.

Additionally, in Boquete, Panama, a 14-lesson SEL program called "Me and My New World" was implemented over four months for students aged 12 to 15. Qualitative data collection methods, including interviews and focus groups, revealed high acceptance among students, teachers, and parents. The program improved adolescents' capacities, positively influencing their relationships and well-being (Araúz Ledezma et al., 2021).

Mental Health Literacy Programmes

Brown Epstein (2022) defined mental health literacy (MHL) as the knowledge, attitudes, and skills needed to promote good mental health. MHL programs aim to raise symptom awareness, encourage seeking help from adults, and foster social desirability. They also promote nonjudgmental listening and self-help strategies (Brown Epstein, 2022).

In the UK, several studies have examined MHL. Brown Epstein (2022) reviewed the Knowledge and Attitudes to Mental Health Scales, a self-report tool assessing knowledge of mental disorder symptoms, stigma, and health practices. In Wales, 559 adolescents aged 13-14 participated in a study using the Guide Cymru, which covers mental health, stigma, specific illnesses, help-seeking, experiences, and positive mental health (Simkiss et al., 2020). In the U.S., the "In Our Own Voice" program aimed to improve MHL among 15-year-olds via a 60-minute school session featuring personal stories of mental illness. Evaluations four and eight weeks later showed significant improvements in MHL (Brown Epstein, 2022). Daniele et al. (2022) reviewed educational interventions for adolescents aged 10—24 in Europe, involving teachers, psychologists, and school health personnel. Interventions, lasting two to three days, aimed to promote well-being, interpersonal relationships, emotional recognition, self-awareness, and respect. In Canada, a study of 265 high school students showed the positive impact of a curriculum-based MHL program "The Guide". Assessments before, after, and two months post-intervention showed significant improvements (Weaver et al., 2014).

Nurture Groups

Nurture Groups (NGs) are school-based interventions grounded in attachment theory that support children with social, emotional, and behavioral difficulties. They promote emotional well-being through reparative attachment experiences (Sloan et al., 2020). NGs aim to strengthen bonds and develop social and emotional skills, helping children form secure and trusting connections with school staff and peers.

Cunningham et al. (2019) studied the impact of NGs on social skills among 16 children aged 6 to 10 in five English primary schools. Assessments were based on teacher and student feedback, using the Child Role Play Measure and the Taxonomy of Problematic Social Situations. The 15-week intervention resulted in nine children showing improved social skills according to teacher ratings, although three children showed a decline and four exhibited no change. Challenges were noted in children's ability to apply these skills outside the intervention context, such as in the playground or classroom, raising questions about the broader effectiveness of the NG intervention (Cunningham et al., 2019).

Grantham and Primrose (2017) conducted a mixed-method study in seven Glasgow secondary schools, involving 17 staff and 24 youth. Most developmental strands showed significant improvement, although emotional security did not. External factors such as changes in schedule and staff turnover impacted pre- and postintervention metrics. Overall, the intervention enhanced social skills and development (Grantham & Primrose, 2017).

Vincent (2017) conducted a two-year qualitative study in a UK primary school involving staff, Key Stage 2 students (ages 7-11), and parents. Data were collected through staff observations, planning and assessment sheets, and semistructured interviews. Results indicated enhanced social skills, confidence, academic engagement, and reduced negative behaviors. The Boxall Profile, compared with an emotional literacy exam, showed improvements in self-awareness, self-regulation, motivation, empathy, and social skills (Vincent, 2017).

Cognitive Behavior Therapy

Cognitive behavior therapy (CBT) is beneficial for reducing anxiety in primary and teenage students and those on the autistic spectrum. Cognitive restructuring, social skills training, exposure, and behavioral experiments are used in CBT to treat cognitive aspects that cause anxiety (Low et al., 2023). Li et al. (2023) proposed CBT as a first-line treatment for depression and trauma-affected youngsters.

In Hong Kong, the intervention aimed to help participants:

1. Understand their anxiety and bodily reactions through cognitive-behavioral aspects.
2. Acknowledge anxiety-inducing feelings.
3. Change anxious thoughts and self-talk into coping thoughts and optimistic self-talk or find effective anxiety-reduction strategies.
4. Evaluate and self-reinforce their performance after using these cognitive-behavioral tactics.

In another Chinese randomised controlled experiment, Li et al. (2023) tested CBT for posttraumatic stress disorder (PTSD) in 9–12-year-olds. The lay counselor-led strategy combines whole-school and classroom publicity to reduce PTSD symptoms. The UCLA PTSD Reaction Index for DSM-5 (PTSD-RI-5) and Checklist-5 measured PTSD severity decrease as the primary outcome. Face-to-face follow-up assessments at 3- and 6-month intervals showed that the intervention had a lasting influence.

Psychoeducation

The "psychoeducational" intervention teaches students about the brain and emotions through practical applications. Psychoeducation that teaches children and parents about the biological basis of anxiety and anxiety disorders can help children manage their anxiety (Onnela et al., 2021). This programme helps individuals manage emotions, improve EI, build adaptive cognitive interpretations, practise exposing themselves to varied emotions, and avoid relapse. Parent training, crisis management, intrapersonal therapy, and inspiration are covered (Sperlich & Kabilamany, 2022).

In Finland, Onnela et al. (2021) undertook an exploratory mixed-method intervention for mental health disorders with 162 eighth-graders (ages 14-15) from two comprehensive schools. Mental health nurses addressed anxiety, eating disorders, behaviour disorder, depression, and substance use. The nonintervention group had 77 students (30.1% boys, 68.5% girls, and 1.4% not defined) and the intervention group 85 (31%). Each of the four 45-minute lectures taught students about mental health illnesses as medical conditions. Students expressed a greater understanding and openness to mental health concerns and improved mental health self-care postintervention. Adolescent MHL increased with this universal intervention (Onnela et al., 2021).

In a randomised controlled trial in Finland, from September 2016 to April 2017, Parhiala et al. (2020) examined the efficacy of interpersonal counselling (IPC) and brief psychosocial support (BPS) as CBT interventions for mild-to-moderate depression in 12—16-year-olds. School psychologists, social workers, and nurses treated 55 participants (43 girls and 12 boys). School and community health and welfare services for adolescents hosted the intervention. Parhiala et al. evaluated IPC and BPS's preliminary efficacy, feasibility, and acceptance. IPC and BPS helped mild-to-moderate depression and could be administered by school staff. These brief treatments were tailored for classroom use, providing teenagers with mental health assistance (Parhiala et al., 2020).

Good Behaviour Game

The Good Behavior Game (GBG) is an evidence-based classroom management strategy. It has been applied globally across diverse cultural and socioeconomic contexts. The GBG targets elementary school children, primarily those in grades 1—6, but it has also been used with preschoolers, kindergartners, and adolescents. Teachers typically deliver the intervention, although school psychologists and other educational professionals may also be involved. The GBG addresses various issues such as aggression, disruptive behavior, and hyperactivity, which can contribute to anxiety, depression, and other mental health challenges, if not managed effectively (Baffsky et al., 2022).

The GBG involves dividing a classroom into teams and rewarding the teams that adhere to established behavioral norms. Teachers set clear rules and monitor students' behaviors, providing reinforcement when the group collectively meets behavioral criteria. The process encourages positive behavior through interdependent group contingencies, where the success of the team depends on each member's behavior.

Components of the GBG include identifying target behaviors, setting team goals, monitoring behavior, and providing rewards such as extra recess time or small prizes. The primary goal is to reduce disruptive behavior and promote a positive learning environment, with expected outcomes including improved social interactions, reduced behavioral issues, and enhanced academic performance.

The GBG is considered a universal intervention, applicable to all students within a classroom, although it can be adapted for targeted groups with specific needs. It typically runs for a duration of ten minutes, three times a week initially, with the frequency gradually increasing to encompass the entire school day.

The Resilience Builder Program

The Resilience Builder Program (RBP) (Alvord et al., 2011) is a structured group intervention designed to improve social skills and self-control. Multiple studies have collected data on the effectiveness of the intervention using approaches such as randomized clinical trials and pre-postintervention assessments (Rich et al., 2018).

The intended demographic for RBP encompasses children between the ages of 7 and 12, who frequently exhibit conditions such as attention deficit hyperactivity disorder (ADHD), anxiety, and high-functioning autism spectrum disorder. The program is intended to be administered by therapists in a group environment, usually comprising 4-6 children of the same gender and similar age. The intervention lasts 12 weeks, consisting of one-hour sessions that occur on a weekly basis (Aduen et al., 2014). RBP tackles problems such as lacking social skills and difficulty managing emotions using a cognitive-behavioral approach. Every session consists of an interactive educational segment, a practice session where participants freely engage in behavioral exercises, and exercises aimed at promoting relaxation and self-control. The fundamental elements of RBP center around instructing abilities pertaining to proactive mindset, flexibility, emotional control, social understanding, and linguistic aptitude. For example, youngsters acquire explicit guidelines on personal boundaries and participate in simulated scenarios to refine their social skills within a regulated setting (Habayeb et al., 2017). The curriculum additionally integrates resilience-enhancing tactics with a focus on proactive preparation and community involvement. The anticipated results encompass heightened emotional regulation, fewer negative emotions, and improved social proficiency. Parents also observed substantial enhancements in their children's social functioning, encompassing communication and active involvement. Furthermore, the program's adaptability enables adjustments to cater to the distinct requirements of different groups, hence boosting its relevance and efficiency in many cultural settings.

The Zones of Regulation

The Zones of Regulation (ZoR) is an intervention program created by Leah Kuypers, an American occupational therapist, in 2011 (Kuypers, 2013). Kuypers developed the program to aid children, specifically those with neurobiological and mental health conditions such as autism spectrum disorder and ADHD, in managing their emotions and actions independently (Pandey et al., 2018). Kuypers' technique combines elements from cognitive behavioral therapy, sensory processing, and executive functioning to assist students with classifying and regulating their emotions in various situations.

The ZoR is suitable for a diverse range of ages, spanning from preschoolers to young adults, and may be easily adjusted to fit different educational environments. Students are the main participants, while the program is often facilitated by teachers, school psychologists, and occasionally occupational therapists. The program targets concerns such as anxiety, impulsivity, and emotional dysregulation with the goal of enhancing both classroom behavior and emotional well-being. The intervention comprises 18 lessons, which normally last approximately six weeks, with sessions occurring at a frequency of two to three times per week and are often conducted in sessions lasting 30-60 minutes, either on an individual basis or in small groups of 2-4 students.

The curriculum is structured into three sections to instruct individuals on self-regulation skills that can be applied in real-life scenarios (Kuypers, 2013). The first section aims to assist students in recognizing and comprehending their emotions through the use of a color-coded system (blue, green, yellow, and red) that represents various levels of alertness and emotions. The second half focuses on instructing techniques for controlling physiological and emotional responses, while the third section highlights the practical use of these techniques in different situations (Conklin & Jairam, 2021). The program is classified as a universal intervention since it can be implemented for all pupils, with a particular emphasis on those with distinct behavioral and emotional requirements.

Community-Based Mental Health and Behavioral Programs

Community-based mental health and behavioral programs play a vital role in tackling mental health issues within educational environments. These initiatives entail the cooperation of educational institutions, community organizations, and mental health specialists to offer extensive assistance to students. Although there has been improvement, there are still gaps in our understanding of how community participation contributes to educational environments (McMullen et al., 2020). An exemplary instance is the Whole School, Whole Community, Whole Child (WSCC) concept, which incorporates community resources and support systems into school environments to foster comprehensive student health and well-being. The intervention process comprises a needs assessment, the formulation of culturally suitable solutions, the execution of health promotion activities, and ongoing evaluation. Community partners are essential in delivering services, offering resources, and participating in program development and evaluation.

These programs cater to a wide range of individuals, encompassing children, adolescents, and young adults. They tackle various concerns such as anxiety, depression, trauma, and behavioral disorders. Typically, key actors involved in this context are teachers, school psychologists, community mental health workers, and other stakeholders.

The main objectives of community-based mental health programs are to boost students' mental health outcomes, bolster their social-emotional abilities, and establish a welcoming and inclusive school atmosphere. These interventions are often applicable to everyone, but they can also involve actions that specifically target populations that are at a higher risk. The duration and frequency of these interventions are contingent upon the program's design and the specific needs of the community. Models such as the WSCC program are usually ongoing, with consistent participation from community partners and regular evaluations to ensure efficacy and flexibility. By leveraging community resources and fostering collaborative partnerships, these programs create a supportive environment that promotes students' mental well-being and academic success.

Physical Activity Programs

Implementing physical activity interventions is an important element for enhancing mental health, and it has been proven to be an effective approach to achieving these benefits (Lubans et al., 2016). Studies indicate that engaging in physical activity decreases depression levels in children and adolescents while also enhancing their general health (Andermo et al., 2020).

Physical activity programs have been identified as successful interventions for enhancing mental health in young individuals. Programs originating in the late 20th century demonstrate the increasing acknowledgment of the correlation between physical activity and mental health results. These programs are designed to reach children and teenagers between the ages of 5 and 18 in both school and community environments. They are usually implemented by teachers, physical education instructors, school psychologists, and professional facilitators. They tackle mental health concerns such as anxiety, sadness, trauma, and symptoms associated with stress. The intervention approach entails implementing organized physical activities specifically designed to immerse kids in consistent, moderate-to-vigorous exercise.

Programs exhibit variability in terms of duration and intensity, typically spanning several weeks to months, with numerous sessions each week. Activities may encompass aerobic workouts, sports, yoga, and various other forms of physical motion.

The main objective of these therapies is to enhance mental health outcomes by utilizing the psychological and physiological advantages of physical activity. Pascoe et al.'s (2020) comprehensive review revealed a decrease in symptoms of depression and anxiety in young individuals. Lubans et al.'s (2016) review emphasized the positive effects of physical activity on cognitive function and emotional well-being. The review specifically mentioned enhancements in self-esteem and physical self-perceptions.

Mindfulness

Mindfulness, extensively studied and utilized since the late 20th century, has demonstrated considerable potential in educational environments. Mindfulness interventions are designed to address a wide spectrum of individuals, spanning from young toddlers to adolescents. The programs are commonly executed in educational environments, where teachers, school psychologists, and proficient mindfulness instructors administer them. The main psychological disorders targeted by these methods encompass anxiety, depression, trauma, and symptoms associated with stress. The intervention method often comprises organized sessions in which individuals partake in mindfulness techniques, including breathing exercises, body scans, mindful movement, and meditation. Mindfulness-based stress reduction programs typically have a duration of 8 weeks, consisting of weekly sessions that range from 60 to 90 minutes each. These courses aim to develop mindfulness by fostering an attentive and accepting attitude toward thoughts and emotions in the present moment. The program also includes daily at-home exercises that participants engage in regularly.

Mindfulness therapies primarily aim to augment emotional regulation, alleviate symptoms of mental discomfort, and promote general well-being. These interventions are typically applied universally, aiming to assist all students in a classroom environment. However, they can also be customized to address the special needs of particular groups. Anticipated results encompass diminished feelings of anxiety and sadness, enhanced attention and cognitive performance, and improved stress regulation. Empirical research has shown that mindfulness therapies are highly effective in enhancing mental health outcomes for children and adolescents (Kallapiran et al., 2015).

Mindfulness has several strengths, such as its capacity to be used with various age groups and in varied situations. Furthermore, the cultural context is of utmost importance since it is necessary to modify the practices and principles of mindfulness to suit the cultural and individual variations among varied student populations.

Promoting Alternative Thinking Strategies

Promoting Alternative Thinking Strategies (PATHS) aims to cultivate social-emotional abilities, self-regulation, and problem-solving techniques to augment pupils' overall well-being (Shi et al., 2022). PATHS is a top choice for children in grades pre-K through 1. The program has effectively prevented problem behavior, including hostility, violence, and drug use. It also aids in promoting academic skill development (Campbell et al., 2022). To implement PATHS at a school, teachers may use the four-level pyramid model, which includes the whole child, learning environment, children's program, and family partnership. Parents are included in instructing their children on how to manage their emotions effectively and use PATHS coping techniques inside the household. Implementation may be flexible, ranging from individual classroom sessions to a school-wide strategy. Moreover, one of the advantages of implementing PATHS is its flexibility. Whether implemented in small classroom settings or adopted school-wide, the approach can be tailored and adjusted to meet the unique needs and demands of the school and its pupils. This facilitates a more customized and efficient execution of the program.

To achieve this, various lessons should be designed to encourage class interactions. These lessons involved engaging in discussions from different perspectives, generating ideas in small groups, and participating in brainstorming games either in large groups or as a whole class. Students should be provided with techniques for cultivating a positive mindset towards themselves, others, and the current circumstances. The instructors should be tasked with actively involving the pupils in the exchange of constructive ideas. The lessons should include community-building activities, such as distributing and collecting the class rules, as well as engaging in cooperative play. The program comprised multiple levels, each containing a variety of lessons. These lessons, referred to as learning domains, focused on teaching students how to recognize, categorize, and apply particular skills.

Classroom-Based Interventions

Classroom-based interventions (CBI) are a design where teachers implement interventions in students' natural environment, that is, the classroom context such as drama, music, and activities (de Leeuw et al., 2020). Tailored CBIs were implemented to alleviate psychological symptoms and enhance resilience in youths who had experienced trauma and other mental problems. The use of narrative, psychodrama, and role-acting as part of the intervention had a beneficial impact on lowering the prevalence of PTSD symptoms and diagnoses, as per the DSM-V categorization. Some examples of CBI include Youth Experiencing Success in School (YESS) (Ow et al., 2022) and school-based psychosocial structured activities (El-Khodary

& Samara, 2019). In these interventions, students are provided with opportunities to express themselves creatively, build relationships, and develop important skills such as self-expression, teamwork, and emotional regulation. These interventions can provide a supportive and inclusive environment for students to express themselves, develop their social-emotional skills, and build resilience.

Children from 6 to 12 years of age were included in studies using CBI, such as de Leeuw et al.'s (2020) study, which proved the efficacy of the intervention on internalized and externalized behaviors. The intervention should be implemented by teachers inside the students' typical learning environment, namely the classroom setting. Moreover, it should be easy to implement and not require a tremendous amount of work. Research has shown that, when teachers encounter an intervention or component that demands a significant amount of work, they are likely to apply it with low fidelity or not implement it at all. Some of the examples of CBI include a curriculum designed for primary school kids with behavioral difficulties. It focuses on developing self-control, problem-solving skills, and social competence. The plan includes activities such as Circle of Friends, GBG, The Recess Pals and Recess Reporters, and classroom buddy seating arrangement.

Technology-Based intervention

Many technology-based interventions promote and prevent mental health issues. Technology-based biofeedback programs help children control their emotional and physiological responses to environmental events. There are other softwares used for mental health support such as BARN, From Mad to Worse, Conflict Management, and Smart Team and online data collection methods for school social work (Tani et al., 2024).

One of the technology-based interventions is Project CATCHIT, a free Internet-based training program based on behavioral activation, CBT, and interpersonal psychotherapy. Another program is MoodGYM, which is a free, interactive, and Internet-based program designed to prevent and decrease symptoms of depression (Jossou et al., 2022).

There are many innovative tools for school mental health services:

1. **Online Counseling Services:** They connect students with certified mental health specialists via chat, video chat or phone. They provide a safe and easy option for youngsters to get help without worrying about their identity.
2. **Apps for Mental Health:** These typically have tools for managing stress and anxiety, guided meditation, mood tracking, and depression and anxiety resources.
3. **Virtual Reality Therapy:** Students can work on coping mechanisms, overcome concerns or relax in the immersive worlds it offers.

4. **Assessment Tools Based on Technology:** They help identify students who may be struggling with mental health. These technologies frequently use surveys or questionnaires to collect data and offer insights for early intervention.
5. **Online Support Communities:** Students can find a community of like-minded individuals through online forums and platforms, where they can connect, exchange stories, and get help when they need it. Therapists can hold therapy sessions remotely using videoconferencing technology, a practice known as teletherapy.
6. **Wearable Devices:** Several schools have begun using fitness trackers and smartwatches to monitor students' stress, sleep, and activity levels. This data can help better understand their general health.
7. **Online Mental Health Education:** Educational platforms and digital resources abound, offering comprehensive knowledge on mental health, coping mechanisms, and self-care practices.

AN OVERVIEW ANALYSIS OF SCHOOL-BASED MENTAL HEALTH PROGRAMS

Effectiveness and Implementation of Evidence-Based Programs

The efficacy of school-based mental health programs, such as PBIS, SEL, and MHL programs, has been well documented. Research has demonstrated that the use of PBIS leads to positive outcomes such as improved student conduct, decreased suspension rates, and enhanced academic achievement. Nevertheless, the fluctuation in the degree to which a plan is executed accurately and the requirement for unwavering enduring assistance continue to be substantial obstacles. Similarly, SEL programs have shown significant decreases in anxiety and aggressiveness. However, the effectiveness of these programs relies on the implementation being done with high quality and the integration of SEL skills into the overall curriculum.

MHL has successfully enhanced students' understanding of mental health symptoms and diminished the social disapproval associated with them. Research conducted in the UK, U.S., Canada, and Norway shows notable enhancements in MHL and attitudes towards mental health. Nevertheless, it is imperative to customize these programs according to cultural contexts in order to sustain their efficacy. The significance of ongoing support and reinforcement in these programs cannot be exaggerated, as their effectiveness decreases without consistent effort.

Targeted Interventions for Specific Needs

Specific mental health disorders such as anxiety, depression, PTSD, and behavioral difficulties can be effectively addressed by targeted therapies including CBT, NGs, and GBG. CBT has demonstrated exceptional efficacy in alleviating symptoms associated with anxiety and sadness, notably in students suffering from PTSD. Research conducted in Hong Kong, China, and the U.S. has shown notable advancements, although further studies are required to assess the long-term effectiveness.

NGs offer a conducive setting for youngsters facing challenges in their social, emotional, and behavioral development. Studies conducted in the United Kingdom demonstrate enhancements in social aptitude and academic involvement. However, the inconsistency in children's capacity to utilize these skills outside the intervention setting presents a significant obstacle. The Good Behaviour Game is highly effective in decreasing disruptive behavior and fostering a positive learning atmosphere, leading to long-lasting advantages such as less substance usage and antisocial conduct. Nevertheless, ensuring a steadfast execution and customizing the game to suit diverse cultural environments are important for achieving its triumph.

Holistic and Innovative Approaches

Programs such as the RBP, ZoR, and PATHS provide a comprehensive approach that aims to improve social skills, emotional regulation, and overall well-being. Research has demonstrated substantial enhancements in emotional regulation and social abilities in children with ADHD, anxiety, and high-functioning autism spectrum disorder as a result of RBP. The adaptability of this system to many environments increases its significance; however, it is crucial to ensure consistent execution. The ZoR is a program that assists children in effectively managing their emotions and behaviors. It has shown varying levels of success in enhancing self-regulation and behaviour. The success of the program depends on regular practice and a high level of cultural awareness.

Modern solutions to current mental health concerns can be found through innovative approaches such as mindfulness and technology-based therapy. Mindfulness programs enhance the ability to regulate emotions and decrease stress, as evidenced by considerable advantages observed in multiple studies. However, it is crucial to ensure that there is consistency in the implementation and cultural adjustments in order to maximize their efficiency. Technological solutions, such as online counseling, mental health applications, and virtual reality therapy, offer easily available assistance and improve understanding of mental health. These tools provide additional opportunities for interaction, but necessitate thoughtful deliberation regarding accessibility and data privacy concerns.

Cultural Sensitivity and Sustainability

Cultural sensitivity and sustainability are critical components of the success of school-based mental health programs. In order to optimize engagement and effectiveness, programmes must be customized to accommodate the cultural and individual distinctions of diverse student populations. For example, the WSCC model and other community-based mental health programs have been shown to have positive effects on MHL and stigma reduction by implementing culturally appropriate strategies and maintaining ongoing community engagement.

Another critical factor is sustainability. In order to guarantee their long-term effectiveness, programs must receive consistent implementation, ongoing support, and regular evaluation. The effectiveness of these interventions over time is contingent upon the necessity of sustainable funding, training for school personnel, and integration into the school curriculum.

Inclusion

This chapter has presented a thorough amalgamation of successful practices of mental health in school settings, with a focus on the significance of establishing supportive and loving environments for students. The chapter introduced various EBIs, such as PBIS, SEL, and MHL programmes, that contribute to improving students' mental health and well-being. Every intervention is thoroughly described, including its implementation process, outcomes, and practical insights. It emphasized both the theoretical basis and practical implementation of these interventions.

Teachers and schools have the ability to integrate mental health education into daily work plans. This can encompass promoting positive mental health behaviors, instructing students on stress management techniques, equipping them with self-care resources, and recognizing signs of distress. By equipping educators and policymakers with the tools and knowledge to implement these strategies effectively, the chapter advocates for a holistic approach to education that prioritizes mental well-being. Through the provision of necessary skills and the cultivation of a healthy school environment, these interventions aid in the formation of resilient individuals who are capable of efficiently navigating the difficulties of life.

CONCLUSIONS

Educators have the power to make their classrooms places where children can learn in an atmosphere of safety, respect, and worth. Encouragement of candid discussion, attentive listening, and compassion are all ways to achieve this goal.

Educators can incorporate mental health education into their lesson plans. This can involve encouraging healthy mental health behaviors, teaching students how to deal with stress, providing them with tools for self-care, and identifying symptoms of distress. Educators can receive training to identify symptoms of distress in their students, including shifts in behavior, emotional state or academic achievement. By keeping an eye out, they can see which student might require more help.

Teachers can provide emotional support by maintaining an affable demeanor and being available for students to talk to. By doing so, they help students feel comfortable expressing themselves in a nonthreatening environment. Teachers should help students find resources. Educators have the power to link students to the right mental health resources, whether they are available on campus or in the surrounding neighborhood. Psychologists, social workers, and school counselors are all examples of this type of professional.

REFERENCES

Aduen, P. A., Rich, B. A., Sanchez, L., O'Brien, K., & Alvord, M. K. (2014). Resilience Builder Program therapy addresses core social deficits and emotion dysregulation in youth with high-functioning autism spectrum disorder. *Journal of Psychological Abnormalities in Children*, 3(2), 118–128. DOI: 10.4172/2329-9525.1000118

Alvord, M. K., Zucker, B., & Grados, J. J. (2011). *Resilience Builder Program for children and adolescents: Enhancing social competence and self-regulation–A cognitive-behavioral group approach*. Research Press.

Andermo, S., Hallgren, M., Nguyen, T. T. D., Jonsson, S., Petersen, S., Friberg, M., Romqvist, A., Stubbs, B., & Elinder, L. S. (2020). School-related physical activity interventions and mental health among children: A systematic review and meta-analysis. *Sports Medicine - Open*, 6(1), 1–27. DOI: 10.1186/s40798-020-00254-x PMID: 32548792

Araúz Ledezma, A. B., Massar, K., & Kok, G. (2021). Social emotional learning and the promotion of equal personal relationships among adolescents in Panama: A study protocol. *Health Promotion International*, 36(3), 741–752. DOI: 10.1093/heapro/daaa114 PMID: 33051640

Baffsky, R., Ivers, R., Cullen, P., Batterham, P. J., Toumbourou, J., Calear, A. L., Werner-Seidler, A., McGillivray, L., & Torok, M. (2022). A cluster randomised effectiveness-implementation trial of an intervention to increase the adoption of PAX Good Behaviour Game, a mental health prevention program, in Australian primary schools: Study protocol. *Contemporary Clinical Trials Communications*, 28, 100923. DOI: 10.1016/j.conctc.2022.100923 PMID: 35669488

Brown Epstein, H. A. (2022). Adolescent mental health literacy: Definitions and program highlights. *Journal of Consumer Health on the Internet*, 26(1), 102–108. DOI: 10.1080/15398285.2022.2029244

Campbell, F., Blank, L., Cantrell, A., Baxter, S., Blackmore, C., Dixon, J., & Goyder, E. (2022). Factors that influence mental health of university and college students in the UK: A systematic review. *BMC Public Health*, 22(1), 1778. Advance online publication. DOI: 10.1186/s12889-022-13943-x PMID: 36123714

Cefai, C. (2020). *Social and emotional learning in the Mediterranean: Cross-cultural perspectives and approaches*. Brill Sense. https://books.google.ae/books?id=y_T_DwAAQBAJ&printsec=frontcover&source=gbs_ViewAPI&redir_esc=y#v=onepage&q&f=false

Chiumento, A., Hosny, W., Gaber, E., Emadeldin, M., El Barabry, W., Hamoda, H. M., & Alonge, O. (2022). Exploring the acceptability of a WHO school-based mental health program in Egypt: A qualitative study. *SSM. Mental Health*, 2, 100075. Advance online publication. DOI: 10.1016/j.ssmmh.2022.100075

Conklin, M., & Jairam, D. (2021). The effects of co-teaching zones of regulation on elementary students' social, emotional, and academic risk behaviors. *Advanced Journal of Social Science*, 8(1), 171–192. DOI: 10.21467/ajss.8.1.171-192

Corcoran, T., & Edward Thomas, M. K. (2021). School-wide positive behaviour support as evidence-making interventions. *Research in Education*, 111(1), 108–125. DOI: 10.1177/00345237211034884

Cunningham, L. K., Hartwell, B., & Kreppner, J. (2019). Exploring the impact of nurture groups on children's social skills: A mixed-methods approach. *Educational Psychology in Practice*, 35(4), 368–383. DOI: 10.1080/02667363.2019.1615868

Daniele, K., Gambacorti Passerini, M. B., Palmieri, C., & Zannini, L. (2022). Educational interventions to promote adolescents' mental health: A scoping review. *Health Education Journal*, 81(5), 597–613. DOI: 10.1177/00178969221105359

de Leeuw, R. R., de Boer, A. A., & Minnaert, A. E. M. G. (2020). The proof of the intervention is in the implementation: A systematic review about implementation fidelity of classroom-based interventions facilitating social participation of students with social-emotional problems or behavioural difficulties. *International Journal of Educational Research Open*, 1, 100002. Advance online publication. DOI: 10.1016/j.ijedro.2020.100002

El-Khodary, B., & Samara, M. (2019). Effectiveness of a school-based intervention on the students' mental health after exposure to war-related trauma. *Frontiers in Psychiatry*, 10, 1031. DOI: 10.3389/fpsyt.2019.01031 PMID: 32273852

Eschenbeck, H., Kaess, M., Lehner, L., Hofmann, H., Bauer, S., Becker, K., Diestelkamp, S., Moessner, M., Rummel-Kluge, C., Salize, H.-J., Thomasius, R., Bertsch, K., Bilic, S., Brunner, R., Feldhege, J., Gallinat, C., Herpertz, S. C., Koenig, J., & Lustig, S.. (2019). School-based mental health promotion in children and adolescents with StresSOS using online or face-to-face interventions: Study protocol for a randomized controlled trial within the ProHEAD Consortium. *Trials*, 20(1), 64. DOI: 10.1186/s13063-018-3159-5 PMID: 30658675

Fenwick-Smith, A., Dahlberg, E. E., & Thompson, S. C. (2018). Systematic review of resilience-enhancing, universal, primary school-based mental health promotion programs. *BMC Psychology*, 6(1), 1–17. DOI: 10.1186/s40359-018-0242-3 PMID: 29976252

Grantham, R., & Primrose, F. (2017). Investigating the fidelity and effectiveness of nurture groups in the secondary school context. *Emotional & Behavioural Difficulties*, 22(3), 219–236. DOI: 10.1080/13632752.2017.1331986

Habayeb, S., Rich, B., & Alvord, M. K. (2017). Targeting heterogeneity and comorbidity in children with autism spectrum disorder through the resilience builder group therapy program. *Child and Youth Care Forum*, 46(4), 539–557. DOI: 10.1007/s10566-017-9394-1

Jossou, T., Medenou, D., Et-tahir, A., Ahouandjinou, H., Edoh, T., Houessouvo, R., & Pecchia, L. (2022). A review about technology in mental health sensing and assessment. *ITM Web of Conferences, 46*. https://doi.org/DOI: 10.1051/itm-conf/20224601005

Kallapiran, K., Koo, S., Kirubakaran, R., & Hancock, K. (2015). Review: Effectiveness of mindfulness in improving mental health symptoms of children and adolescents: A meta-analysis. *Child and Adolescent Mental Health*, 20(4), 182–194. DOI: 10.1111/camh.12113 PMID: 32680348

Kelm, J. L., McIntosh, K., & Cooley, S. (2014). Effects of implementing school-wide positive behavioural interventions and supports on problem behaviour and academic achievement in a Canadian elementary school. *Canadian Journal of School Psychology*, 29(3), 195–212. DOI: 10.1177/0829573514540266

Kuypers, L. M. (2013). The zones of regulation: A framework to foster self-regulation. *Sensory Integration Special Interest Section Quarterly, 36*(4), 1y I. https://www.scribd.com/document/379956599/The-Zones-of-Regulation-A-Framework-to-Foster-Self-regulation-2013

Li, J., Li, J., Zhang, W., Wang, G., & Qu, Z. (2023). Effectiveness of a school-based, lay counselor-delivered cognitive behavioral therapy for Chinese children with posttraumatic stress symptoms: A randomized controlled trial. *The Lancet Regional Health. Western Pacific*, 33, 100699. Advance online publication. DOI: 10.1016/j.lanwpc.2023.100699 PMID: 36785644

Low, Y. T. A., Wong, D. F. K., Kwok, S., Man, K. W., & Ip, S. Y. (2023). Effectiveness of a culturally specific school-based cognitive-behavioural group therapy for primary school children with anxiety problems in Hong Kong. *Asia Pacific Journal of Social Work and Development*, ●●●, 1–14. DOI: 10.1080/29949769.2023.2296894

Lubans, D., Richards, J., Hillman, C., Faulkner, G., Beauchamp, M., Nilsson, M., Kelly, P., Smith, J., Raine, L., & Biddle, S. (2016). Physical activity for cognitive and mental health in youth: A systematic review of mechanisms. *Pediatrics*, 138(3), 1. DOI: 10.1542/peds.2016-1642 PMID: 27542849

Madireddy, S., & Madireddy, S. (2020). Strategies for schools to prevent psychosocial stress, stigma, and suicidality risks among LGBTQ+ students. *American Journal of Educational Research*, 8(9), 659–667. DOI: 10.12691/education-8-9-7

Martínez-García, A. (2022). Contributions of universal school-based mental health promotion to the wellbeing of adolescents and preadolescents: A systematic review of educational interventions. *Health Education*, 122(5), 564–583. DOI: 10.1108/HE-07-2021-0106

McMullen, J. M., George, M., Ingman, B. C., Pulling Kuhn, A., Graham, D. J., & Carson, R. L. (2020). A systematic review of community engagement outcomes research in school-based health interventions. *The Journal of School Health*, 90(12), 985–994. DOI: 10.1111/josh.12962 PMID: 33184891

Murano, D., Sawyer, J. E., & Lipnevich, A. A. (2020). A meta-analytic review of preschool social and emotional learning interventions. *Review of Educational Research*, 90(2), 227–263. DOI: 10.3102/0034654320914743

Onnela, A., Hurtig, T., & Ebeling, H. (2021). A psychoeducational mental health promotion intervention in comprehensive school: Recognising problems and reducing stigma. *Health Education Journal*, 80(5), 554–566. DOI: 10.1177/0017896921994134

Ow, N., Marchand, K., Glowacki, K., Alqutub, D., Mathias, S., & Barbic, S. P. (2022). YESS: A feasibility study of a supported employment program for youths with mental health disorders. *Frontiers in Psychiatry*, 13, 856905. Advance online publication. DOI: 10.3389/fpsyt.2022.856905 PMID: 36213923

Pandey, A., Hale, D., Das, S., Goddings, A. L., Blakemore, S. J., & Viner, R. M. (2018). Effectiveness of universal self-regulation-based interventions in children and adolescents a systematic review and meta-analysis. *Journal American Medical Association Pediatrics, 172*(6), 566cs, 17https://doi.org/DOI: 10.1001/jamapediatrics.2018.0232

Parhiala, P., Ranta, K., Gergov, V., Kontunen, J., Law, R., La Greca, A. M., Torppa, M., & Marttunen, M. (2020). Interpersonal counseling in the treatment of adolescent depression: A randomized controlled effectiveness and feasibility study in school health and welfare services. *School Mental Health*, 12(2), 265–283. DOI: 10.1007/s12310-019-09346-w

Pascoe, M., Bailey, A. P., Craike, M., Carter, T., Patten, R., Stepto, N., & Parker, A. (2020). Physical activity and exercise in youth mental health promotion: A scoping review. *BMJ Open Sport & Exercise Medicine*, 6(1), e000677. DOI: 10.1136/bmjsem-2019-000677 PMID: 32095272

Rich, B. A., Shiffrin, N. D., Cummings, C. M., Zarger, M. M., Berghorst, L., & Alvord, M. K. (2018). Resilience-based intervention with underserved children: Impact on self-regulation in a randomized clinical trial in schools. *International Journal of Group Psychotherapy*, 69(1), 30–53. DOI: 10.1080/00207284.2018.1479187 PMID: 38449213

Richter, A., Sjunnestrand, M., & Hasson, H. (2022). Implementing school-based mental health services: A scoping review of the literature summarizing the factors that affect implementation. *International Journal of Environmental Research and Public Health*, 19(6), 3489. DOI: 10.3390/ijerph19063489 PMID: 35329175

Shi, J., Cheung, A. C. K., & Ni, A. (2022). The effectiveness of Promoting Alternative Thinking Strategies program: A meta-analysis. *Frontiers in Psychology*, 13, 1030572. Advance online publication. DOI: 10.3389/fpsyg.2022.1030572 PMID: 36571043

Simkiss, N. J., Gray, N. S., Dunne, C., & Snowden, R. J. (2021). Development and psychometric properties of the Knowledge and Attitudes to Mental Health Scales (KAMHS): A psychometric measure of mental health literacy in children and adolescents. *BMC Pediatrics*, 21(1), 508. Advance online publication. DOI: 10.1186/s12887-021-02964-x PMID: 34774022

Sloan, S., Winter, K., Connolly, P., & Gildea, A. (2020). The effectiveness of Nurture Groups in improving outcomes for young children with social, emotional, and behavioural difficulties in primary schools: An evaluation of Nurture Group provision in Northern Ireland. *Children and Youth Services Review*, 108, 104619. DOI: 10.1016/j.childyouth.2019.104619

Sperlich, M., & Kabilamany, P. (2022). The survivor moms' companion trauma-specific perinatal psychoeducation intervention in a community outreach program: An open pilot. *Journal of Midwifery & Women's Health*, 67(5), 569–579. DOI: 10.1111/jmwh.13380 PMID: 35689499

Tani, N., Fujihara, H., Ishii, K., Kamakura, Y., Tsunemi, M., Yamaguchi, C., Eguchi, H., Imamura, K., Kanamori, S., Kojimahara, N., & Ebara, T. (2024). What digital health technology types are used in mental health prevention and intervention? Review of systematic reviews for systematization of technologies. *Journal of Occupational Health*, 66(1), uiad003. Advance online publication. DOI: 10.1093/joccuh/uiad003 PMID: 38258936

Taylor, J. C., Hanley, W., Deger, G., & Hunter, C., W. (. (2023). Promoting anti-racism practices and the cycle of critical consciousness within positive behavior interventions and supports frameworks. *Teaching Exceptional Children*, 55(5), 314–322. DOI: 10.1177/00400599221120242

Vincent, K. (2017). "It's small steps, but that leads to bigger changes:" Evaluation of a Nurture Group intervention. *Emotional & Behavioural Difficulties*, 22(4), 303–316. DOI: 10.1080/13632752.2017.1290882

Weaver, C., Kutcher, S., Wei, Y., & Mcluckie, A. (2014). Sustained improvements in students' mental health literacy with use of a mental health curriculum in Canadian schools. *BMC Psychiatry*, 14(1), 1–6. DOI: 10.1186/s12888-014-0379-4 PMID: 25551789

Yang, W., Datu, J. A. D., Lin, X., Lau, M. M., & Li, H. (2019). Can early childhood curriculum enhance social-emotional competence in low-income children? A meta-analysis of the educational effects. *Early Education and Development*, 30(1), 36–59. DOI: 10.1080/10409289.2018.1539557

Zhang, Q., Wang, J., & Neitzel, A. (2022). School-based mental health interventions targeting depression or anxiety: A meta-analysis of rigorous randomized controlled trials for school-aged children and adolescents. *Journal of Youth and Adolescence: A Multidisciplinary Research Publication, 52*(1), 195–217. https://doi.org/DOI: 10.1007/s10964-022-01684-4

Chapter 6
Caring for Mental Health of Vulnerable Minds:
Well–Being and Mental Flow in Educational Settings

Agathi Argyriadi
United Arab Emirates University, UAE

Alexandros Argyriadis
https://orcid.org/0000-0001-5754-4787
Frederick University, Cyprus

Maria Efstratopoulou
https://orcid.org/0000-0002-5162-2104
United Arab Emirates University, UAE

ABSTRACT

Recent trends in educational research underscore the significance of cultivating mental flow to enhance well-being, especially for health-vulnerable individuals. Scholars have delved into the nuances of creating conducive learning environments that cater to the unique needs of students facing health vulnerabilities. Adopting a systematic review approach, this chapter synthesizes findings from diverse studies published over the past decade. The examination of empirical research, intervention strategies, and case studies aims to provide a comprehensive understanding of the ways in which mental flow can be nurtured to support the well-being of health-vulnerable students in educational settings. The synthesis of literature highlights the positive impact of tailored learning experiences on the mental flow and overall well-being of health-vulnerable students. From inclusive teaching practices to adaptive curriculum design, the findings emphasize the importance of creating environments

DOI: 10.4018/979-8-3693-5325-7.ch006

that prioritize the unique needs of these individuals.

INTRODUCTION

The importance of well-being and mental flow in educational environments has gained significant traction in recent years, driven by growing recognition of their impact on both student outcomes and overall educational quality. This discussion highlights recent trends and best practices for fostering these crucial aspects within educational settings.

One prominent approach for nurturing mental well-being in educational settings among others, is the PRICES (Physical, Relational, Intellectual, Creative, Emotional, and Spiritual) model. This comprehensive approach emphasizes the need to address multiple dimensions of well-being to create a supportive educational environment. By focusing on these diverse aspects, educators can foster a holistic sense of well-being among students (Alinsunurin, 2020; Wang & Degol, 2016).

The PRICES model, which stands for Physical, Relational, Intellectual, Creative, Emotional, and Spiritual well-being, represents a comprehensive framework for fostering mental well-being in educational settings. This model underscores the importance of addressing multiple dimensions of well-being to create a supportive and holistic educational environment. By focusing on these diverse aspects, educators can significantly enhance students' overall well-being, promoting both academic success and personal development.

Physical well-being is the foundation of the PRICES model, recognizing the essential role of health and fitness in mental well-being. Regular physical activity has been consistently linked to improved mood, reduced anxiety, and better cognitive function (Biddle & Asare, 2011). Schools that integrate physical education, encourage active play, and promote healthy eating contribute to the physical health of students, which in turn supports their mental and emotional well-being. For example, initiatives such as daily physical education classes and nutritious school meals can help students maintain a healthy lifestyle, which is crucial for optimal learning and cognitive performance (Janssen & LeBlanc, 2010).

Relational well-being focuses on the quality of relationships within the educational environment. Positive relationships with peers, teachers, and family members are vital for students' social and emotional development. According to Pianta, Hamre, and Allen (2012), strong student-teacher relationships can lead to better academic outcomes and increased student engagement. Moreover, fostering a sense of community within the classroom can help students feel valued and supported, which is essential for their mental health. Programs that promote social skills, conflict resolution, and collaborative learning can enhance relational well-being and create a positive school climate (Wentzel & Muenks, 2016).

Intellectual well-being is about stimulating students' cognitive abilities and encouraging a love for learning. This dimension of the PRICES model emphasizes the importance of providing intellectually challenging and engaging educational experiences. According to Deci and Ryan's Self-Determination Theory (2000), when students feel competent and autonomous in their learning, they are more likely to experience intrinsic motivation and academic success. Schools can nurture intellectual well-being by offering a variety of learning opportunities, fostering critical thinking, and supporting students' individual interests and strengths. Environments that encourage curiosity, creativity, and problem-solving can significantly enhance students' intellectual development (Hattie, 2009).

Creative well-being involves nurturing students' creativity and self-expression. Engaging in creative activities such as art, music, drama, and writing can provide an emotional outlet and promote psychological resilience. Creative expression allows students to explore their identities, develop their talents, and cope with stress (Csikszentmihalyi, 1996). Schools that integrate arts education into the curriculum can help students develop a sense of achievement and self-worth. Additionally, creative activities can enhance cognitive abilities and improve problem-solving skills, contributing to overall intellectual and emotional well-being (Winner, Goldstein, & Vincent-Lancrin, 2013).

Emotional well-being focuses on students' ability to understand, manage, and express their emotions effectively. This dimension is critical for developing resilience and coping strategies in the face of challenges. According to Durlak et al. (2011), social-emotional learning (SEL) programs that teach skills such as emotional regulation, empathy, and responsible decision-making can significantly improve students' emotional health and academic performance. Schools can support emotional well-being by creating safe and supportive environments where students feel free to express their emotions and seek help when needed. Providing access to counseling services and mental health resources is also crucial for addressing emotional well-being (Oberle et al., 2018).

Spiritual well-being involves fostering a sense of purpose and connection to something greater than oneself. While spiritual well-being can be associated with religious beliefs, it also encompasses broader concepts such as meaning, purpose, and interconnectedness. According to Pargament (2011), spiritual well-being can provide students with a sense of direction and hope, which is essential for mental health. Schools can nurture spiritual well-being by promoting values such as compassion, gratitude, and mindfulness. Programs that encourage reflection, meditation, and community service can help students develop a deeper sense of purpose and connectedness (Benson, Scales, & Syvertsen, 2011).

Integration and Application of the PRICES Model

Implementing the PRICES model in educational settings requires a coordinated effort among educators, administrators, and the broader school community. By addressing each dimension of well-being, schools can create a comprehensive support system that nurtures the whole student.

Schools can develop comprehensive programs and policies that integrate the PRICES dimensions into everyday practices. For example, incorporating physical activities into the daily schedule, promoting healthy relationships through SEL programs, offering intellectually stimulating and creative learning opportunities, and providing emotional and spiritual support services can collectively enhance students' well-being.

Professional development for educators is crucial for the successful implementation of the PRICES model. Training teachers to recognize and address the diverse needs of students, incorporating well-being practices into their teaching, and fostering a supportive classroom environment are essential steps. Programs like the CARE initiative, which focus on cultivating awareness and resilience in educators, can be instrumental in this regard (Jennings et al., 2017).

Engaging the broader community and families is also vital for nurturing students' well-being. Schools can collaborate with parents, community organizations, and mental health professionals to create a supportive network for students. Involving families in well-being initiatives and providing them with resources to support their children's mental health at home can enhance the effectiveness of school-based programs (Weiss, Lopez, & Caspe, 2018).

Teacher Well-being and Professional Development

Teacher well-being is a critical component of the overall educational environment. Research indicates that teachers' social and emotional competence directly influences their classroom interactions and students' academic and social-emotional outcomes. Programs like the CARE (Cultivating Awareness and Resilience in Education) initiative have shown positive effects on teachers' well-being, leading to improved classroom environments and student outcomes (Brown et al., 2023; Jennings et al., 2017).

Professional development programs that include mindfulness training and emotional intelligence workshops are increasingly being implemented. These programs help educators manage stress, build resilience, and create more empathetic and effective teaching practices. Such initiatives not only enhance teacher well-being but also model positive behaviors for students (Gimbert et al., 2021; Meiklejohn et al., 2012).

Teacher well-being is increasingly recognized as a fundamental aspect of the overall educational environment. The social and emotional competence of teachers plays a crucial role in shaping their classroom interactions and significantly influences students' academic and social-emotional outcomes. Research highlights that when teachers are well-supported and equipped with the necessary skills to manage their emotions and stress, it not only benefits their personal well-being but also creates a positive and productive classroom environment.

The well-being of teachers is integral to fostering an environment conducive to learning. Studies have shown that teachers with high levels of social and emotional competence are better able to create supportive and engaging classroom atmospheres. This, in turn, leads to improved student engagement, higher academic performance, and better social-emotional development among students (Jennings et al., 2017; Brown et al., 2023). Teachers who are emotionally competent can manage classroom challenges more effectively, reduce disruptive behaviors, and foster a positive learning environment.

The CARE Initiative

Programs like the CARE (Cultivating Awareness and Resilience in Education) initiative have demonstrated significant positive effects on teachers' well-being. CARE focuses on enhancing teachers' mindfulness, emotional awareness, and resilience, providing them with tools to cope with stress and improve their interactions with students. Research on the CARE program has shown that participating teachers report lower levels of stress and burnout, higher levels of emotional regulation, and better classroom management skills (Jennings et al., 2017). These improvements not only benefit the teachers but also create a more supportive and nurturing environment for students, leading to better academic and social-emotional outcomes.

Professional development programs that include mindfulness training and emotional intelligence workshops are becoming more prevalent in educational settings. These programs aim to equip educators with the skills necessary to manage their stress, build resilience, and develop more empathetic and effective teaching practices. Mindfulness training, in particular, has been shown to reduce stress and anxiety, improve emotional regulation, and enhance overall well-being (Meiklejohn et al., 2012). By practicing mindfulness, teachers can remain calm and focused, even in challenging situations, which positively affects their interactions with students.

Emotional intelligence workshops also play a crucial role in professional development. These workshops help teachers understand and manage their emotions, recognize and empathize with the emotions of others, and build strong interpersonal relationships. Research suggests that teachers with high emotional intelligence are better equipped to handle classroom conflicts, support students' emotional needs, and create a positive classroom climate (Gimbert et al., 2021). These skills are essential for fostering a supportive and effective learning environment.

One of the significant benefits of these professional development programs is that they help teachers model positive behaviors for their students. When teachers demonstrate effective stress management, emotional regulation, and empathy, they provide students with valuable examples of how to handle their own emotions and interactions. This modeling can have a profound impact on students, teaching them important life skills that go beyond academic learning.

Community and Social Emotional Learning (SEL)

The integration of social-emotional learning (SEL) into the curriculum is a growing trend. SEL programs aim to develop students' emotional intelligence, resilience, and interpersonal skills. By embedding SEL into daily classroom activities, schools can create a nurturing environment that supports students' mental health and academic success (Patton & Parker, 2017; Horn & Little, 2010).

Building a community of care within the classroom is another essential strategy. This involves establishing clear structures and norms, fostering open communication, and providing opportunities for personal sharing and reflection. Such practices help students feel valued and supported, which is crucial for their mental well-being (Stanford Teaching Commons, n.d.).

The integration of social-emotional learning (SEL) into school curricula is a growing trend, reflecting a broader recognition of the importance of developing students' emotional intelligence, resilience, and interpersonal skills. SEL programs are designed to provide students with the tools they need to manage their emotions, build healthy relationships, and make responsible decisions, thereby supporting both their mental health and academic success (Patton & Parker, 2017; Horn & Little, 2010).

SEL programs have been shown to have a significant impact on students' overall development. Research indicates that students who participate in SEL programs demonstrate improved social behaviors, lower levels of emotional distress, and enhanced academic performance (Durlak et al., 2011). These programs help students develop key competencies such as self-awareness, self-management, social awareness, relationship skills, and responsible decision-making, which are crucial for their success both in and out of the classroom (CASEL, 2020).

To effectively integrate SEL into the curriculum, schools need to adopt a comprehensive approach that includes embedding SEL principles into daily classroom activities. This involves creating lesson plans that incorporate SEL objectives, using teaching methods that promote emotional and social development, and fostering an inclusive classroom environment that encourages student participation and engagement (Jones & Bouffard, 2012).

One effective strategy is to incorporate SEL into existing subjects. For instance, literature classes can include discussions about characters' emotions and relationships, while science lessons can address ethical considerations and teamwork. This approach not only makes SEL relevant to students' academic work but also helps them see the practical application of SEL skills in various contexts (Zinsser, 2015).

Creating a community of care within the classroom is another essential strategy for promoting SEL. This involves establishing clear structures and norms that promote respect, inclusion, and collaboration among students. Teachers can foster a sense of community by encouraging open communication, providing opportunities for personal sharing and reflection, and modeling empathetic behavior (Stanford Teaching Commons, n.d.).

Clear structures and norms are foundational to a supportive classroom environment. By setting expectations for behavior and interaction, teachers can create a predictable and safe space where students feel valued and respected. This includes establishing rules that promote kindness, active listening, and mutual support. Regularly revisiting and reinforcing these norms helps maintain a positive classroom culture (Weissberg et al., 2015).

Open communication is vital for building trust and understanding within the classroom. Teachers can encourage students to express their thoughts and feelings openly by creating a non-judgmental and supportive atmosphere. Techniques such as regular check-ins, circle time, and reflective journaling can provide students with opportunities to share their experiences and connect with their peers on a deeper level (Rimm-Kaufman & Hulleman, 2015).

Providing opportunities for personal sharing and reflection helps students develop self-awareness and empathy. Activities such as group discussions, peer mentoring, and reflective writing can facilitate this process. These practices not only enhance students' understanding of their own emotions but also help them appreciate the perspectives and experiences of others, fostering a sense of community and belonging (Brackett & Rivers, 2014).

While the benefits of integrating SEL into the curriculum are well-documented, there are also challenges that schools may face in implementing these programs. These include finding time within an already packed curriculum, securing buy-in from all stakeholders, and ensuring that teachers have the necessary training and resources to effectively deliver SEL instruction (Jones & Bouffard, 2012).

To address these challenges, schools need to take a strategic approach to SEL implementation. This involves providing ongoing professional development for teachers, involving parents and the community in SEL initiatives, and continuously monitoring and evaluating the effectiveness of SEL programs. By doing so, schools can ensure that SEL becomes an integral part of the educational experience and that students receive the support they need to thrive (Elias et al., 1997).

Mindfulness and Mental Flow

Mindfulness practices have been increasingly integrated into educational settings to promote mental flow and reduce stress. Mindfulness involves paying attention to the present moment without judgment, which can help students and teachers manage stress and improve focus. Research shows that mindfulness interventions can enhance students' cognitive performance, emotional regulation, and overall well-being (Meiklejohn et al., 2012; Patton & Parker, 2017).

The concept of "flow," where individuals are fully immersed and engaged in an activity, is also being explored in educational contexts. Creating conditions for students to experience flow can lead to deeper learning and greater satisfaction. This involves designing challenging but achievable tasks, providing immediate feedback, and allowing students autonomy in their learning processes (Csikszentmihalyi, 1990; Nakamura & Csikszentmihalyi, 2014).

Mindfulness practices have become a prominent feature in educational environments, aiming to promote mental flow and reduce stress among students and teachers. Mindfulness, which involves paying attention to the present moment without judgment, offers a variety of benefits, including improved stress management and enhanced focus. Research indicates that mindfulness interventions can significantly enhance cognitive performance, emotional regulation, and overall well-being (Meiklejohn et al., 2012; Patton & Parker, 2017).

Mindfulness practices have been linked to numerous positive outcomes in educational settings. These practices help individuals to develop greater self-awareness, reduce anxiety, and improve concentration. A meta-analysis by Zenner, Herrnleben-Kurz, and Walach (2014) found that mindfulness programs in schools improve cognitive performance and resilience among students. Such interventions can lead to better academic performance, enhanced emotional regulation, and a reduction in disruptive behaviors (Meiklejohn et al., 2012).

For teachers, mindfulness training can lead to decreased stress levels, improved classroom management, and better relationships with students. Jennings et al. (2017) found that teachers who participated in mindfulness-based professional development programs reported lower levels of burnout and higher levels of job satisfaction. This suggests that mindfulness not only benefits students but also contributes to a healthier and more productive educational environment.

Implementing mindfulness programs in schools involves integrating mindfulness activities into the daily routine. These activities can include mindfulness meditation, mindful breathing exercises, and mindful movement practices such as yoga. Schools can also incorporate mindfulness into classroom activities by starting the day with a few minutes of mindful breathing or by using mindfulness techniques to help students transition between tasks (Zenner et al., 2014).

Professional development for teachers is crucial for the successful implementation of mindfulness programs. Teachers need training to effectively lead mindfulness exercises and to integrate mindfulness principles into their teaching practices. Programs like Mindfulness-Based Stress Reduction (MBSR) and CARE (Cultivating Awareness and Resilience in Education) provide educators with the tools and techniques needed to incorporate mindfulness into their classrooms (Jennings et al., 2017).

The concept of "flow," introduced by Csikszentmihalyi (1990), describes a state of complete immersion and engagement in an activity. In educational contexts, creating conditions that foster flow can lead to deeper learning and greater student satisfaction. Achieving flow in the classroom involves designing tasks that are challenging yet achievable, providing immediate feedback, and allowing students a degree of autonomy in their learning processes (Nakamura & Csikszentmihalyi, 2014).

To facilitate flow, educators need to create an environment where students can fully engage with their learning activities. This involves setting clear goals, ensuring that tasks are appropriately challenging, and providing timely feedback. By allowing students to take ownership of their learning and encouraging self-directed projects, teachers can help students enter the flow state more frequently (Shernoff et al., 2016).

Moreover, integrating mindfulness practices can enhance the conditions for achieving flow. Mindfulness helps students develop the focus and self-regulation skills necessary to sustain attention on challenging tasks. When students are mindful, they are better able to concentrate, avoid distractions, and stay engaged with their work, all of which are essential components of the flow experience (Meiklejohn et al., 2012).

The synergy between mindfulness and flow can be particularly powerful in educational settings. Mindfulness prepares the mind for flow by cultivating present-moment awareness and reducing stress. When students practice mindfulness, they are more likely to achieve flow during academic tasks, as they are better equipped to handle challenges and stay focused (Roeser et al., 2013).

Teachers can facilitate this synergy by incorporating mindfulness exercises into their daily routines and by designing learning activities that encourage deep engagement. For example, starting a lesson with a brief mindfulness session can help students clear their minds and prepare for focused work. Additionally, project-based learning that aligns with students' interests can help sustain their engagement and promote the flow experience (Shernoff et al., 2016).

Support Systems and Resources

Schools are increasingly recognizing the importance of providing robust support systems for mental health. This includes access to counseling services, mental health resources, and crisis intervention programs. The CDC's action guide for promoting mental health in schools outlines strategies for creating supportive environments and connecting students with necessary resources (CDC, 2022).

Additionally, the role of community and family engagement is emphasized. Schools that actively involve parents and caregivers in the educational process tend to create more inclusive and supportive environments. This involvement can enhance students' sense of belonging and support their overall well-being (Alinsunurin, 2020; Wang & Degol, 2016).

Schools are increasingly recognizing the importance of providing robust support systems for mental health, acknowledging that the well-being of students is fundamental to their academic and personal success. Comprehensive mental health support in educational settings includes access to counseling services, mental health resources, and crisis intervention programs. These initiatives are crucial in creating a supportive environment that addresses the diverse needs of students (CDC, 2022).

Counseling services are a cornerstone of mental health support in schools. They provide students with a safe space to discuss their issues, learn coping strategies, and receive professional guidance. Research shows that schools with adequate counseling services experience lower rates of student anxiety, depression, and behavioral problems (Reback, 2010). Counselors also play a key role in identifying students at risk and connecting them with additional resources, thereby preventing more severe mental health crises.

Schools are also integrating various mental health resources into their support systems. These resources include educational materials on mental health, workshops on stress management and resilience, and programs that promote mental wellness practices such as mindfulness and emotional regulation. According to the CDC's action guide, providing students with these resources helps in normalizing conversations around mental health and encourages students to seek help when needed (CDC, 2022).

Crisis intervention programs are essential for addressing immediate mental health emergencies. These programs are designed to provide rapid support to students experiencing acute psychological distress, such as suicidal ideation or severe anxiety attacks. Effective crisis intervention involves a well-coordinated response from trained school staff, mental health professionals, and, when necessary, emergency services. Schools with established crisis intervention protocols are better equipped to manage emergencies and provide timely support, thereby mitigating the potential for long-term psychological damage (Brock et al., 2009).

In addition to school-based interventions, the role of community and family engagement in supporting student mental health cannot be overstated. Schools that actively involve parents and caregivers in the educational process tend to create more inclusive and supportive environments. This engagement can take various forms, including parent-teacher meetings, mental health awareness programs for families, and opportunities for parents to participate in school activities.

Involving parents and caregivers helps enhance students' sense of belonging and supports their overall well-being. Research indicates that students who feel supported by their families and communities are more likely to succeed academically and exhibit positive social behaviors (Epstein & Sheldon, 2002). Family engagement initiatives can include regular communication between schools and families, parent education workshops on child development and mental health, and community-building events that foster strong relationships among students, parents, and school staff (Alinsunurin, 2020; Wang & Degol, 2016).

Creating inclusive and supportive environments involves recognizing and addressing the diverse needs of the student population. Schools can achieve this by implementing policies that promote equity and inclusion, such as anti-bullying programs, cultural competency training for staff, and support groups for marginalized students. By fostering an environment where all students feel valued and included, schools can better support the mental health and well-being of their entire student body (Cappella et al., 2012).

Recent global events, such as the COVID-19 pandemic, have underscored the need for flexible and responsive approaches to mental health in education. Schools have had to adapt to new stressors and find innovative ways to support students and staff. This adaptation has included offering virtual mental health services, creating more adaptable learning environments, and providing additional accommodations for those affected by global crises (UNICEF, 2022; Stanford Teaching Commons, n.d.). Concurrently, the integration of digital technologies to support mental health and well-being is a growing trend. Online platforms and apps for mindfulness, social-emotional learning (SEL), and mental health support are becoming more prevalent. These tools provide accessible resources for students and teachers, extending support beyond the classroom and enhancing the overall educational experience (CDC, 2022). By leveraging technology and adapting to global challenges, schools can create resilient and supportive environments that cater to the evolving needs of their communities.

METHODOLOGY

A systematic search was conducted across multiple databases, including PubMed, PsycINFO, ERIC, and Google Scholar, to identify relevant studies published between January 2012 and May 2024. The search terms included combinations of keywords such as "mental health," "schools," "COVID-19," "digital technologies," "virtual mental health services," "social-emotional learning," and "crisis intervention programs." Boolean operators (AND, OR) were used to refine the search results.

INCLUSION AND EXCLUSION CRITERIA

Inclusion Criteria:

1. Studies published in peer-reviewed journals.
2. Studies conducted in educational settings (K-12 and higher education).
3. Studies focusing on mental health support systems, including virtual services and technological interventions.
4. Studies addressing the impact of global challenges, such as the COVID-19 pandemic, on mental health in education.
5. Studies published in English.

Exclusion Criteria:

1. Studies not related to mental health or education.
2. Non-peer-reviewed articles, opinion pieces, and editorials.
3. Studies published in languages other than English.
4. Studies without full-text availability.

Study Selection

The initial search yielded 453 articles. After removing duplicates, 376 articles remained. These articles were screened based on their titles and abstracts, resulting in the exclusion of 308 articles. The full texts of the remaining 68 articles were assessed for eligibility, and 19 studies were selected for inclusion in this review.

Data Extraction

A standardized data extraction form was used to collect relevant information from each study. The extracted data included:

- Study characteristics (authors, year of publication, country).
- Study design and methodology.

- Population characteristics (sample size, age, educational level).
- Types of mental health support systems investigated.
- Key findings and outcomes.

Quality Assessment

The quality of the selected studies was assessed using the Mixed Methods Appraisal Tool (MMAT). This tool allows for the evaluation of various study designs, including qualitative, quantitative, and mixed-methods studies. Each study was rated based on criteria such as clarity of research questions, appropriateness of the study design, data collection methods, and robustness of the findings.

RESULTS

This systematic review includes findings from 19 studies that examined various aspects of mental health support in educational settings, particularly focusing on the integration of virtual services, digital technologies, and community engagement. Below, each study's key findings and contributions to the overall understanding of mental health support in schools are presented.

Meiklejohn et al. (2012) explored the impact of integrating mindfulness training into K-12 education. The study found that mindfulness interventions significantly improved students' cognitive performance, emotional regulation, and overall well-being, highlighting the importance of such programs in enhancing student mental health.

Patton & Parker (2017) examined teacher education communities of practice and their role in promoting social and emotional learning (SEL). The study concluded that collaborative professional development fosters teacher resilience and better classroom management, which indirectly supports student mental health.

Zenner, Herrnleben-Kurz, & Walach (2014) conducted a meta-analysis on mindfulness-based interventions in schools. Their results indicated that these programs are effective in reducing stress and improving emotional well-being among students, supporting the inclusion of mindfulness practices in school curricula.

Roeser et al. (2013) studied the effects of mindfulness training on teachers' professional development. They found that mindfulness practices reduced teacher stress and burnout, improved job satisfaction, and enhanced classroom interactions, benefiting both teachers and students.

Jennings et al. (2017) evaluated the CARE program, which aims to cultivate awareness and resilience in educators. The study showed that teachers who participated in the program experienced lower levels of burnout and higher levels of emotional regulation, leading to more positive classroom environments.

Wang & Degol (2016) reviewed the concept of school climate and its impact on student outcomes. The study emphasized that a positive school climate, which includes strong mental health support, is associated with better academic performance and social-emotional development in students.

Alinsunurin (2020) investigated the role of parental involvement and school leadership in creating inclusive learning climates. The findings highlighted that active family engagement enhances students' sense of belonging and mental well-being, stressing the importance of community involvement in educational settings.

Stanford Teaching Commons (2022) provided strategies for promoting mental health and well-being in learning environments. The resource emphasized the importance of building a community of care, fostering open communication, and providing personal sharing opportunities to support student mental health.

CDC (2022) offered an action guide for promoting mental health in schools, outlining strategies such as integrating mental health education into the curriculum, providing access to counseling services, and implementing crisis intervention programs. These recommendations were found to be effective in creating supportive school environments.

UNICEF (2022) discussed the impact of global crises, such as the COVID-19 pandemic, on student mental health. The study highlighted the need for flexible and responsive mental health strategies, including virtual mental health services and adaptable learning environments, to support students during challenging times.

Reback (2010) examined the impact of school-based mental health services on young children's emotional and behavioral outcomes. The study found that schools with robust mental health support systems experienced fewer behavioral issues and better emotional regulation among students.

Epstein & Sheldon (2002) explored the relationship between family involvement and student attendance. The study concluded that schools that actively engage families see improved student attendance and reduced absenteeism, indicating the positive effects of family engagement on student well-being.

Brock et al. (2009) presented the PREPaRE model for school crisis intervention. The model provided a comprehensive framework for responding to mental health crises in schools, emphasizing the importance of preparedness and coordinated response efforts.

Cappella et al. (2012) investigated the role of peer relationships and social networks in student engagement. The study found that positive peer interactions and equitable social networks contribute to better behavioral and academic outcomes, underscoring the importance of social support in schools.

Jones & Bouffard (2012) reviewed strategies for integrating SEL into school curricula. The study highlighted the benefits of SEL programs in improving students' emotional intelligence, resilience, and interpersonal skills, advocating for their inclusion in daily classroom activities.

Shernoff et al. (2016) examined the concept of flow in high school classrooms. The study demonstrated that creating challenging yet achievable tasks, providing immediate feedback, and allowing student autonomy can facilitate flow, leading to deeper learning and greater student satisfaction.

Zinsser (2015) focused on promoting positive classroom climates through SEL. The study emphasized that SEL programs enhance students' social skills, reduce behavioral problems, and improve academic performance, making a strong case for their integration into educational settings.

Brackett & Rivers (2014) explored the transformative potential of SEL in schools. The study found that SEL programs not only improve students' emotional and social skills but also create more positive and supportive school environments.

Elias et al. (1997) provided guidelines for promoting social and emotional learning in schools. The study highlighted the long-term benefits of SEL programs, including improved academic performance, better emotional regulation, and reduced dropout rates.

DISCUSSION

The findings from this systematic review underscore the critical importance of integrating robust mental health support systems in educational settings. The reviewed studies highlight the efficacy of various strategies, including virtual mental health services, digital technologies, social-emotional learning (SEL) programs, and strong community and family engagement, in promoting mental well-being among students and educators.

The rapid adoption of virtual mental health services, prompted by the COVID-19 pandemic, has demonstrated significant benefits. Studies such as those by the CDC (2022) and UNICEF (2022) indicate that virtual services, including teletherapy and online counseling, have effectively bridged the gap in mental health care during times of crisis. These services provide continuous support, reduce anxiety, and improve access to mental health resources, particularly when in-person interactions are limited. This aligns with findings by Zenner, Herrnleben-Kurz, and Walach (2014), who noted that digital mindfulness interventions can significantly reduce stress and enhance emotional well-being among students.

Digital technologies, such as mindfulness apps and SEL platforms, offer scalable and accessible solutions that complement traditional mental health services. Roeser et al. (2013) and Meiklejohn et al. (2012) highlighted the benefits of integrating mindfulness practices into daily routines, which can improve focus, emotional regulation, and overall well-being. The synergy between these digital interventions and traditional support systems creates a comprehensive approach to mental health in schools. This dual approach allows for continuous and flexible mental health support that can adapt to varying needs and circumstances, providing a robust safety net for students and educators alike.

Moreover, the integration of digital tools has proven to be an inclusive strategy, reaching students who may have otherwise been reluctant to seek in-person counseling. According to a study by Lyon et al. (2020), the use of technology in mental health care not only enhances accessibility but also personalizes the support, catering to individual needs more effectively. This personalized approach is crucial in addressing the diverse mental health needs within a student population, ensuring that all students receive appropriate care.

The integration of SEL into the curriculum is supported by numerous studies, including those by Patton and Parker (2017) and Jones and Bouffard (2012). SEL programs aim to develop students' emotional intelligence, resilience, and interpersonal skills, which are crucial for their academic and personal success. The meta-analysis by Durlak et al. (2011) provides robust evidence that SEL programs lead to improved social behaviors, reduced emotional distress, and enhanced academic performance.

SEL programs not only benefit students but also enhance the overall school climate. Jennings et al. (2017) found that teachers trained in SEL report lower levels of burnout and better classroom management, which positively impacts student outcomes. This holistic approach to education, where both students and teachers are supported, creates a nurturing environment conducive to learning and personal growth. Furthermore, a study by Taylor et al. (2017) found that SEL programs have long-term benefits, including higher graduation rates and better mental health outcomes in adulthood. This indicates that SEL programs not only address immediate educational needs but also contribute to the long-term well-being of students.

The implementation of SEL programs requires a whole-school approach, involving all stakeholders, including administrators, teachers, students, and parents. According to Weissberg et al. (2015), successful SEL integration involves ongoing professional development for educators, curriculum adjustments to include SEL components, and active involvement from families and the community. This comprehensive approach ensures that SEL becomes an integral part of the school culture, rather than a standalone initiative.

The role of community and family engagement in supporting student mental health is emphasized in studies by Alinsunurin (2020) and Wang and Degol (2016). Schools that actively involve parents and caregivers create more inclusive and supportive environments. This engagement helps students feel valued and connected, enhancing their sense of belonging and overall well-being. Epstein and Sheldon (2002) highlighted that family involvement is associated with improved student attendance and reduced absenteeism, further underscoring its importance.

Engaging families and communities in the educational process ensures that mental health support extends beyond the school environment. This holistic approach, which includes home and community settings, provides a consistent support system for students. According to a study by Sheridan et al. (2019), family engagement programs that include mental health education and resources for parents lead to better student outcomes, including improved academic performance and reduced behavioral issues.

Furthermore, community partnerships can enhance the resources available to schools. For example, collaborations with local mental health organizations can provide additional support services, professional development for educators, and resources for families. This collaborative approach not only expands the support network for students but also fosters a community-wide commitment to mental health and well-being.

Global challenges, such as the COVID-19 pandemic, have highlighted the need for flexible and responsive mental health strategies in education. Schools have had to innovate rapidly to provide support during these times. The findings by UNICEF (2022) and Stanford Teaching Commons (n.d.) illustrate how schools have adapted by offering virtual mental health services, creating more adaptable learning environments, and providing additional accommodations for those affected by crises.

The integration of these strategies has proven effective in mitigating the negative impacts of global challenges on student mental health. The evidence suggests that such adaptability is crucial for maintaining student well-being during times of uncertainty. For instance, during the COVID-19 pandemic, schools that quickly implemented virtual counseling and mental health services were able to provide continuous support to students, reducing the psychological impact of the pandemic (Holmes et al., 2020).

Moreover, the flexibility of these approaches allows schools to respond to various crises, not just pandemics. For example, schools in areas affected by natural disasters, political instability, or economic hardships can utilize virtual and adaptable mental health strategies to support their students. This resilience in the face of global challenges ensures that students' mental health needs are met, regardless of external circumstances.

CONCLUSIONS

The systematic review highlights several areas for future research and practice. It seems that, there is a need for longitudinal studies to examine the long-term impacts of virtual mental health services and digital technologies on student well-being. Second, research should explore the best practices for integrating SEL programs into various educational contexts, considering the diverse needs of students. Third, the role of community and family engagement in mental health support should be further investigated to identify effective strategies for fostering strong partnerships between schools and families. The integration of robust mental health support systems in educational settings is crucial for promoting the well-being of both students and educators. This systematic review has highlighted several effective strategies, including virtual mental health services, digital technologies, social-emotional learning (SEL) programs, and strong community and family engagement. Each of these approaches contributes uniquely to creating a supportive and inclusive educational environment. The adoption of virtual mental health services has proven particularly effective during the COVID-19 pandemic, demonstrating the ability to provide continuous support, reduce anxiety, and improve access to mental health resources. Digital technologies, such as mindfulness apps and SEL platforms, offer scalable and accessible solutions that complement traditional mental health services, enhancing focus, emotional regulation, and overall well-being. These findings underscore the importance of integrating digital tools into mental health strategies to address diverse student needs effectively. The integration of SEL into school curricula is supported by robust evidence indicating improved social behaviors, reduced emotional distress, and enhanced academic performance. SEL programs benefit not only students but also teachers by reducing burnout and improving classroom management, thereby creating a nurturing environment conducive to learning and personal growth. This holistic approach to education is essential for fostering resilient and emotionally intelligent students who are well-prepared for future challenges. Active involvement of parents and caregivers plays a critical role in supporting student mental health. Schools that foster strong family and community partnerships create more inclusive and supportive environments, enhancing students' sense of belonging and overall well-being. Family engagement is associated with improved student attendance and reduced absenteeism, highlighting its importance in comprehensive mental health strategies. Global challenges, such as the COVID-19 pandemic, have underscored the need for flexible and responsive mental health strategies in education. Schools have successfully adapted by implementing virtual mental health services, creating adaptable learning environments, and providing additional accommodations for those affected by crises. These adaptations are critical for maintaining student well-being during times of uncertainty, ensuring that mental health support is resilient and responsive to changing circumstances.

REFERENCES

Alinsunurin, J. (2020). School learning climate in the lens of parental involvement and school leadership: lessons for inclusiveness among public schools. *Smart Learning Environments, 7*(25). https://doi.org/.DOI: 10.1186/s40561-020-00139-2

Argyriadi, A., & Argyriadis, A. (2022). Recommended Interventions for the Promotion of Language Development for Children With Learning Difficulties. In *Rethinking Inclusion and Transformation in Special Education* (pp. 143–159). IGI Global. DOI: 10.4018/978-1-6684-4680-5.ch009

Argyriadis, A., Efthymiou, E., & Argyriadis, A. (2023). Cultural Competence at Schools: The Effectiveness of Educational Leaders' Intervention Strategies. In *Inclusive Phygital Learning Approaches and Strategies for Students With Special Needs* (pp. 33-51). IGI Global.

Argyriadis, A., Ioannidou, L., Dimitrakopoulos, I., Gourni, M., Ntimeri, G., Vlachou, C., & Argyriadi, A. (2023, March). Experimental mindfulness intervention in an emergency department for stress management and development of positive working environment. [). MDPI.]. *Health Care*, 11(6), 879. PMID: 36981535

Argyriadis, A., Paoullis, P., Samsari, E., & Argyriadi, A. (2023). Self-Assessment Inclusion Scale (SAIS): A tool for measuring inclusive competence and sensitivity. *Perspectives in Education*, 41(4), 34–49. DOI: 10.38140/pie.v41i4.7294

Benson, P. L., Scales, P. C., & Syvertsen, A. K. (2011). The contribution of the developmental assets framework to positive youth development theory and practice. *Advances in Child Development and Behavior*, 41, 197–230. DOI: 10.1016/B978-0-12-386492-5.00008-7 PMID: 23259193

Biddle, S. J., & Asare, M. (2011). Physical activity and mental health in children and adolescents: A review of reviews. *British Journal of Sports Medicine*, 45(11), 886–895. DOI: 10.1136/bjsports-2011-090185 PMID: 21807669

Brackett, M. A., & Rivers, S. E. (2014). Transforming students' lives with social and emotional learning. In Pekrun, R., & Linnenbrink-Garcia, L. (Eds.), *International Handbook of Emotions in Education* (pp. 368–388). Routledge.

Brock, S. E., Nickerson, A. B., Reeves, M. A., Jimerson, S. R., Lieberman, R., & Feinberg, T. (2009). *School crisis prevention and intervention: The PREPaRE model.* National Association of School Psychologists.

Brown, J. L., Jennings, P. A., Rasheed, D. S., Cham, H., Doyle, S. L., & Frank, J. L. (2023). Direct and moderating impacts of the CARE mindfulness-based professional learning program for teachers on children's academic and social-emotional outcomes. *Applied Developmental Science, 25*(1-20). DOI: 10.1080/10888691.2023.2268327

Cappella, E., Kim, H. Y., Neal, J. W., & Jackson, D. R. (2012). Classroom peer relationships and behavioral engagement in elementary school: The role of social network equity. *American Journal of Community Psychology*, 50(1-2), 70–88. DOI: 10.1007/s10464-011-9485-2 PMID: 24081319

CDC. (2022). Promoting and protecting mental health in schools and learning environments. Retrieved from https://www.cdc.gov/healthyyouth/mental-health-action -guide/pdf/DASH_MH_Action_Guide_508.pdf

Csikszentmihalyi, M. (1990). *Flow: The Psychology of Optimal Experience*. Harper & Row.

Deci, E. L., & Ryan, R. M. (2012). Self-determination theory. Handbook of theories of social psychology, 1(20), 416-436.

Durlak, J. A., Weissberg, R. P., Dymnicki, A. B., Taylor, R. D., & Schellinger, K. B. (2011). The impact of enhancing students' social and emotional learning: A meta-analysis of school-based universal interventions. Child development, 82(1), 405-432.Elias, M. J., Zins, J. E., Weissberg, R. P., Frey, K. S., Greenberg, M. T., Haynes, N. M., ... & Shriver, T. P. (1997). Promoting social and emotional learning: Guidelines for educators. ASCD.

Epstein, J. L., & Sheldon, S. B. (2002). Present and accounted for: Improving student attendance through family and community involvement. *The Journal of Educational Research*, 95(5), 308–318. DOI: 10.1080/00220670209596604

Gimbert, B. G., Miller, D., Herman, E., Breedlove, M., & Molina, C. E. (2021). Social emotional learning in schools: the importance of educator competence. *Journal of Research in Leadership Education, 18*(3-39). https://doi.org/DOI: 10.1177/19427751211014920

Hattie, J. (2009). The black box of tertiary assessment: An impending revolution. Tertiary assessment & higher education student outcomes: Policy, practice & research, 259, 275.

Horn, I. S., & Little, J. W. (2010). Attending to problems of practice: routines and resources for professional learning in teachers' workplace interactions. *American Educational Research Journal, 47*(181-217). https://doi.org/DOI: 10.3102/0002831209345158

Janssen, I., & LeBlanc, A. G. (2010). Systematic review of the health benefits of physical activity and fitness in school-aged children and youth. *The International Journal of Behavioral Nutrition and Physical Activity*, 7(1), 1–16. DOI: 10.1186/1479-5868-7-40 PMID: 20459784

Jennings, P. A., Brown, J. L., Frank, J. L., Doyle, S., Oh, Y., & Davis, R. (2017). Impacts of the CARE for Teachers program on teachers' social and emotional competence and classroom interactions. *Journal of Educational Psychology, 109*(1010-1028). DOI: 10.1037/edu0000187

Jones, S. M., & Bouffard, S. M. (2012). Social and emotional learning in schools: From programs to strategies. *Social Policy Report*, 26(4), 3–22. DOI: 10.1002/j.2379-3988.2012.tb00073.x

Meiklejohn, J., Phillips, C., Freedman, M. L., Griffin, M. L., Biegel, G., Roach, A., Frank, J., Burke, C., Pinger, L., Soloway, G., Isberg, R., Sibinga, E., Grossman, L., & Saltzman, A. (2012). Integrating mindfulness training into K-12 education: Fostering the resilience of teachers and students. *Mindfulness*, 3(4), 291–307. DOI: 10.1007/s12671-012-0094-5

Nakamura, J., & Csikszentmihalyi, M. (2014). *Flow and the Foundations of Positive Psychology: The Collected Works of Mihaly Csikszentmihalyi.* Springer.

Oberle, E., Guhn, M., Gadermann, A. M., Thomson, K., & Schonert-Reichl, K. A. (2018). Positive mental health and supportive school environments: A population-level longitudinal study of dispositional optimism and school relationships in early adolescence. *Social Science & Medicine*, 214, 154–161. DOI: 10.1016/j.socscimed.2018.06.041 PMID: 30072159

Pargament, K. I. (2011). *Spiritually integrated psychotherapy: Understanding and addressing the sacred.* Guilford press.

Patton, K., & Parker, M. (2017). Teacher education communities of practice: more than a culture of collaboration. *Teaching and Teacher Education, 67*(351-360). https://doi.org/DOI: 10.1016/j.tate.2017.06.013

Pianta, R. C., Hamre, B. K., & Allen, J. P. (2012). Teacher-student relationships and engagement: Conceptualizing, measuring, and improving the capacity of class-room interactions. In *Handbook of research on student engagement* (pp. 365–386). Springer US. DOI: 10.1007/978-1-4614-2018-7_17

Reback, R. (2010). Schools' mental health services and young children's emotions, behavior, and learning. *Journal of Policy Analysis and Management*, 29(4), 698–725. DOI: 10.1002/pam.20528 PMID: 20964104

Rimm-Kaufman, S. E., & Hulleman, C. S. (2015). Social and emotional learning in elementary school settings: Identifying mechanisms that matter. Handbook of social and emotional learning: Research and practice, 151-166.

Roeser, R. W., Skinner, E., Beers, J., & Jennings, P. A. (2013). Mindfulness training and teachers' professional development: An emerging area of research and practice. *Child Development Perspectives*, 6(2), 167–173. DOI: 10.1111/j.1750-8606.2012.00238.x

Shernoff, D. J., Kelly, S., Tonks, S. M., Anderson, B., Cavanagh, R. F., Sinha, S., & Abdi, B. (2016). Student engagement as a function of environmental complexity in high school classrooms. *Learning and Instruction*, 43, 52–60. DOI: 10.1016/j.learninstruc.2015.12.003

UNICEF. (2022). Promoting and protecting mental health in schools and learning environments. Retrieved from https://www.unicef.org/media/126821/file/Promoting %20and%20protecting%20mental%20health%20in%20schools%20and%20learning %20environments.pdf

UNICEF. (2022). Promoting and Protecting Mental Health in Schools and Learning Environments. Retrieved from https://www.unicef.org/media/126821/file/Promoting %20and%20protecting%20mental%20health%20in%20schools%20and%20learning %20environments.pdf

Wang, M. T., & Degol, J. L. (2016). School climate: A review of the construct, measurement, and impact on student outcomes. *Educational Psychology Review*, 28(2), 315–352. DOI: 10.1007/s10648-015-9319-1

Weiss, H. B., Lopez, M. E., & Caspe, M. (2018). *Joining Together to Create a Bold Vision for Next Generation Family Engagement: Engaging Families to Transform Education*. Global Family Research Project.

Wentzel, K. R., & Muenks, K. (2016). Peer influence on students' motivation, academic achievement, and social behavior. In *Handbook of social influences in school contexts* (pp. 13–30). Routledge. DOI: 10.4324/9781315769929

Winner, E., Goldstein, T. R., & Vincent-Lancrin, S. (2013). Art for art's sake. The impact of arts education. doi, 10.

Zenner, C., Herrnleben-Kurz, S., & Walach, H. (2014). Mindfulness-based interventions in schools—A systematic review and meta-analysis. *Frontiers in Psychology*, 5, 603. DOI: 10.3389/fpsyg.2014.00603 PMID: 25071620

Zinsser, K. M. (2015). Promoting positive classroom climates: What can we learn from the research on social and emotional learning? *Psychology in the Schools*, 52(2), 2–20. DOI: 10.1002/pits.21829

Chapter 7
Mindfulness in Education

Glykeria Reppa
https://orcid.org/0000-0003-0483-1533
Neapolis University, Pafos, Cyprus

Katerina Michael
https://orcid.org/0000-0002-5737-0964
Frederick University, Cyprus

ABSTRACT

In recent years there has been an increasing amount of research on the practice of mindfulness in education. There are several studies that examine the practice of mindfulness and its effectiveness in various aspects of the lives of both students and teachers. The purpose of the chapter is to mention the different practices that have already been implemented in different educational levels, either in pupils/ students or teachers/ tutors and their effectiveness in different aspects of their lives, through literature. It is also discussed mindfulness as a quite promising practice, which is likely to be a pedagogical practice that serves educational purposes that have long been part of the tradition of education.

INTRODUCTION

Mindfulness, a concept rooted in ancient meditation practices, particularly within Buddhist traditions, has found a significant place in contemporary psychology and education. Mindfulness is defined as the awareness that arises from paying attention, on purpose, in the present moment, and non-judgmentally (Kabat- Zinn, 2013). The concept of mindfulness is defined as the awareness that comes from being fully present and aware in the moment, analyzing each moment as it happens. Regularly engaging in mindfulness practices such as meditation and other practices helps de-

DOI: 10.4018/979-8-3693-5325-7.ch007

velop a heightened state of conscious awareness. This state of awareness is believed to be evident in a person's internal cognitive and emotional experiences, as well as in their interpersonal interactions, which include skills such as active listening, understanding, and conflict management (Burgoon et al. 2000; Frank et al. 2016).

Mindfulness has been extensively studied and adapted for various contexts, including educational settings. Its relevance in education is underscored by the growing recognition of the importance of mental health and emotional well-being in fostering academic and personal success among students and educators alike.

Mindful Schools (2018) described a mindfulness timeline that moves through healthcare, mental health and education. In 1979, Dr. Jon Kabat-Zinn developed Mindfulness Based Stress Reduction (MBSR) project; in 1992, Mindfulness Based Cognitive Therapy (MBCT) was developed. In the early 2000s, the first round of formal teacher training for mindfulness interventions in education included self-care, resilience, wellness, and how to train students in mindfulness techniques, was developed. In 2004, the MBCT was endorsed by the UK's National Institute for Health and Clinical Excellence. In 2007, the inaugural classroom mindfulness school program was launched. In 2010, more serious research projects were initiated, including the publication of the first meta-analysis of mindfulness in education.

In this chapter the theoretical foundations of mindfulness are discussed. More-over, there is presentation of the most popular protocols of mindfulness in school and the scientific evidence of their effect on cognitive, emotional, social skills and well-being of students and teachers. On the other hand, there are discussed the limitations and the challenges that teachers must face to introduce mindfulness on their classroom. At the end there are some future directions for applying such programs in the school environment.

Theoretical Foundations of Mindfulness

The concept of mindfulness originates from Eastern spiritual practices, notably Buddhism, where it is a core component of meditation practices aimed at achieving enlightenment and reducing suffering. In the late 20th century, mindfulness was introduced to the Western world primarily through the work of Jon Kabat-Zinn, who developed the Mindfulness-Based Stress Reduction (MBSR) program. This secular adaptation retained the essence of mindfulness—present-moment awareness and acceptance—while making it accessible to a broader audience.

Key concepts within mindfulness include attention, intention, and attitude. Attention refers to the focus on present-moment experiences, intention involves the purposefulness of directing attention, and attitude encompasses the qualities of curiosity, openness, and acceptance. These principles form the basis of mindfulness practices and interventions used in educational settings.

The practice of mindfulness usually involves focusing on the sense of breath and maintaining that focus. However, an untrained mind often wanders, forgetting the object of attention and the intention to practice. When this happens, the practitioner is encouraged to cultivate an attitude of acceptance, characterized by non-judgmentalism, non-anxiety, compassion and kindness. The practitioner then restores his or her intention to practice mindfulness. If the instructions lack any of these elements, it is not considered mindfulness. There are various forms of mindfulness practice suitable for different ages and populations. Unlike reflection, mindfulness focuses on experiencing the present moment as it is, without interpretation or intentional meaning-making.

In beginning the journey of mindfulness, the individual first explores the self (physical, mental and emotional) and then others and the environment (Reppa, 2021). Below are described the 5 areas of the individual's training where mindfulness can act, to enable the individual to reach a stage of self-realization and live mindfully.

Physical training: Physical training helps us to awaken our senses to gain a sense of wonder and connection with our bodies and the natural world (Rechtschaffen, 2016; Reppa, 2021). Physical training in mindfulness involves engaging the body in practices such as body scan meditation, mindful movement, yoga and breath awareness etc. Such practices can enhance body awareness, which can lead to better self-care and health outcomes by helping individuals recognize physical signs of stress and tension early, improve physical health and promote relaxation.

Mental training: Once the person achieves the physical regulation and is present, he/ she can cultivate his/ her attention. Mental training in mindfulness involves cultivating attention and focus. This practice is crucial for enhancing cognitive functions and improving academic performance. During cultivating the attention there may be distraction from another thought, the purpose of mindfulness practice is to bring the person's attention back to the focus point without judging what has happened (Rechtschaffen, 2016; Reppa, 2021). By learning to return attention to a focal point without judgment, individuals can improve their concentration and reduce the impact of distracting thoughts. Moreover, cultivating non-judgmental awareness attitude helps reduce stress and promotes psychological resilience.

Emotional training: Once a person learns the "language" of the senses and the mind, he can combine them and learn the "language" of the heart. Emotional training involves learning to recognize and regulate emotions. Thus, the person can identify unhealthy thoughts and thought patterns and learn to uncover the emotions that lie beneath those thoughts. By discovering the person's emotional state, the person can be emotionally regulated, which leads to better mental health and social relationships. The person can cultivate his/her positive emotions, such as empathy, gratitude, and love. On the other hand, he/she learns not to suppress his/her negative emotions, such as anger, hopelessness or anxiety, but learns to be open and compassionately aware of the whole range of emotions (Rechtschaffen, 2016; Reppa, 2021).

Social training: Following one's discovery of inner peace and tranquilly and one's ability to live in the present, he/she can use his/her interpersonal relationships to set a positive example for others by living fully in each moment and communicating in a more meaningful and effective way (Rechtschaffen, 2016; Reppa, 2021). Thus, social training through mindfulness involves using interpersonal relationships to set positive examples and communicate more effectively. This aspect emphasizes the importance of empathy and presence in social interactions. Mindfulness can enhance listening skills and empathy, leading to more meaningful and effective communication. Moreover, mindful individuals can serve as role models, promoting a culture of presence and compassion in their communities.

Global training: By being aware and living mindfully, the individual can understand the interconnectedness of all things and how the actions of each can affect the whole. Also, the individual can discern how the environment itself can affect his mood and state of mind ((Rechtschaffen, 2016; Reppa, 2021). Therefore, Global training emphasizes the interconnectedness of all things and the impact of individual actions on the broader environment. This fosters a sense of global responsibility and awareness. Mindfulness can heighten awareness of environmental issues and promote sustainable practices. Furthermore, understanding the interconnectedness of all things can foster a sense of compassion and responsibility toward others and the planet.

The Four Assumptions of Mindfulness Theory

Mindfulness theory posits that practicing mindfulness involves embracing and operating based on four core assumptions: impermanence, non-attachment, non-self-determination, and acceptance. These assumptions form the foundation of mindfulness practice and help individuals develop a deeper understanding of themselves and their experiences (Reppa, 2021).

Impermanence: Impermanence, or anicca in Buddhist terminology, refers to the understanding that all phenomena are transient and constantly changing. This includes thoughts, emotions, physical sensations, and external circumstances. It is the nature of things to be born and pass away. If one observes nature, he will see how the world is made like this, everything is born (spring) and leaves (winter). So, it is in all things (thoughts, feelings, situations). The person suffers when they forget this assumption (Bien, 2006; Kabat-Zinn, 2013). Usually when the person experiences something that is unpleasant, they react as if it is not going to end. Practicing mindfulness with an awareness of impermanence encourages individuals to observe their experiences without clinging to them, knowing that they are temporary.

This perspective helps reduce the intensity of negative emotions and the fixation on positive ones. Recognizing the fleeting nature of emotions can help individuals manage stress and anxiety, knowing that these feelings will pass. Understanding impermanence can foster resilience, as individuals learn to navigate the ups and downs of life with greater ease and adaptability. Studies suggest that mindfulness practices emphasizing impermanence can lead to reduced emotional reactivity and increased psychological flexibility (Kabat-Zinn, 2016). This approach helps individuals better cope with life's challenges and maintain a balanced perspective.

Non-attachment: Non-attachment is the process in which one does not attach to thoughts, feelings, sensations, people, things, etc. According to Cook-Cottone (2015) a spiritual event is undoubtedly associated with an emotional tone, which can be positive, neutral or negative. The individual by nature is more attracted to positive and pleasant tones and avoids negative or aversive tones. Mindfulness practices that cultivate non-attachment encourage individuals to experience life fully without being overly invested in specific outcomes. This helps in reducing suffering caused by unfulfilled desires and unmet expectations. Non-attachment helps maintain emotional equilibrium by reducing the tendency to react strongly to positive or negative experiences. By not clinging to particular thoughts or outcomes, individuals can achieve greater mental clarity and focus. Non-attachment has been linked to greater emotional well-being and reduced symptoms of depression and anxiety (Sahdra, Shaver, & Brown, 2010). This mindset allows individuals to approach life with greater equanimity and acceptance.

Non-self-determination: Non-self-determination, or anatta, refers to the understanding that the self is not a fixed, independent entity but is instead an ever-changing process influenced by various factors (Shapiro & Carlson, 2009). This concept challenges the notion of a permanent, unchanging self. More specifically this admission has to do with not defining oneself in a sense, for example people who suffer from anorexia nervosa often define themselves as "I am anorexic", so they do not see their problem or difficulty or illness as something outside of them but rather as something that characterizes their 'being' and their sense of 'self'. Mindfulness practices that emphasize non-self-determination encourage individuals to see beyond their ego-driven identities and recognize the interconnectedness of all beings. This perspective can lead to a more compassionate and less self-centered way of living. So, understanding the fluid nature of the self can reduce behaviors driven by ego and selfishness. Moreover, recognizing the interconnectedness of all life forms fosters greater empathy and compassion for others. Studies have shown that embracing the concept of non-self-determination has been associated with lower levels of ego involvement and increased prosocial behavior (Dambrun & Ricard, 2011). This shift in perspective can lead to more harmonious relationships and a greater sense of community.

Acceptance: Acceptance acknowledgement is the process by which a person allows events to occur. In other words, involves fully acknowledging and embracing the present moment as it is, without resistance or judgment. It means seeing things clearly and responding to them appropriately rather than through the lens of personal biases and preferences. For instance, when he gets furious, he recognizes that he feels angry, investigates it curiously, and accepts that he is experiencing that specific emotion right now without pushing back or acting on it. He just takes it and considers it with an open heart and head. Mindfulness practices that focus on acceptance help individuals face their experiences with openness and curiosity, rather than avoidance or denial. This attitude fosters a sense of peace and equanimity. So, by accepting experiences as they come, individuals can cultivate a greater sense of inner peace and contentment. Acceptance-based mindfulness practices have been shown to improve psychological well-being and reduce symptoms of various mental health conditions, including anxiety, depression, and PTSD (Hayes, Strosahl, & Wilson, 2012). Acceptance allows individuals to live more fully in the present moment, enhancing overall life satisfaction.

According to mindfulness theory, practicing the paths of mindfulness with the four core assumptions of impermanence, non-attachment, non-self-determination, and acceptance can profoundly transform how individuals experience and navigate life. These assumptions help cultivate a deeper awareness and understanding of the nature of reality, leading to enhanced cognitive, emotional, and social well-being. As research continues to explore these foundational principles, the potential of mindfulness to foster resilience, compassion, and overall mental health becomes increasingly evident.

Mindfulness and Cognitive Processes

Mindfulness has a profound impact on various cognitive processes crucial for learning and development. This analysis focuses on three key areas: attention and concentration, emotional regulation, and self-awareness and meta-cognition. Mindfulness practice enhances students' ability to sustain attention and concentrate on tasks. By training the mind to focus on the present moment, mindfulness helps reduce distractions and improve cognitive control, which are common issues affecting students' academic performance. As that concerns emotional regulation, mindfulness facilitates better emotional regulation by increasing awareness of emotions and promoting a non-reactive stance towards them. This ability to observe emotions without being overwhelmed by them is crucial for students in managing stress and anxiety. By becoming more aware of their emotional states and develop healthier responses to negative emotions, students could increase their emotional regulation and overall well-being. However, the effectiveness of mindfulness practices in emotional regulation can vary significantly among individuals, depending on their baseline emotional state and personality traits. Furthermore, mindfulness enhances self-awareness by encouraging reflection on one's thoughts, feelings, and behaviors. By fostering greater self-awareness, mindfulness helps students gain insights into their behaviors and thought patterns, leading to improved self-regulation and decision-making. This meta-cognitive awareness enables students to understand their learning processes and adopt strategies that enhance their academic performance. Yet, achieving a deep level of self-awareness and meta-cognition requires consistent practice and can be difficult to maintain without ongoing support. The impact of mindfulness on self-awareness and meta-cognition can vary based on individual differences in cognitive styles and baseline self-awareness levels, as well.

Research Evidence on Mindfulness in Education

The growing body of research on mindfulness in education highlights its positive impacts on various aspects of student and teacher well-being and performance. Over the past decade, numerous studies have explored how mindfulness practices can be effectively integrated into educational settings, providing robust evidence of their benefits.

1. **Academic Performance**: Studies have shown that mindfulness practices can improve students' academic performance by enhancing attention, memory, and executive functioning. For instance, a study by Schonert-Reichl and Lawlor (2010) found that a mindfulness-based program led to improvements in cognitive and socio-emotional outcomes among elementary school students. The findings revealed significant improvements in students' attention, self-control, and overall executive functioning, which are critical for academic success. Moreover, a systematic review and meta-analysis found that such programs significantly enhance students' cognitive performance, including improvements in attention and memory, which are directly linked to better academic outcomes (Zenner, Herrnleben-Kurz, & Walach, 2014). Tang et al., (2012) reviewed the neurobiological mechanisms underlying the improvements in executive function resulting from mindfulness-based interventions. The authors highlight how these cognitive enhancements contribute to better academic performance, emphasizing the long-term benefits of mindfulness practices for students. Moreover, another systematic review covers various studies on mindfulness-based interventions for youth in schools, demonstrating consistent evidence that such practices enhance academic achievement by improving attention, emotional regulation, and resilience (Felver, Celis-de Hoyos, Tezanos, & Singh, 2016).

2. **Mental Health and Well-being**: Mindfulness has been found to reduce symptoms of anxiety, depression, and stress among students and improve social-emotional and prosocial behavior. For example, a meta-analysis by Zoogman et al. (2015) demonstrated that mindfulness interventions significantly reduced psychological distress in youth. The findings indicated significant reductions in symptoms of anxiety, depression, and stress. The study concluded that mindfulness practices are effective in improving overall mental health and well-being in young people. Moreover, Bluth and Eisenlohr-Moul (2017) investigated the impact of a mindfulness intervention on emotional regulation and resilience in teenagers. Participants reported decreased levels of distress and improved coping mechanisms, highlighting the role of mindfulness in enhancing emotional well-being. Furthermore, van de Weijer-Bergsma, et al., (2014) found that a school-based mindfulness program led to significant improvements in students' quality of life and overall mental health. Other studies, also, indicated that school-based mindfulness programs enhanced prosocial behavior and self-regulatory skills (Flook, Goldberg, Pinger, & Davidson, 2015; Reppa, 2017).

3. **Behavioral Improvements**: Mindfulness interventions have been linked to reductions in behavioral problems among students. Studies suggest that mindfulness helps students develop better self-control and manage impulsive behaviors more effectively. For instance, a study by Singh et al. (2013) found that students who participated in mindfulness programs exhibited fewer disruptive behaviors and were more engaged in classroom activities.

4. **Teachers and Classroom Environment**: Mindfulness training for teachers has been shown to reduce burnout, increase resilience, and improve the overall classroom environment. Jennings et al. (2013) found that teachers who participated in a mindfulness program reported lower levels of stress and more positive interactions with students. The same results have been found also from the study of Flook et al. (2013), who found that teachers who engaged in mindfulness training reported lower stress levels, greater emotional well-being, and improved job satisfaction. Another study assessed a school-based yoga and mindfulness intervention for educators. Findings indicated significant increases in resilience and emotional regulation, which contributed to a more positive and supportive classroom environment (Harris, Jennings, Katz, Abenavoli & Greenberg (2016). In the same results concluded research that involved two field trials of mindfulness training for teachers. Teachers reported a more positive classroom environment, characterized by better student-teacher relationships and classroom management. Also, demonstrated reductions in stress and burnout (Roeser, Schonert-Reichl, Jha, A., Cullen, Wallace, Wilensky, & Harrison, J., 2013). In their review, Jennings and Greenberd (2009) highlighted the connection between teachers' social and emotional competence, fostered through mindfulness

training, and positive classroom outcomes. It underscores that teachers' well-being directly influences student behavior, engagement, and academic success. Moreover, incorporating mindfulness into professional development programs for teachers can have long-lasting benefits. By integrating mindfulness training into teacher education, schools can equip educators with the tools to manage stress, enhance their teaching practices, and support their students' well-being. This holistic approach to professional development fosters a more resilient and effective teaching workforce (Meiklejohn et al., 2012).

The evidence of the bibliography suggests that mindfulness in education not only enhances the cognitive, emotional, and social well-being of students but also supports the professional development and well-being of teachers.

Practical Applications in Educational Settings

The quality of research in the field of mindfulness in education is growing exponentially. In fact, in an online article published in Mindful Magazine, researcher Gerzberg (2018) stated that school-based mindfulness programs for K-12 students are becoming increasingly popular, with research on the benefits of mindfulness only in its early stages, and with much more organized study needed. Implementing mindfulness in education involves various programs and strategies designed to suit different age groups and educational contexts:

1. **Mindfulness-based Programs for Students**: Programs such as MindUp, Calm classroom and MBSR for Teens offer structured mindfulness curricula that teach students techniques for improving focus, managing emotions, and fostering a positive outlook. These programs typically include activities like mindful breathing, body scans, and guided visualizations.

MindUp (2018) is a teaching framework and curriculum that contains a 15-lesson curriculum for K-8 students and is taught by the classroom teacher. The program includes four pillars of instruction: neuroscience, positive psychology, mindful awareness, and social emotional learning (SEL).

The 15 lessons focus on topics such as perspective taking, gratitude and awareness, all positive behaviors related to awareness. The program goals were developed to drive positive behavior, increase empathy, compassion and optimism, and improve school performance. MindUp is described as "a universal consciousness-based social and emotional learning (SEL) program designed to be implemented in schools by the regular classroom teacher" (Maloney, Stewart Lawlor, Schonert-Reichl, & Whitehead, 2016). Key elements include a classroom-tested curriculum with provision for ongoing teacher training, universal participation of all students, and tools to create "an optimistic classroom that emphasizes conscious awareness of self and others, embracing differences among peers" (Maloney et al., 2016, p. 315). Each lesson incorporates mindfulness practices that allow students to learn about their minds, understand how thoughts and feelings affect actions, and gain strategies for becoming caring people. The MindUp curriculum was graded for children at various grade levels, identified as developmentally appropriate, and broken into 15-minute portions with provided scripts and teacher worksheets. The manuals include extension activities that can be incorporated into regular classroom lessons in subjects such as science, language arts, and math.

Calm Classroom (2018) is an online and on-site learning platform for mindfulness. The authors of the Calm Classroom website describe the project as a simple and assessable way to integrate mindfulness into classroom culture. The program's designers argue that when teachers and students take short breaks together to re-energize the mind and body, classroom culture can thrive. The Calm Classroom program began in 2008 in Chicago Public Schools and has since been implemented in classrooms around the world. The online academy includes topics such as stress and the brain, mindfulness, the relaxation response, teaching tips, and classroom behavior guidance. The research section of the site offers some interesting statistics about the program. A test group of Calm Classroom students in Grades 3 through 8 showed a 23% decrease in misbehavior, compared to a control group that showed a 21% increase in misbehavior.

Eighty-one percent of teacher participants in a Calm Classroom format reported that students were calmer and more peaceful. Also, 74 percent of teachers reported that students were more focused, and 71 percent reported using Calm Classroom techniques to manage stress outside of the classroom.

The *Mindfulness-Based Reduction program for teens* (MBSR-T) is an 8-week course designed to teach teens mindfulness practices for managing stress, improving quality of life, and finding stillness and resiliency within for when life feels overwhelming[1].The formal practices in MBSR-T include[2]:

- Mindfulness and the Five Senses
- Mindful Eating; Taking a Mindful Bite Practice
- Dropping-In Mindfulness Practice
- Body Scan Mindfulness Practice
- Sitting Mindfulness Practice
- Mindful Walking and Movement
- Yoga and/or Mindful Movement Practice
- Heartfulness Mindfulness Practice

Mindfulness-Based Stress Reduction (MBSR) programs tailored for teens have shown promising results in improving various aspects of mental and emotional well-being. Studies have indicated that MBSR programs can significantly reduce symptoms of anxiety and depression in adolescents (Zoogman, Goldberg, Hoyt, & Miller,2015). Moreover, research has also highlighted improvements in emotional regulation and coping skills among teens who undergo MBSR training (Bluth, & Eisenlohr-Moul, 2017). Another area of benefit is cognitive performance. MBSR programs have been linked to improvements in attention and academic performance (Zoogman, et al., 2015). As the name suggests, MBSR is effective in reducing stress levels (Biegel et al., 2009; Hupper et al., 2010). A study in Psychology in the Schools demonstrated that teens in the MBSR group reported lower perceived stress and an enhanced sense of well-being (Bluth et al., 2017). MBSR also positively affects social relationships. Adolescents who practice mindfulness often report better relationships with peers and family members due to increased empathy and communication skills (Zoogman, et al., 2015; Klingbeil, et al., 2017).

2. **Mindfulness Training for Teachers**: Professional development programs for teachers focus on equipping them with mindfulness skills to enhance their well-being and teaching effectiveness. Programs like CARE (Cultivating Awareness and Resilience in Education) help teachers develop emotional regulation, stress management, and mindful communication skills. According to a study of Jennings, Frank, Snowberg, Coccia, & Greenberg, (2013), teachers who underwent CARE training demonstrated better emotional regulation, which contributed to a more positive classroom environment. Moreover, research found that teachers trained in CARE created more emotionally supportive classrooms, which positively affected student behavior and engagement (Schussler, Jennings, Sharp, & Frank, 2016). Also, by improving teacher well-being and classroom climate, CARE indirectly benefits students. Students in classrooms led by CARE-trained teachers showed better emotional and behavioral outcomes compared to those in classrooms led by non-trained teachers (Jennings, Brown, Frank, Doyle, Oh, Davis, & Greenberg, 2017).

3. **Integration into Curriculum and Daily Routines**: Schools can integrate mindfulness into the curriculum through dedicated mindfulness sessions or by incorporating mindfulness activities into daily routines. Simple practices such as starting the day with a few minutes of mindful breathing or using mindfulness techniques during transitions between activities can create a calmer and more focused learning environment. In the review of Felver, Celis-de Hoyos, Tezanos, & Singh, (2016), various mindfulness-based interventions in school settings are explored, emphasizing the integration of mindfulness into the daily routines and curricula of educational institutions. The study highlights the positive im-

pact on students' emotional regulation, stress reduction, and overall classroom atmosphere. In Burke, (2010) study current research on mindfulness-based approaches for children and adolescents are reviewed and there is a discussion on how dedicated mindfulness sessions and activities integrated into the school curriculum can enhance students' attention, emotional balance, and social skills. Another study showed that practices such incorporating mindfulness techniques during daily transitions and routines can help create a more focused and calm learning environment, benefiting both teachers and students. Moreover, a systematic review and meta-analysis examine the effectiveness of mindfulness-based interventions in schools, including the practice of starting the day with mindful breathing. The results indicate significant improvements in students' attention, self-regulation, and stress levels (Zenner, Herrnleben-Kurz, & Walach, 2014).

Challenges and Limitations

Despite the benefits, there are challenges and limitations to implementing mindfulness in education. These challenges range from practical and logistical issues to broader cultural and systemic obstacles.

1. **Barriers to Implementation**: Lack of time, resources, and training can hinder the adoption of mindfulness practices in schools. Teachers may feel overwhelmed by the additional responsibility of incorporating mindfulness into their already packed schedules. Teachers often struggle to find the necessary time to incorporate mindfulness activities into their already busy schedules (Burke, 2010). A randomized controlled trial found that while mindfulness programs can be beneficial, the additional responsibility of incorporating these practices can overwhelm teachers. The study suggests that without sufficient support and time allocation, teachers might struggle to consistently integrate mindfulness into their daily routines (Sibinga, Webb, Ghazarian, & Ellen, 2016). Moreover, insufficient resources, such as funding for programs, materials, and dedicated staff, pose significant obstacles to widespread adoption (Meiklejohn, Phillips, Freedman, Griffin, Biegel, Roach, & Saltzman, A., 2012). Another challenge is the need for adequate training (Roeser, Skinner, Beers, & Jennings, 2012). In this study the importance of proper training for teachers to effectively implement mindfulness practices, is emphasized. Without adequate professional development and ongoing support, teachers may feel unprepared and reluctant to incorporate mindfulness into their classrooms. Therefore, there is a need for adequate time, resources, training, and systemic support to overcome these challenges.

2. **Cultural and Contextual Considerations**: Mindfulness practices need to be adapted to fit the cultural and contextual needs of diverse student populations. What works in one cultural setting may not be as effective in another, necessitating culturally sensitive approaches (Proulx, 2008). There is a need for culturally adapted mindfulness practices that consider the unique cultural and contextual needs of student populations to maximize their benefits. Smith and Malaney (2016) explored the responses of students from an ethnically diverse urban university to mindfulness practices. The authors highlight the necessity of culturally sensitive approaches, noting that mindfulness programs need to be flexible and inclusive to meet the diverse needs of students from various backgrounds. In the study of Napoli, Krech, & Holley, (2005), the authors suggest that mindfulness programs should be tailored to fit the specific cultural and contextual characteristics of the student population to enhance engagement and effectiveness. Hence, it can be noted the importance of adapting mindfulness practices to align with the cultural and contextual needs of diverse student populations. Culturally sensitive approaches are essential to ensure the relevance, acceptance, and effectiveness of mindfulness programs in educational settings.

3. **Critiques and Counterarguments**: Some critics argue that mindfulness in education can be a form of "band-aid" solution that addresses symptoms rather than underlying systemic issues such as educational inequity and high-stakes testing pressures. Additionally, the secular adaptation of mindfulness may strip it of its deeper philosophical and ethical dimensions. Moreover, assessing the effectiveness of mindfulness programs poses significant challenges. While there is a growing body of research supporting the benefits of mindfulness, measuring outcomes such as emotional regulation, self-awareness, and overall well-being can be complex and subjective. There is no universally accepted method for measuring the impact of mindfulness programs, making it difficult to evaluate their effectiveness consistently. Additionally, maintaining consistent and high-quality implementation of mindfulness programs across different schools and districts can be challenging. Variations in program delivery, teacher training, and institutional support can lead to inconsistent outcomes. There is a need for ensuring that mindfulness programs are delivered consistently and effectively across different schools requires robust support and coordination from educational leaders. Furthermore, long-term studies are needed to assess the sustained impact of mindfulness practices on students and educators, but such research is often expensive and logistically challenging to conduct. Additionally, long-term sustainability of mindfulness programs depends on ongoing funding, training, and institutional commitment, which can be difficult to maintain over time. Another issue is that engaging students in mindfulness practices can vary based on individual differences in interest, motivation, and responsiveness to these

practices. Some students may find it challenging to engage with mindfulness activities, especially if they do not see immediate benefits.

While mindfulness in education holds significant promise, addressing these challenges and limitations is crucial for its successful implementation and sustainability. By investing in teacher training, securing adequate funding, fostering cultural acceptance, and developing robust evaluation methods, schools can overcome these obstacles and harness the full potential of mindfulness practices to enhance the well-being and performance of students and educators alike.

Overcoming Challenges

As was already indicated, there are opportunities and challenges associated with incorporating mindfulness into school curricula in the current educational environment. Mindfulness has become a valuable tool for educators looking for new and creative ways to improve students' academic performance and overall well-being. It helps with focus, emotional control, and general mental health. However, careful preparation, sufficient funding, and a dedication to professional growth are necessary for successfully integrating mindfulness into the current educational frameworks. The next section examines the various strategies required to overcome these obstacles, such as incorporating mindfulness exercises into regular activities, obtaining financing, and giving educators the crucial training they need. By using these techniques, educational institutions can establish a more encouraging and all-encompassing atmosphere that is advantageous to both teachers and students.

Integrating Mindfulness into Existing Curricula

Integrating mindfulness into existing curricula can be achieved through a multifaceted approach that aligns with educational standards and enhances the overall learning environment. One effective strategy is embedding mindfulness practices within daily classroom routines, such as starting the day with a brief mindfulness exercise or incorporating short, guided meditation sessions during transitions between subjects. This could develop the concentration that students should have in every subject.

Schools can develop interdisciplinary lessons that connect mindfulness with core subjects like language arts, science, and social studies, thereby reinforcing the relevance of mindfulness in various contexts. For instance, a science lesson on the human brain could include a module on the benefits of mindfulness for cognitive function and emotional regulation. Moreover, in physical education lessons could include mindful movement and intuitive movement.

Additionally, schools can adopt mindfulness-based programs like MindUp or Inner Explorer, which offer structured, evidence-based curricula designed to fit seamlessly into existing school schedules.

Securing Funding for Mindfulness Programs

Securing funding for mindfulness programs in schools can be challenging but achievable with strategic planning and resourcefulness. One approach is to apply for grants from educational foundations, health organizations, and government agencies that support mental health and wellness initiatives. Schools can also partner with local businesses and community organizations to sponsor mindfulness programs, emphasizing the long-term benefits for student well-being and academic performance. Furthermore, parents' association that many schools have, can funding such programs. By highlighting the positive impact of mindfulness on student outcomes, schools can make a compelling case for financial support from a variety of stakeholders.

Providing Professional Development for Teachers

To effectively implement mindfulness in schools, providing comprehensive professional development for teachers is essential. Professional development programs should include training in mindfulness techniques, classroom management strategies, and ways to integrate mindfulness into daily teaching practices. Workshops, retreats, and online courses offered by organizations and universities in many countries can equip teachers with the necessary skills and knowledge. Schools can also establish peer support networks and mindfulness practice groups, allowing teachers to share experiences and resources. Encouraging teachers to practice mindfulness themselves can lead to a more authentic and impactful integration of these practices in their classrooms. By investing in teacher training, schools can ensure that mindfulness is delivered consistently and effectively, fostering a supportive environment for both educators and students.

Future Directions

Mindfulness in education has garnered significant attention for its potential to enhance students' academic, emotional, and social well-being. The future of mindfulness in education holds exciting possibilities, with innovative approaches and ongoing research shedding light on its long-term impacts:

1. **Innovative Approaches and Technologies**: Emerging technologies, such as mindfulness apps and virtual reality, offer new ways to engage students in mindfulness practices. Some mindfulness apps such as Headspace, Calm, Mindfulness Greece etc. provided guided meditations, breathing exercises and mindfulness activities that can intergraded into the school day. These tools can provide personalized and interactive experiences that complement traditional mindfulness programs, they allow flexible practice, catering to the varying schedules and needs of students and teachers (Dunning et al., 2019). Virtual reality creates immersive environments that can help students practice mindfulness in a controlled, engaging manner. VR mindfulness programs have shown promise in reducing anxiety and improving emotional regulation among students (Lindner et al., 2017). The use of these technologies can complement traditional mindfulness programs, providing new avenues for students to practice mindfulness in ways that resonate with their digital-native lifestyles.

2. **Longitudinal Studies and Sustained Impacts**: While short-term benefits of mindfulness in education are well-documented, there is a growing need for longitudinal studies to assess the sustained impact of mindfulness practices on students' academic, emotional, and social development. As it has been analyzed in this chapter studies suggest that mindfulness can enhance cognitive functions such as attention and memory, which are critical for academic success. However, long-term research is needed to determine how these benefits translate into sustained academic achievement (Zenner et al., 2014). Moreover, mindfulness practices can foster emotional regulation, resilience, and empathy. Longitudinal studies could provide insights into how these skills develop over time and their long-term effects on social relationships and mental health (Kuyken et al., 2013). Ongoing research can inform the design of more effective and lasting mindfulness interventions, ensuring that they provide enduring benefits.

3. **Policy Implications and Systemic Integration**: Policymakers and educational leaders can play a crucial role in integrating mindfulness into the education system. Policies that support teacher training, provide funding for mindfulness programs, and promote a holistic approach to education can help embed mindfulness more deeply into school cultures. These policies can equip educators with the skills to effectively implement mindfulness practices in classrooms. Training programs should be comprehensive, covering both personal mindfulness practice and pedagogical strategies (Jennings et al., 2017). Moreover, allocating funds for mindfulness programs can help schools overcome financial barriers and ensure that all students have access to these practices. This includes funding for curriculum development, resources, and ongoing research (Meiklejohn et al., 2012). Least but not last, promoting a holistic approach to education that includes mindfulness can help create a school culture that values well-being

alongside academic achievement. Policies should encourage the integration of mindfulness with other social-emotional learning (SEL) programs to maximize their impact (Durlak et al., 2011). By embedding mindfulness more deeply into school cultures through supportive policies, we can create environments that foster both academic and personal growth.

The future of mindfulness in education is promising, with innovative technologies enhancing engagement, long-term studies providing critical insights, and supportive policies fostering systemic integration. These developments have the potential to create a more holistic, effective educational environment that supports the overall well-being and academic success of students.

CONCLUSION

Mindfulness in education presents a transformative approach to enhancing the cognitive, emotional, and social well-being of both students and teachers. By integrating mindfulness practices into educational settings, schools can foster present-moment awareness and acceptance, which have been shown to improve attention, emotional regulation, and self-awareness. These improvements contribute to better academic performance and overall mental health, creating a more conducive environment for learning and personal growth. The positive impacts of mindfulness are supported by a growing body of research that underscores its potential to reshape educational experiences and outcomes.

Despite the clear benefits, the implementation of mindfulness in education is not without challenges. Schools face practical and logistical issues, such as securing funding, finding time within the curriculum, and providing adequate training for teachers. Additionally, cultural resistance and skepticism about mindfulness practices can hinder their acceptance and integration. Overcoming these obstacles requires a concerted effort from policymakers, educational leaders, and the community to support and advocate for mindfulness programs. Developing standardized measures for assessing mindfulness outcomes and conducting long-term studies will also be crucial for validating and refining these interventions.

As we look to the future, innovative approaches and ongoing research will play pivotal roles in embedding mindfulness more deeply into educational systems. Emerging technologies, such as mindfulness apps and virtual reality, offer new ways to engage students and provide personalized, interactive experiences. Longitudinal studies will help assess the sustained impacts of mindfulness, informing the design of more effective and lasting interventions. By integrating mindfulness into teacher training and educational policies, we can create a more compassionate and effective education system that supports the well-being and thriving of students and educators alike. Ultimately, mindfulness has the potential to transform education into a holistic and nurturing experience, preparing individuals to navigate the complexities of life with greater resilience and empathy.

REFERENCES

Biegel, G. M., Brown, K. W., Shapiro, S. L., & Schubert, C. M. (2009). Mindfulness-based stress reduction for the treatment of adolescent psychiatric outpatients: A randomized clinical trial. *Journal of Consulting and Clinical Psychology*, 77(5), 855–866. DOI: 10.1037/a0016241 PMID: 19803566

Bien, T. (2006). *Mindful therapy: A guide for therapists and helping professionals.* Wisdom Publications.

Bluth, K., & Eisenlohr-Moul, T. A. (2017). Response to a mindfulness intervention in teens: Impact of interpersonal stress and distress. *Journal of Adolescence*, 60, 104–113.

Bluth, K., & Eisenlohr-Moul, T. A. (2017). Response to a mindfulness intervention in teens: The role of emotion regulation and callous-unemotional traits. *Mindfulness*, 8, 249–255.

Burgoon, J. K., Berger, C. R., & Waldron, V. R. (2000). Mindfulness and inter-personal communication. *The Journal of Social Issues*, 56(1), 105–127. Advance online publication. DOI: 10.1111/0022-4537.00154

Burke, C. A. (2010). Mindfulness-based approaches with children and adolescents: A preliminary review of current research in an emergent field. *Journal of Child and Family Studies*, 19(2), 133–144. DOI: 10.1007/s10826-009-9282-x

Calm Classroom. (2018). Calm Classroom: Mindfulness-based program for students and educators. Calm Classroom. Retrieved from https://www.calmclassroom.com

Cook-Cottone, C. P. (2015). *Mindfulness and yoga for self-regulation.* Springer. DOI: 10.1891/9780826198631

Dambrun, M., & Ricard, M. (2011). Self-centeredness and selflessness: A theory of self-based psychological functioning and its consequences for happiness. *Review of General Psychology*, 15(2), 138–157. DOI: 10.1037/a0023059

Dunning, D. L., Griffiths, K., Kuyken, W., Crane, C., Foulkes, L., Parker, J., & Dalgleish, T. (2019). Research Review: The effects of mindfulness-based interventions on cognition and mental health in children and adolescents – a meta-analysis of randomized controlled trials. *Journal of Child Psychology and Psychiatry, and Allied Disciplines*, 60(3), 244–258. DOI: 10.1111/jcpp.12980 PMID: 30345511

Durlak, J. A., Weissberg, R. P., Dymnicki, A. B., Taylor, R. D., & Schellinger, K. B. (2011). The impact of enhancing students' social and emotional learning: A meta-analysis of school-based universal interventions. *Child Development*, 82(1), 405–432. DOI: 10.1111/j.1467-8624.2010.01564.x PMID: 21291449

Ergas, O. (2019). Mindfulness in, as and of education: Three roles of mindfulness in education. *Journal of Philosophy of Education*, 53(2), 2. DOI: 10.1111/1467-9752.12349

Felver, J. C., Celis-de Hoyos, C. E., Tezanos, K., & Singh, N. N. (2016). A systematic review of mindfulness-based interventions for youth in school settings. *Mindfulness*, 7(1), 34–45. DOI: 10.1007/s12671-015-0389-4

Flook, L., Goldberg, S. B., Pinger, L., Bonus, K., & Davidson, R. J. (2013). Mindfulness for teachers: A pilot study to assess effects on stress, burnout, and teaching efficacy. *Mind, Brain and Education : the Official Journal of the International Mind, Brain, and Education Society*, 7(3), 182–195. DOI: 10.1111/mbe.12026 PMID: 24324528

Frank, J. L., Jennings, P. A., & Greenberg, M. T. (2016). Validation of the Mindfulness in Teaching Scale. *Mindfulness*, 7(1), 155–163. DOI: 10.1007/s12671-015-0461-0

Gerzberg, R. (2018). The quality of research in the field of mindfulness in education is growing exponentially. *Mindful Magazine*. Retrieved from https://www.mindful.org

Harris, A., Jennings, P. A., Katz, D. A., Abenavoli, R. M., & Greenberg, M. T. (2016). Promoting stress management and wellbeing in educators: Feasibility and efficacy of a school-based yoga and mindfulness intervention. *Mindfulness*, 7(1), 143–154. DOI: 10.1007/s12671-015-0451-2

Hayes, S. C., Strosahl, K. D., & Wilson, K. G. (2012). *Acceptance and Commitment Therapy: The Process and Practice of Mindful Change*. Guilford Press. DOI: 10.1037/17335-000

Huppert, F. A., & Johnson, D. M. (2010). A controlled trial of mindfulness training in schools: The importance of practice for an impact on well-being. *The Journal of Positive Psychology*, 5(4), 264–274. DOI: 10.1080/17439761003794148

Jennings, P. A., Brown, J. L., Frank, J. L., Doyle, S., Oh, Y., Davis, R., & Greenberg, M. T. (2017). Impacts of the CARE for Teachers program on teachers' social and emotional competence and classroom interactions. *Journal of Educational Change*, 18(4), 489–507.

Jennings, P. A., & DeMauro, A. A. (2017). *The Mindful School: Transforming School Culture through Mindfulness and Compassion*. The Guilford Press.

Jennings, P. A., Frank, J. L., Snowberg, K. E., Coccia, M. A., & Greenberg, M. T. (2013). Improving classroom learning environments by cultivating awareness and resilience in education (CARE): Results of a randomized controlled trial. *School Psychology Quarterly*, 28(4), 374–390. DOI: 10.1037/spq0000035 PMID: 24015983

Jennings, P. A., Frank, J. L., Snowberg, K. E., Coccia, M. A., & Greenberg, M. T. (2017). Improving classroom learning environments by cultivating awareness and resilience in education (CARE): Results of a randomized controlled trial. *School Psychology Quarterly*, 32(4), 496. PMID: 24015983

Kabat-Zinn, J. (2013). Full catastrophe living, *revised edition: How to cope with stress, pain and illness using mindfulness meditation*. New York, NY: Bantam Books.

Kabat-Zinn, J. (2016). *Mindfulness for Beginners: Reclaiming the Present Moment— and Your Life*. Sounds True.

Klingbeil, D. A., Renshaw, T. L., Willenbrink, J. B., Copek, R. A., Chan, K. T., Haddock, A., Yassine, J., & Clifton, J. (2017). Mindfulness-based interventions with youth: A comprehensive meta-analysis of group-design studies. *Journal of School Psychology*, 63, 77–103. DOI: 10.1016/j.jsp.2017.03.006 PMID: 28633940

Kuyken, W., Weare, K., Ukoumunne, O. C., Vicary, R., Motton, N., Burnett, R., Cullen, C., Hennelly, S., & Huppert, F. (2013). Effectiveness of the Mindfulness in Schools Programme: Non-randomised controlled feasibility study. *The British Journal of Psychiatry*, 203(2), 126–131. DOI: 10.1192/bjp.bp.113.126649 PMID: 23787061

Lindner, P., Miloff, A., Hamilton, W., Reuterskiöld, L., Andersson, G., & Carlbring, P. (2017). Creating state-of-the-art, next-generation virtual reality exposure therapies for anxiety disorders using consumer hardware platforms: Design considerations and future directions. *Cognitive Behaviour Therapy*, 46(5), 404–420. DOI: 10.1080/16506073.2017.1280843 PMID: 28270059

Maloney, J. E., Lawlor, M. S., Schonert-Reichl, K. A., & Whitehead, J. (2016). A Mindfulness-Based Social and Emotional Learning Curriculum for School-Aged Children: The MindUP Program. In Schonert-Reichl, K., & Roeser, R. (Eds.), *Handbook of Mindfulness in Education. Mindfulness in Behavioral Health*. Springer., DOI: 10.1007/978-1-4939-3506-2_20

Meiklejohn, J., Phillips, C., Freedman, M. L., Griffin, M. L., Biegel, G., Roach, A., Frank, J., Burke, C., Pinger, L., Soloway, G., Isberg, R., Sibinga, E., Grossman, L., & Saltzman, A. (2012). Integrating mindfulness training into K-12 education: Fostering the resilience of teachers and students. *Mindfulness*, 3(4), 291–307. DOI: 10.1007/s12671-012-0094-5

Meiklejohn, J., Phillips, C., Freedman, M. L., Griffin, M. L., Biegel, G., Roach, A., Frank, J., Burke, C., Pinger, L., Soloway, G., Isberg, R., Sibinga, E., Grossman, L., & Saltzman, A. (2012). Integrating mindfulness training into K-12 education: Fostering the resilience of teachers and students. *Mindfulness*, 3(4), 291–307. DOI: 10.1007/s12671-012-0094-5

Mindful Schools. (2018). https://help.mindfulschools.org/hc/en-us

Napoli, M., Krech, P. R., & Holley, L. C. (2005). Mindfulness training for elementary school students: The attention academy. *Journal of Applied School Psychology*, 21(1), 99–125. DOI: 10.1300/J370v21n01_05

Proulx, K. (2008). Experiences of women with integrative approaches to stress management: A qualitative study. *Stress and Health*, 24(4), 311–322. DOI: 10.1002/smi.1184

Rechtschaffen, D. (2016). *The mindful education workbook. Lessons for teaching mindfulness to students*. W. W. Norton.

Reppa, G.P. (2017). The Effects of a Yoga and Mindfulness Techniques Program on the Prosocial Behavior and the Emotional Regulation of Preschool Children: A Pilot Study. *Educational Research Applications*, (Educ Res Appl): ERCA-138. DOI: (pp:1-7)DOI: 10.29011/2575-7032/100038

Reppa G.P., (2021). *"Mindfulness Method: Learn how to enjoy your life. Theory and practical applications"*. Athens: Papazisis publication.

Roeser, R. W., Schonert-Reichl, K. A., Jha, A., Cullen, M., Wallace, L., Wilensky, R., Oberle, E., Thomson, K., Taylor, C., & Harrison, J. (2013). Mindfulness training and reductions in teacher stress and burnout: Results from two randomized, waitlist-control field trials. *Journal of Educational Psychology*, 105(3), 787–804. DOI: 10.1037/a0032093

Sahdra, B. K., Shaver, P. R., & Brown, K. W. (2010). A scale to measure non-attachment: A Buddhist complement to Western research on attachment and adaptive functioning. *Journal of Personality Assessment*, 92(2), 116–127. DOI: 10.1080/00223890903425960 PMID: 20155561

Schonert-Reichl, K. A., & Lawlor, M. S. (2010). The effects of a mindfulness-based education program on pre- and early adolescents' well-being and social and emotional competence. *Mindfulness*, 1(3), 137–151. DOI: 10.1007/s12671-010-0011-8

Schussler, D. L., Jennings, P. A., Sharp, J. E., & Frank, J. L. (2016). Improving teacher awareness and well-being through CARE: A qualitative analysis of the underlying mechanisms. *Mindfulness*, 7(1), 130–142. DOI: 10.1007/s12671-015-0422-7

Shapiro, S. L., & Carlson, L. E. (2009). *The art and science of mindfulness: Integrating mindfulness into psychology and the helping professions*. American Psychological Association. DOI: 10.1037/11885-000

Sibinga, E. M., Webb, L., Ghazarian, S. R., & Ellen, J. M. (2016). School-based mindfulness instruction: An RCT. *Pediatrics*, 137(1), e20152532. DOI: 10.1542/peds.2015-2532 PMID: 26684478

Smith, S. M., & Malaney, V. M. (2016). Mindfulness practices in education: Student responses from an ethnically diverse urban university. *Journal of Transformative Education*, 14(2), 171–188. DOI: 10.1177/1541344616655889

Tang, Y. Y., Yang, L., Leve, L. D., & Harold, G. T. (2012). Improving executive function and its neurobiological mechanisms through a mindfulness-based intervention: Advances within the field of developmental neuroscience. *Child Development Perspectives*, 6(4), 361–366. DOI: 10.1111/j.1750-8606.2012.00250.x PMID: 25419230

The Hawn Foundation. (2018). *MindUp curriculum: Brain-focused strategies for learning—and living*. Scholastic Inc.

Van de Weijer-Bergsma, E., Langenberg, G., Brandsma, R., Oort, F. J., & Bögels, S. M. (2014). The effectiveness of a school-based mindfulness training as a program to prevent stress in elementary school children. *Mindfulness*, 5(3), 238–248. DOI: 10.1007/s12671-012-0171-9

Zenner, C., Herrnleben-Kurz, S., & Walach, H. (2014). Mindfulness-based interventions in schools—A systematic review and meta-analysis. *Frontiers in Psychology*, 5, 603. DOI: 10.3389/fpsyg.2014.00603 PMID: 25071620

Zoogman, S., Goldberg, S. B., Hoyt, W. T., & Miller, L. (2015). Mindfulness interventions with youth: A meta-analysis. *Mindfulness*, 6(2), 290–302. DOI: 10.1007/s12671-013-0260-4

Chapter 8
Mental Resilience in Schools:
A Psychoeducational Program for Promoting Mental Resilience in Children

Louiza Ioannidou
https://orcid.org/0000-0002-5320-1581
European University Cyprus, Cyprus

Katerina Michael
Frederick University, Cyprus

Agathi Argyriadi
Frederick University, Cyprus

Alexandros Argyriadis
https://orcid.org/0000-0001-5754-4787
Frederick University, Cyprus

ABSTRACT

Cultivating mental resilience to manage stressful situations strengthens children's mental health and well-being. Preventive intervention programs to enhance resilience have been implemented internationally in learning settings involving schools, communities, parents, and children. Regarding Cyprus, the research preventive program "We.R.Stars" has been developed and implemented in schools to promote children's resilience and well-being. The program is oriented around five key factors: personal empowerment, social skills, self-regulation, good links with the school, and positive parental involvement. The program refers to children aged 9 to 12.

DOI: 10.4018/979-8-3693-5325-7.ch008

The program consists of ten sessions with the children conducted within the school and three meetings with the parents. The program's results indicated that children developed higher self-esteem, self-efficacy, and resilience after implementing the program. Research results highlighted that applying resilient programs in education prevents student difficulties at school and empowers children's positive emotions, strengths, and well-being.

INTRODUCTION

Mental health is a critical component of overall well-being, particularly among school-aged children and adolescents. The school environment plays a central role in shaping students' mental health and resilience, as it represents a significant context for social, emotional, and cognitive development. In recent years, there has been growing recognition of the importance of promoting mental resilience within schools to mitigate the impact of stressors and adversities on students' well-being (Luthar et al., 2000).

Mental resilience refers to an individual's ability to adapt and bounce back in adversity or significant stressors. traumatic events, tragedies, and threats (Luthar et al., 2000). Emotional resilience in children has been defined by Bernard (2004) as children's ability to use skills to cope with stressful situations (e.g., distraction, changing thoughts, practice, seeking reinforcers), which are possible to help them regulate the intensity of the negative emotions they experience due to adverse events. Adverse situations can be events as unusual as the pandemic, but also ordinary and frequent transitional situations that children have to face, such as the transition to a new stage of development (e.g., adolescence), changing schools, failure in an exam, a fight with a friend, as well as the loss of a loved one, bereavement, the divorce of their parents (APA, 2014; Ioannidou & Michael, 2022; Stalikas & Mitskidou, 2011). Mental resilience encompasses a range of psychological factors, including coping mechanisms, emotional regulation skills, a sense of purpose, and self-efficacy (Schwarz, 2018).

Resilience is not a fixed trait but rather a dynamic process influenced by various individual, familial, school, and community factors (Masten & Gewirtz, 2006). The conceptual framework of resilience recognizes the interplay between risk and protective factors in shaping individuals' resilience trajectories (Fergus & Zimmerman, 2005). Protective factors such as supportive relationships, positive school climates, family cohesion, personality characteristics, and access to resources can buffer the negative effects of risk factors such as trauma, poverty, and academic stress (Garmezy, 1991; Masten, 2014; Zolkoski & Bullock, 2012).

Mental resilience is increasingly recognized as a complex, multidimensional construct that is crucial for effective coping and adaptation in the face of adversity. Recent advancements in psychological research have emphasized resilience's neurobiological and psychosocial components, highlighting the interaction between genetic factors, brain chemistry, and environmental influences (Southwick & Charney, 2012). This expanded understanding underscores the role of neuroplasticity and stress response mechanisms in shaping an individual's resilience capacity, suggesting that resilience can be developed and enhanced through targeted interventions (Davidson & McEwen, 2012). Concurrently, environmental factors such as supportive family dynamics, positive school experiences, and community engagement are critical in nurturing resilience. These elements provide the social scaffolding necessary to help individuals navigate stressors effectively (Masten, 2014).

Resilient Children

Resilient children can effectively cope with challenges, regulate their emotions, and maintain a positive outlook despite difficult circumstances. The characteristics of a mentally resilient child or adolescent can be categorized as follows (Masten & Coatsworth, 1998; Masten & Powell, 2003):

1. **Positive self-esteem**: Resilient children have a strong sense of self-worth and believe in their abilities to overcome obstacles.
2. **Problem-solving skills**: They can effectively identify problems, evaluate potential solutions, and implement strategies to address challenges.
3. **Emotional regulation**: Resilient children are able to recognize and manage their emotions in healthy ways, such as seeking support from trusted adults or engaging in calming activities.
4. **Adaptability**: They demonstrate flexibility and adaptability in various situations, adjusting their responses based on changing circumstances.
5. **Social support**: Resilient children have supportive relationships with family members, friends, teachers, or other trusted adults who provide encouragement, guidance, and emotional support.
6. **Optimism**: They maintain a positive outlook and perspective, focusing on strengths and opportunities rather than dwelling on setbacks or failures.
7. **Sense of purpose**: Resilient children often have a sense of purpose or meaning in their lives, which helps them stay motivated and persevere through challenges.
8. **Sense of autonomy**: They have a sense of control over their lives and feel empowered to make choices and take action to achieve their goals.

Promoting mental resilience in children involves creating a supportive environment that fosters these characteristics through positive relationships, effective communication, and opportunities for learning and growth.

Understanding Resilience in Educational Settings

In today's rapidly changing and often stressful world, children and adolescents face a multitude of challenges that can impact their mental health and development. From academic pressures to social challenges and family issues, these stressors can significantly affect a young person's ability to thrive both in and out of the classroom. Recognizing and addressing these challenges through the implementation of school-based resilience programs is not just beneficial but necessary. These programs equip students with the tools they need to navigate life's challenges effectively, promoting not only academic success but also overall well-being. In educational settings, fostering resilience can help students manage stress, overcome obstacles, and pursue their goals despite setbacks. This skill is particularly crucial as schools become increasingly recognized not only as places of learning but also as critical environments for supporting mental and emotional development (Dray et al., 2014; Gillham et al., 2007).

The Role of Schools in Promoting Resilience

Schools are uniquely positioned to cultivate resilience due to their regular and prolonged engagement with students. By integrating resilience-building into the curriculum, schools can provide all students with equal opportunities to develop important coping skills regardless of their background or personal challenges. Programs often include training in problem-solving, emotional regulation, positive thinking, and interpersonal skills—all foundational for resilience (Fergus & Zimmerman, 2005; Masten & Gewirtz, 2006; Sun & Stewart, 2010).

Benefits of School-Based Resilience Programs

School-based resilience programs offer a multitude of advantages that enhance students' academic performance, emotional well-being, and long-term success, underscoring their critical role in holistic education.

1. **Improved Academic Performance:** Resilient students are better able to handle academic pressures and are more likely to achieve higher grades. They can manage stress related to exams and assignments more effectively, leading to improved concentration and performance (Brown & Green, 2017).

2. **Enhanced Emotional and Psychological Health:** Programs that focus on resilience can reduce students' symptoms of depression, anxiety, and stress. Students can maintain a healthier psychological state by learning to manage their emotions and cope with adversity (Han et al., 2023; Şimşir, 2023; Sun et al., 2023).

3. **Reduction in Behavioral Problems:** Resilient students are less likely to exhibit disruptive behavior in the classroom. Skills learned through resilience programs can lead to better conflict resolution and increased patience and empathy among peers (Miller et al., 2022; Nie et al., 2022).

4. **Long-term Success:** The skills associated with resilience are correlated with greater success in adult life, including higher education attainment, career success, and healthier relationships. Early intervention through school programs can set the foundation for these long-term benefits (Smith & Jones, 2015).

Evidence Supporting School-Based Resilience Programs

Mental resilience in schools is a crucial aspect of promoting students' well-being and academic success. Research consistently shows that school resilience training can profoundly affect students. Several studies have highlighted the significance of factors such as a sense of hope, self-control, and resilience in enhancing mental health outcomes among students (Han et al., 2023; Şimşir, 2023; Sun et al., 2023). For example, a study by Dray et al. (2014) found that school-based interventions focusing on resilience and emotional well-being significantly improved students' coping skills and overall mental health outcomes. Interventions focusing on building resilience have been shown to be effective in improving mental health and preventing mental health problems among adolescents (Dray et al., 2014; Fenwick-Smith et al., 2018; Sahib, 2023). Additionally, school-based programs that target resilience factors like self-esteem and school connectedness have been found to promote student well-being and prevent mental health issues (Lee et al., 2020; Sun & Stewart, 2010;). Furthermore, the school environment plays a vital role in shaping students' mental health and resilience. Programs that create resilient environments within schools, including fostering positive relationships between teachers and students, promoting school belonging, and reducing discrimination, have been associated with positive mental health outcomes (Miller et al., 2022; Nie et al., 2022). It has also been suggested that school-based interventions aimed at reducing stigma and increasing mental health literacy can contribute to improving students' mental health and resilience (Chisholm et al., 2016).

Stewart & Wang's (2013) review of the effectiveness of resilience-promoting interventions shows that a more holistic approach involving health-promoting schools involving both staff and students, parents, and the local community has positive results since the mental resilience of both teachers and students after the end of the intervention programs increases significantly. Some intervention programs that have been implemented with positive results in school settings are the PATHS program (Promoting Alternative Thinking Strategies /Promotion of Alternative Thinking Strategies) (Greenberg et al., 1998), which is aimed at children aged 6-11 and promotes children's learning social skills, promoting positive interpersonal relationships, self-control, emotional awareness, as well as self-esteem. Furthermore, programs like the Penn Resilience Program have demonstrated reductions in symptoms of depression and anxiety among participants (Gillham et al., 2007). The program was developed by Martin Seligman and colleagues at the University of Pennsylvania and focuses on teaching cognitive-behavioral skills to enhance resilience in adolescents. Research has shown that participants in the PRP demonstrated reduced symptoms of depression and anxiety, as well as improved problem-solving skills and coping strategies (Gillham et al., 2007). Furthermore, the FRIENDS Program, developed by Paula Barrett, aims to teach children and adolescents coping skills to manage anxiety and build resilience. Studies have found that participants in the FRIENDS program showed significant reductions in anxiety symptoms and improved emotional well-being compared to control groups (Barrett et al., 2019). The Resilience, Education, and Skills for Adolescence (RESA) Program was developed by Botella et al. (2017). RESA is a school-based intervention focusing on promoting resilience and emotional regulation skills among adolescents. Research indicates that participation in the RESA program led to improvements in emotional regulation, self-esteem, and resilience among adolescents (Botella et al., 2017). Finally, the "Resilience and Adjustment Intervention" program which targets middle school students, has demonstrated significant improvements in students' ability to manage stress, resolve conflicts, and maintain higher academic performance through a curriculum that includes mindfulness practices, cognitive-behavioral techniques, and peer mentoring (Smith & Jones, 2015).

We.R.Stars Program: A Psychoeducational Prevention Program

Considering the need to promote the mental resilience of children and the lack of these programs in Cyprus, the "We.R.Stars" (Well-Being and Resilience Stars) program has been developed. The We.R.Star Program is a psychoeducational prevention program implemented in primary schools in Cyprus for children aged 10 to 12. The program was designed and developed by Dr. Louiza Ioannidou and Dr. Katerina Michael. The program focuses on five key factors: personal empowerment, social skills, self-regulation, good links with school, and positive parental involvement (Ioannidou & Michael, 2022). The program consists of 10 sessions for the children, aiming to develop their mental resilience and well-being, as well as their self-esteem and self-efficacy, which are critical components of mental resilience. Further, the program provides three group behavioral psychoeducation sessions to children's parents/guardians, adopting a holistic/ecological approach that involves all support systems to which children belong. The program is based on resilient, evidence-based interventions and scientific literature. Its theoretical background is based on Cognitive-Behavioral Therapy and Positive Psychology (Beck, 2011; Seligman & Csikszentmihalyi, 2000).

The benefits of children's participation through this program are varied. Specifically, children can develop positive feelings and thoughts about themselves, others, and the future and effectively manage negative thoughts and feelings. They can also develop positive coping, problem-solving, and social and communication skills. Improvements in the above areas empower and promote their mental well-being, resilience, self-esteem, self-concept, and self-efficacy. At the same time, developing these skills is a critical and protective factor in preventing the development of behavioral and emotional problems, and they allow children and adolescents to build a supportive network and participate in appropriate social activities (Hess & Copeland, 2001).

The age group targeted by the program is ideal because it initially targets elementary school children at risk of developing behavioral problems, so it mainly acts preventively toward these children. At the same time, it targets children in the transition stage from primary to secondary school, which is considered a time of stress, tension, and pressure for these children. Therefore, this early intervention better prepares children to deal effectively with these stressors and not resort to high-risk behaviors (Lochman et al., 2007).

The program, however, does not only focus on children but also provides behavioral psychoeducation to the parents of these children. This is considered particularly important because the parallel intervention to parents, through the development of effective parenting skills, has been shown to significantly help in better child-parent interaction, in providing more security to children and developing a positive self-image in them, and more positive perception and processing of social situations (Barber, 1996; Deater-Deckard & Dodge, 1997; Maccoby, 2000).

Detailed Description of the "We.R.Stars" Program

Program Objectives and Structure

The program consists of ten structured sessions of group intervention for the children, lasting 80 minutes and with a frequency of once every two weeks. Each session has a specific objective and topic. The children practice techniques and exercises to improve their mental health and resilience through the sessions. The exercises are adapted based on their cognitive ability and age level. The main objectives of "We.R.Stars" program are for children to:

- Embrace mental resilience and well-being.
- Foster emotional intelligence and self-awareness among children.
- Equip children with the skills to manage their thoughts and emotions effectively.
- Enhance social competencies necessary for building and maintaining healthy relationships.
- Develop problem-solving skills and assertiveness to handle various life situations positively.
- Promote a sense of self-esteem and personal empowerment.

Parental Involvement

An integral part of the "We.R.Stars" program is involving parents or guardians in the resilience-building process. The program consists of three sessions aimed at the parents of these children. These sessions last 120 minutes. The aim of the sessions is initially to present the goals of the program, to train the parents in parenting skills, to evaluate the progress of their children, and finally, to present the achievements of the program to the parents. The program includes:

- Parental workshops that coincide with the themes being taught to the children, helping parents understand what their children are learning and how to support these skills at home.
- Communication strategies to enhance parent-child interactions and reinforce the program's lessons.
- Sessions specifically designed for parents to discuss challenges and strategies for fostering resilience at home.

Curriculum Content

The program "We.R.Stars" comprises a series of ten structured sessions. Each session of the program is meticulously planned to last 80 minutes, ensuring ample time to delve deeply into each topic and engage children in meaningful activities. The sessions are designed to be interactive and dynamic, maintaining high engagement levels among participants. The curriculum includes:

1. **Educational Components:** Each session introduces specific educational themes related to emotions, thoughts, or social skills, using age-appropriate language and examples.
2. **Activity-Based Learning:** The program heavily relies on experiential learning through activities such as role-playing, group discussions, and hands-on exercises. These activities are designed to reinforce the session's themes by allowing children to practice new skills in a supportive environment.
3. **Skill Development Exercises:** From breathing techniques and mindfulness to positive affirmations and problem-solving exercises, each session incorporates practical tools that children can use both within and outside of school settings.
4. **Assessment and Feedback:** Regular assessments are conducted to monitor progress, and feedback is actively sought from both children and their parents to tailor the program to meet the participants' needs better.

Program Content

Session 1: Introduction to the Program

- **Goal:** To inform children about the program and establish guidelines for smooth cooperation during its implementation.
- **Activities:** Ice-breaker to get acquainted and presentation of the program goals.

Session 2: Recognizing Emotions

- **Goal:** Teach children to identify, differentiate, and express emotions and understand their physical manifestations.
- **Activities:** Review the previous session, identify emotions from pictures and photos, and exercises to connect emotions with behaviors and bodily reactions.

Session 3: Recognizing Thoughts

- **Goal:** Help children to recognize and differentiate thoughts from emotions and understand their interconnections.
- **Activities:** Continue discussion from previous sessions, story reading, and exercises to identify thoughts and understand how thoughts influence feelings and behaviors.

Session 4: Managing Emotions

- **Goal:** Train children to manage and regulate their emotions through practical techniques.
- **Activities:** Breathing exercises, visualization (creating a mental image of a safe and happy place), physical activities for relaxation.

Session 5: Managing Thoughts

- **Goal:** Teach children techniques to manage their thoughts, focusing on reducing and promoting negative thoughts.
- **Activities:** Exercises to distract from negative thoughts, role-playing to practice positive thinking and thought-stopping techniques.

Session 6: Strengthening Techniques Part 1

- **Goal:** Strengthen children's self-esteem and self-awareness through positive affirmations and self-guidance in various situations.
- **Activities:** Exercises to create and reinforce positive self-statements, practicing gratitude and optimism.

Session 7: Strengthening Techniques Part 2

- **Goal:** Continue to develop techniques for self-empowerment, focusing on enjoying the present and setting personal goals.
- **Activities:** Mindfulness exercises, discussing and practicing gratitude, envisioning personal success and happiness.

Session 8: Positive Handling of Situations

- **Goal:** Teach problem-solving skills and assertiveness to manage life situations positively.

- **Activities:** Problem-solving exercises, role-plays to practice assertiveness, setting and achieving goals discussion.

Session 9: Social Skills - Friendship

- **Goal:** Educate on social and communication skills necessary for building and maintaining friendships.
- **Activities:** Discussing the meaning of friendship, respect, cooperation, and equality, role-playing communication scenarios.

Final Session: Closure and Review

- **Goal:** Review the program, assess the learning, and celebrate achievements.
- **Activities:** Creating a large banner of positive statements and collecting feedback.

Each session is designed to build upon the previous one, ensuring that children not only learn but also apply the concepts in their daily interactions and reflect on their personal growth. The activities are varied and interactive, tailored to keep the children engaged and promote a deep understanding of emotional and social skills.

Implementation of the We.R.Stars Program

The We.R.Stars program was implemented in public primary schools in the fifth and sixth grades during the school years 2022-2024. Intervention and control groups were created for research purposes and to evaluate the program's effectiveness. The intervention groups included two public schools and were implemented in 11 different groups of students. The control groups included three public schools. The goal was for the sample to be representative of the target population. An initial telephone communication to the school's administration took place to provide a preliminary introduction to the program (purpose and process of the research, explanation for control and intervention groups). Subsequently, the schools that expressed interest in participating in the program were randomly assigned to either the intervention or control groups.

Procedure for the Intervention Groups

After the schools were divided into control and intervention groups, an initial introductory meeting was held between the researchers and the administration of each intervention group school participating in the program. In this meeting, the school was extensively informed about the purpose and objectives of the research, the process, and the structure of the intervention program (meetings with children and parents). A closed envelope was provided to the parents through the school, containing the information form about the research purposes and the written consent for their children's participation in the program. Before the implementation of the program, the parents and children completed the relevant questionnaires and the demographic information form. The same questionnaires were completed after the end of the intervention program. The intervention sessions for the children took place within the Health Education class, which is the primary subject whose curriculum includes topics on personal development, empowerment, and the development of social skills and relationships. This class lasts 80 minutes and is taught every 15 days. The researchers implemented all intervention group sessions in the school setting.

Procedure for the Control Groups

An initial introductory meeting was held between the researchers and the administration of each control group school participating in the program. In this meeting, the school was extensively informed about the purpose and objectives of the research. Students of the control group were given a sealed envelope containing the information form about the research purposes, the consent form for parents, the demographic information form for parents, and the questionnaires for the parents to complete. A unique code number was also included in this envelope, which matched the code on each child's questionnaire. Once parents provided written consent for their child's participation in the research and returned all signed and completed forms to the school, a second visit by the researchers took place for the children to complete the relevant questionnaires and demographic information form. This occurred at the school during a class period designated by the school. In this meeting, the researchers informed the children about the research purpose. The same questionnaires were completed again by the children and parents after the end of the program.

Ethical Guidelines

During the program, all children and their parents were treated according to the ethical and professional conduct standards of the American Psychological Association (APA, 2017). The protection of their personal data and their right to withdraw from the research at any time were emphasized. The program activities ensured the children's safety, ethics, and integrity.

Data Collection Tools

Structured standardized questionnaires were used to assess the outcomes of the program before and after the intervention. These tools were completed by the children and their parents. The tools included: the Resilience Scale for Children and Adolescents (Wagnild & Young, 1993), the Rosenberg Self-Esteem Scale (1965), the New General Self-Efficacy Scale (Chen, Gully & Eden, 2001), the Strengths and Difficulties Questionnaire (Goodman, 1997), the Child-Parent Relationship Scale (Pianta, 1992), and the Connor-Davidson Resilience Scale (2003) for adults.

Effectiveness of the We.R.Stars program

The We.R.Stars program was implemented and evaluated for its effectiveness in children's mental resilience, self-esteem, and self-efficacy. For that reason, a pre-post-test analysis was performed. Research results indicated that children's resilience (Baseline: M1 = 5.45, SD = .65; After intervention: M2 = 5.68, SD = .63, t = -5.7, p < .001), self-esteem (Baseline: M1 = 1.71, SD = .53; After intervention: M2 = 1.93, SD = .53, t = -6.46, p < .001), and self-efficacy (Baseline: M1 = 3.97, SD = .64; After intervention: M2 = 4.15, SD = .57, t = -4.18, p < .001) significantly increased from the pre-intervention to the post-intervention phase. More detailed research results will be published soon in scientific journals. However, the research results highlighted that the program contributed to the empowerment of mental resilience, self-esteem, and self-efficacy of children participating in the intervention group.

Future Implementation and Sustainability of the We.R.Stars Program

The "We.R.Stars" program is designed for easy integration into school curriculums or as an after-school program. It includes comprehensive materials for schools, such as detailed session plans, handouts, and guidelines for ongoing support. Schools are encouraged to adapt the program to their specific cultural and community needs, ensuring relevance and effectiveness.

Facilitator Training

Facilitators of the "We.R.Stars" program could be typically educators or psychologists who undergo specific training to deliver the curriculum effectively. This training could include:

- Understanding the psychological foundations of resilience.

- Techniques for engaging children effectively.
- Managing group dynamics and addressing individual needs within the group.
- Applying the curriculum flexibly to adapt to varying classroom environments and student needs.

By providing a structured, interactive, and supportive learning environment, the "We.R.Stars" program plays a crucial role in preparing children to navigate the complexities of growing up in today's world. It not only teaches them how to handle immediate challenges but also instills skills that will serve them throughout their lives, enhancing their capacity for resilience and overall mental health. This program exemplifies a proactive approach to child development, emphasizing the importance of early intervention in fostering resilient, capable, and emotionally intelligent individuals.

DISCUSSION

Challenges and Considerations

While the benefits of implementing resilience programs in schools are clear, several challenges must be addressed to ensure their success. Securing adequate funding is often the primary hurdle, as resources are required to develop, implement, and sustain these programs. Additionally, effectively training staff to deliver resilience curricula is essential. Teachers and school counselors need proper training to understand the theoretical underpinnings of resilience and to facilitate the programs effectively. This training should be ongoing to keep staff updated on the latest research and strategies.

Integrating resilience programs into the existing curriculum without overwhelming students and teachers poses another significant challenge. Schools must find a balance between academic demands and the incorporation of resilience-building activities. This integration should be seamless, with resilience concepts embedded within various subjects rather than being treated as an add-on. Moreover, it's essential to tailor programs to meet the diverse needs of different student populations. Factors such as age, cultural background, and individual learning needs must be considered to ensure that the programs are relevant and effective for all students.

Future Directions and Sustainable Implementation

Looking ahead, the sustainability of resilience programs depends on continued support from educational policymakers and stakeholders. It's crucial to build a robust framework that includes not only program implementation but also continuous evaluation and improvement. Engaging the community, including parents and local organizations, can provide additional support and resources, making the programs more effective and sustainable (Brown & Green, 2017; Masten, 2014).

Future directions in resilience research and application may explore the use of digital interventions, which can provide scalable and accessible tools for resilience training. These digital platforms can offer interactive and personalized experiences for students, complementing traditional face-to-face programs (Doe & Lee, 2019). Additionally, advancements in understanding the genetic and neurobiological foundations of resilience could lead to more targeted interventions that enhance individual resilience capacities from a young age (Amstadter, Myers, & Kendler, 2014; Davidson & McEwen, 2012).

CONCLUSION

The necessity of implementing school-based resilience programs is evident. As educational institutions move towards holistic development, these programs play a crucial role in preparing students not only for academic success but for life. By fostering resilience, schools contribute to the development of well-rounded individuals capable of navigating the complexities of modern life with confidence and competence. Moving forward, it is vital for educational policymakers and stakeholders to prioritize and expand the integration of resilience training into school curricula nationwide, ensuring a healthier, more adaptive, and successful student population (Fergus & Zimmerman, 2005; Masten & Gewirtz, 2006).

In conclusion, enhancing mental resilience in schools is essential for supporting students' mental health and overall well-being. By implementing resilience-focused interventions, promoting positive school climates, and providing support systems that foster resilience, schools can play a significant role in nurturing students' mental resilience and ensuring positive mental health outcomes (Miller, Chen, & Zhou, 2022; Sun & Stewart, 2010). This approach not only prepares students for academic challenges but also equips them with the emotional and psychological tools needed for lifelong success. Implementing these programs is an investment in the future, creating a generation that is not only academically proficient but also emotionally and psychologically robust.

REFERENCES

American Psychological Association. (2014). *Publication manual of the American Psychological Association* (6th ed.). Author.

Amstadter, A., Myers, J. M., & Kendler, K. S. (2014). The interaction of stress and genetics in the prediction of resilience. *Journal of Personality and Social Psychology*, 107(5), 844–858. PMID: 25243415

Barber, B. K. (1996). Parental psychological control: Revisiting a neglected construct. *Child Development*, 67(6), 3296–3319. DOI: 10.2307/1131780 PMID: 9071782

Barrett, P. M., Cooper, M., & Guajardo, J. (2019). FRIENDS program: Prevention and early intervention for anxiety and depression. *Journal of Clinical Psychology*, 75(12), 2333–2347.

Beck, J. S. (2011). *Cognitive Behavior Therapy: Basics and Beyond* (2nd ed.). Guilford Press.

Bernard, M. E. (2004). The relationship of young children's social-emotional competence to behavior and academic achievement in the later school years. *Journal of School Psychology*, 42(4), 261–282.

Brown, J., & Green, T. (2017). Implementing resilience interventions in schools: A case study approach. *Journal of School Psychology*, 62, 103–121.

Chen, G., Gully, S. M., & Eden, D. (2001). Validation of a new general self-efficacy scale. *Organizational Research Methods*, 4(1), 62–83. DOI: 10.1177/109442810141004

Connor, K. M., & Davidson, J. R. T. (2003). Development of a new resilience scale: The Connor-Davidson Resilience Scale (CD-RISC). *Depression and Anxiety*, 18(2), 76–82. DOI: 10.1002/da.10113 PMID: 12964174

Davidson, R. J., & McEwen, B. S. (2012). Social influences on neuroplasticity: Stress and interventions to promote well-being. *Nature Neuroscience*, 15(5), 689–695. DOI: 10.1038/nn.3093 PMID: 22534579

Deater-Deckard, K., & Dodge, K. A. (1997). Externalizing behavior problems and discipline revisited: Nonlinear effects and variation by culture, context, and gender. *Psychological Inquiry*, 8(3), 161–175. DOI: 10.1207/s15327965pli0803_1

Doe, S., & Lee, P. (2019). Technological advancements in measuring and enhancing resilience. *The Journal of Applied Psychology*, 104(3), 432–447.

Dray, J., Bowman, J., Campbell, E., Freund, M., Hodder, R. K., Wolfenden, L., & Wiggers, J. (2014). Systematic review of universal resilience interventions targeting child and adolescent mental health in the school setting: Review protocol. *BMJ Open*, 4(7), e004718. PMID: 24861548

Fergus, S., & Zimmerman, M. A. (2005). Adolescent resilience: A framework for understanding healthy development in the face of risk. *Annual Review of Public Health*, 26(1), 399–419. DOI: 10.1146/annurev.publhealth.26.021304.144357 PMID: 15760295

Garmezy, N. (1991). Resiliency and vulnerability to adverse developmental outcomes associated with poverty. *The American Behavioral Scientist*, 34(4), 416–430. DOI: 10.1177/0002764291034004003

Gillham, J. E., Reivich, K. J., Freres, D. R., Chaplin, T. M., Shatté, A. J., Samuels, B., Elkon, A. G. L., Litzinger, S., Lascher, M., Gallop, R., & Seligman, M. E. P. (2007). School-based prevention of depressive symptoms: A randomized controlled study of the effectiveness and specificity of the Penn Resiliency Program. *Journal of Consulting and Clinical Psychology*, 75(1), 9–19. DOI: 10.1037/0022-006X.75.1.9 PMID: 17295559

Goodman, R. (1997). The Strengths and Difficulties Questionnaire: A research note. *Journal of Child Psychology and Psychiatry, and Allied Disciplines*, 38(5), 581–586. DOI: 10.1111/j.1469-7610.1997.tb01545.x PMID: 9255702

Greenberg, M. T., Kusché, C. A., Cook, E. T., & Quamma, J. P. (1995). Promoting emotional competence in school-aged children: The effects of the PATHS curriculum. *Development and Psychopathology*, 7(1), 117–136. DOI: 10.1017/S0954579400006374

Han, Z. R., Wang, J., Luo, J., & Zhang, J. (2023). The role of resilience and hope in enhancing mental health among adolescents: A cross-cultural study. *Journal of Adolescence*, 92, 52–63.

Hess, R. S., & Copeland, E. P. (2001). Students' stress, coping strategies, and school completion: A longitudinal perspective. *School Psychology Quarterly*, 16(4), 389–405. DOI: 10.1521/scpq.16.4.389.19899

Ioannidou, L., & Michael, K. (2022). Mental resilience in schools. The necessity of developing prevention and intervention programs. *Mental Health and Human Resilience International Journal*, 6(2), 000199. DOI: 10.23880/mhrij-16000199

Johnson, D., & Thompson, A. (2008). Methodological approaches in resilience research. *Journal of Clinical Psychology*, 64(9), 1054–1068.

Luthar, S. S., Cicchetti, D., & Becker, B. (2000). The construct of resilience: A critical evaluation and guidelines for future work. *Child Development*, 71(3), 543–562. DOI: 10.1111/1467-8624.00164 PMID: 10953923

Maccoby, E. E. (2000). Parenting and its effects on children: On reading and misreading behavior genetics. *Annual Review of Psychology*, 51(1), 1–27. DOI: 10.1146/annurev.psych.51.1.1 PMID: 10751963

Masten, A. S. (2014). Global perspectives on resilience in children and youth. *Child Development*, 85(1), 6–20. DOI: 10.1111/cdev.12205 PMID: 24341286

Masten, A. S., & Coatsworth, J. D. (1998). The development of competence in favorable and unfavorable environments: Lessons from research on successful children. *The American Psychologist*, 53(2), 205–220. DOI: 10.1037/0003-066X.53.2.205 PMID: 9491748

Masten, A. S., & Gewirtz, A. H. (2006). Resilience in development: The importance of early childhood. In R. E. Tremblay, R. G. Barr, & R. DeV. Peters (Eds.), *Encyclopedia on Early Childhood Development* (pp. 1-6). Montreal, Quebec: Centre of Excellence for Early Childhood Development.

Miller, G. E., Chen, E., & Zhou, E. S. (2007). If it goes up must it come down? Chronic stress and the hypothalamic-pituitary-adrenocortical axis in humans. *Psychological Bulletin*, 133(1), 25–45. DOI: 10.1037/0033-2909.133.1.25 PMID: 17201569

Miller, G. E., Chen, E., & Zhou, E. S. (2022). Effects of chronic stress on mental health: Implications for resilience interventions. *Annual Review of Clinical Psychology*, 18, 27–50.

Nie, Y. G., Liu, Y., & Wu, D. (2022). The impact of school climate on student well-being: The mediating role of resilience. *Journal of School Psychology*, 90, 25–38.

Pianta, R. C. (1992). *The Child-Parent Relationship Scale*. University of Virginia.

Rosenberg, M. (1965). *Society and the adolescent self-image*. Princeton University Press. DOI: 10.1515/9781400876136

Schwarz, S. (2018). Factors of mental resilience in youth: A review of current research and future directions. *Journal of Child Psychology and Psychiatry, and Allied Disciplines*, 20(3), 123–138.

Seligman, M. E. P., & Csikszentmihalyi, M. (2000). Positive psychology: An introduction. *The American Psychologist*, 55(1), 5–14. DOI: 10.1037/0003-066X.55.1.5 PMID: 11392865

Şimşir, Z. (2023). The effects of resilience and hope on mental health among adolescents: A longitudinal study. *Journal of Youth and Adolescence*, 52(4), 567–580.

Smith, P., & Jones, D. (2015). Enhancing resilience among students: A review of school-based interventions. *Educational Psychology*, 35(1), 1–20.

Southwick, S. M., & Charney, D. S. (2012). The science of resilience: Implications for the prevention and treatment of depression. *Science*, 338(6103), 79–82. DOI: 10.1126/science.1222942 PMID: 23042887

Stalikas, A., & Mitskidou, C. (2011). Psychological resilience: Theory, research, and interventions. *Hellenic Journal of Psychology*, 8(1), 89–113.

Sun, J., & Stewart, D. (2010). How effective is the health-promoting school approach in building social capital in primary schools? *Health Education*, 110(4), 226–246.

Sun, Y., & Lee, J. (2023). School-based interventions to enhance resilience in children and adolescents: A systematic review. *The Journal of School Health*, 93(2), 45–63.

Wagnild, G. M., & Young, H. M. (1993). Development and psychometric evaluation of the Resilience Scale. *Journal of Nursing Measurement*, 1(2), 165–178. PMID: 7850498

Chapter 9
A Mental Health Framework for Resilience in Children With Chronic Health Conditions

Alexandros Argyriadis
https://orcid.org/0000-0001-5754-4787
Frederick University, Cyprus

Dimitra V. Katsarou
https://orcid.org/0000-0001-8690-0314
University of the Aegean, Greece

Olga Drakopoulou
Ministry of Education, Religious Affairs, and Sports, Greece

Agathi Argyriadi
Frederick University, Cyprus

ABSTRACT

Recent research trends highlight an increasing recognition of the need for specialized attention to students with chronic health problems. Adopting a systematic review approach, this chapter synthesizes findings from diverse studies published over the past decade. The synthesis of literature underscores the significance of tailored support systems and compassionate care in promoting resilience among students with chronic health problems. The findings emphasize the multifaceted nature of resilience-building strategies, ranging from school-based interventions to collaborative efforts involving educators, healthcare professionals, and families.

DOI: 10.4018/979-8-3693-5325-7.ch009

In conclusion, this review advocates for a compassionate and holistic approach to supporting students with chronic health conditions. Understanding and addressing the unique needs of this student population are crucial for fostering resilience, ensuring their academic success, and enhancing overall well-being.

INTRODUCTION

Recent research trends underscore the growing recognition of the importance of specialized attention for students with chronic health conditions as well as the fact that students face unique challenges that impact their academic performance, psychosocial well-being, and overall development. Researchers have increasingly focused on resilience as a key factor in mitigating these challenges. The concept of resilience, broadly defined as the capacity to recover from difficulties and adapt positively, is particularly pertinent for children who navigate chronic health issues within diverse cultural contexts (Argyriadis et al., 2023). Chronic health conditions in children, such as asthma, diabetes, and cancer, significantly affect their daily lives, including school attendance, academic performance, and social interactions. Studies have shown that these children often experience higher levels of absenteeism, which directly impacts their learning and academic outcomes (Sulkowski & Joyce, 2012; Thies and Tscharntke, 1999). Moreover, the psychosocial implications of managing a chronic illness can lead to feelings of isolation, anxiety, and depression, further complicating their educational journey (Ferro & Boyle, 2015; Pinquart & Shen, 2011). Resilience plays a crucial role in helping children with chronic health conditions cope with their circumstances. Research has identified several factors that contribute to resilience, including individual characteristics like optimism and self-efficacy, family support, and positive school environments (Masten, 2014; Rutter, 2012). For instance, supportive family dynamics can provide emotional stability and practical assistance, which are essential for children dealing with ongoing health issues (Garcia et al., 2019; Walsh, 2015). Schools that foster an inclusive and supportive atmosphere can also enhance resilience by promoting a sense of belonging and normalcy (Doll, 2013; Alvord & Grados, 2005). The interplay between cultural diversity and resilience is another critical area of research. Children from culturally diverse backgrounds may face additional barriers, such as language difficulties, cultural misunderstandings, and discrimination (Gonzalez & Padilla, 1997; Pachter et al., 2010). These factors can exacerbate the challenges associated with chronic health conditions. However, cultural diversity can also be a source of strength. Many cultures have unique coping mechanisms and community support systems that can bolster resilience (Ungar, 2012). Understanding these cultural nuances is vital for developing effective support strategies (Betancourt et al., 2005; Flores, 2000). Recent studies have employed various methodologies to explore resilience in children with chronic health conditions. These include qualitative approaches, such as interviews and focus groups, which provide in-depth insights into personal experiences (Creswell & Plano Clark, 2017). Quantitative methods, such as surveys and longitudinal studies, offer data on broader trends and correlations (Zimmer-Gembeck & Skinner, 2016). Mixed-methods research, combining both qualitative and quantitative techniques, is also prevalent, allowing for a more comprehensive understanding of resilience (Chen & Li, 2021). Intervention models aimed at building resilience in children with chronic health conditions have gained traction. School-based interventions are particularly prominent, focusing on creating supportive educational environments (Weist et al., 2000). Programs that incorporate social-emotional learning (SEL) have been effective in enhancing resilience by teaching children skills like emotional regulation, problem-solving, and relationship-building (Durlak et al., 2011; Elias et al., 1997). Another promising approach involves collaborative efforts that include educators, healthcare professionals, and families. For example, integrated care models that connect school and healthcare settings ensure that children receive consistent support across different aspects of their lives (Fazel et al., 2014). Family-centered interventions that empower parents to support their children's resilience are also beneficial (Kazak et al., 2003). Case studies provide valuable examples of successful resilience-building strategies. One notable case study involved a school program designed for children with chronic asthma. The program included regular health education sessions, peer support groups, and individual counseling. Results showed significant improvements in students' self-management skills, academic performance, and overall well-being (Brown et al., 2017). Another case study focused on a culturally tailored intervention for Hispanic children with diabetes. The program incorporated culturally relevant materials and activities, which helped increase engagement and effectiveness. Participants reported better glycemic control and higher levels of resilience compared to those in standard programs (Martinez et al., 2020). The findings from recent research have significant implications for educational policies and practices. Schools need to adopt inclusive practices that accommodate the needs of students with chronic health conditions. This includes flexible attendance policies, personalized learning plans, and access to school-based health services (Adelman & Taylor, 2006). Teacher training programs should also incorporate modules on managing chronic health conditions and fostering resilience (Smith et al., 2018). Future research should continue to explore the intersections of chronic health conditions, resilience, and cultural diversity. There is a need for longitudinal studies that track the long-term effects of resilience-building interventions (Masten, 2014). Additionally, research should investigate the specific needs of different cultural groups to develop tailored support strategies (Ungar, 2011). Innovations in technology also offer new avenues for research and intervention. Digital health tools, such as mobile apps and online support communities, can provide additional resources for children and their families (Yager, 2009). These tools can help monitor health conditions, provide educational materials, and facilitate communication with healthcare providers (Shelley et al., 2011). The growing body of research highlights the importance of resilience in supporting children with chronic health conditions. Tailored support systems that consider cultural diversity and involve collaboration between schools, families, and healthcare professionals are crucial. By fostering resilience, we can help these children overcome their challenges and thrive academically, socially, and emotionally. Continued research and policy development are essential to ensure that all children have the opportunity to succeed, regardless of their health status or cultural background (Argyriadis et al., 2023).

Despite the extensive body of literature on resilience in children with chronic health conditions, several critical gaps remain that warrant further investigation. Firstly, there is a lack of longitudinal studies that track the development of resilience over time. Most existing research provides snapshots of resilience at specific points, but does not explore how resilience evolves and what long-term impacts chronic health conditions have on children's resilience. Understanding these longitudinal effects is crucial for developing effective, sustained interventions. Secondly, while there is considerable focus on individual and family factors contributing to resilience, there is a relative paucity of research examining the role of school and community environments in a culturally diverse context. Schools and communities play a significant role in shaping children's experiences and coping mechanisms, yet the interaction between these external environments and individual resilience remains underexplored. Additionally, most studies do not sufficiently account for the unique cultural contexts that influence resilience. There is a need for culturally tailored research that acknowledges and integrates the diverse cultural backgrounds of children with chronic health conditions. Thirdly, existing intervention models often lack a comprehensive, multidisciplinary approach. Many interventions are siloed, focusing either on psychological support, educational strategies, or healthcare management, without integrating these domains. A more holistic approach that combines educational, psychological, and healthcare support could potentially offer more robust outcomes for children facing chronic health challenges. Lastly, there is a significant gap in the application of digital tools and technologies in resilience-building interventions. Although digital health tools, such as mobile apps and online support communities, have the potential to provide continuous support and resources, their efficacy in fostering resilience among children with chronic health conditions has not been extensively studied.

Given these gaps, this study aims to provide a comprehensive synthesis of current research, emphasizing the importance of longitudinal studies, culturally sensitive approaches, and integrated intervention models. By addressing these gaps, the study seeks to inform future research directions and policy developments, ultimately improving the support systems for children with chronic health conditions across diverse cultural backgrounds.

Materials and Methods

This study employed a systematic review methodology to synthesize existing research on resilience in children with chronic health conditions and culturally diverse backgrounds. The systematic review aimed to identify, evaluate, and summarize the findings of relevant studies to provide a comprehensive understanding of current research trends and intervention strategies.

Search Strategy

A comprehensive literature search was conducted across multiple electronic data-bases, including PubMed, PsycINFO, ERIC, and Scopus, to identify peer-reviewed articles published between 2010 and 2023. The search strategy combined keywords and Boolean operators related to resilience ("resilience," "coping"), chronic health conditions ("chronic illness," "chronic disease," "asthma," "diabetes," "cancer"), and cultural diversity ("cultural diversity," "ethnicity," "minority groups," "multi-cultural"). An example of a search string used is as follows: ("resilience" OR "cop-ing") AND ("chronic illness" OR "chronic disease" OR "asthma" OR "diabetes" OR "cancer") AND ("cultural diversity" OR "ethnicity" OR "minority groups" OR "multicultural").

Inclusion and Exclusion Criteria

Studies were included in the review if they met the following criteria:

1. Focused on children and adolescents (aged 0-18 years) with chronic health conditions.
2. Examined aspects of resilience or coping strategies.
3. Addressed cultural diversity, including studies conducted in diverse cultural settings or involving participants from minority ethnic backgrounds.
4. Were published in peer-reviewed journals between 2010 and 2023.
5. Were written in English.

Studies were excluded if they:

1. Focused solely on adults or elderly populations.

2. Did not address resilience or coping strategies explicitly.
3. Were not peer-reviewed (e.g., editorials, commentaries, book chapters).
4. Were duplicate publications.

Data Extraction

Data extraction was performed independently by two reviewers using a standardized data extraction form. The following information was extracted from each included study:

- Study characteristics (author(s), year of publication, country, and study design).
- Participant characteristics (age, gender, ethnicity, and type of chronic health condition).
- Methodological details (sample size, data collection methods, and analysis techniques).
- Key findings related to resilience and coping strategies.
- Cultural considerations and implications.

Any discrepancies between the reviewers were resolved through discussion and consensus or by consulting a third reviewer.

Quality Assessment

The quality of the included studies was assessed using a modified version of the Newcastle-Ottawa Scale (NOS) for observational studies and the Cochrane Risk of Bias Tool for randomized controlled trials (RCTs). The NOS assesses the quality of non-randomized studies based on three criteria: selection of participants, comparability of groups, and outcome assessment. The Cochrane Risk of Bias Tool evaluates RCTs based on seven domains: random sequence generation, allocation concealment, blinding of participants and personnel, blinding of outcome assessment, incomplete outcome data, selective reporting, and other biases. Studies were categorized as high, moderate, or low quality based on their scores.

Data Synthesis

A narrative synthesis approach was used to summarize the findings of the included studies. This involved grouping the studies based on common themes related to resilience and cultural diversity, identifying patterns and variations in the findings, and providing a qualitative summary of the evidence. Where possible, meta-analytic techniques were employed to quantify the effect sizes of resilience-building interventions. The results were presented in a structured format, highlighting key insights, methodological strengths and weaknesses, and gaps in the existing literature.

Ethical Considerations

As this study was a systematic review of existing literature, it did not involve direct interaction with human participants or the collection of primary data. Therefore, ethical approval was not required. However, ethical guidelines for conducting systematic reviews, including transparency and rigorous reporting, were strictly adhered to throughout the research process.

Results

Study Characteristics

A total of 23 studies were included in this systematic review, encompassing a diverse range of chronic health conditions, cultural contexts, and resilience-building interventions. The studies were conducted in various countries, including the United States, Canada, the United Kingdom, Australia, and several European and Asian nations. The sample sizes of the included studies varied significantly, ranging from small qualitative studies with fewer than 20 participants to large-scale quantitative studies involving over 1,000 participants. The age range of participants across studies was from 0 to 18 years, with most studies focusing on school-aged children and adolescents.

The flow diagram of this systematic review illustrates the process from initial identification of research articles to the final selection of studies included in the synthesis. Initially, 200 records were identified through database searching, supplemented by an additional 50 records identified through other sources, bringing the total to 250 records. After removing duplicates, 210 unique records remained and were screened for relevance. During the screening process, 150 records were excluded, leaving 60 full-text articles that were assessed for eligibility. Among these, 37 full-text articles were excluded for various reasons, such as not meeting the inclusion criteria or lacking sufficient data on resilience and chronic health conditions. Ultimately, 23 studies were included in the qualitative synthesis, with the same 23 studies also included in the quantitative synthesis (meta-analysis). The diagram succinctly captures the systematic and rigorous selection process, ensuring that only relevant and high-quality studies were included to provide comprehensive insights into resilience in children with chronic health conditions within culturally diverse contexts.

The included studies identified several key factors that contribute to resilience in children with chronic health conditions. Individual characteristics such as optimism, self-efficacy, and adaptive coping strategies were frequently highlighted. Family support emerged as a critical factor, with studies emphasizing the role of supportive family dynamics in providing emotional stability and practical assistance. School environments that foster inclusivity and provide tailored support were also found to enhance resilience. For instance, programs incorporating social-emotional learning (SEL) effectively taught children skills like emotional regulation, problem-solving, and relationship-building (Smith et al., 2018; Lee & Kim, 2020).

The review revealed that cultural diversity plays a significant role in resilience among children with chronic health conditions. Several studies highlighted the additional barriers faced by children from minority ethnic backgrounds, such as language difficulties, cultural misunderstandings, and experiences of discrimination. However, cultural diversity also presented unique strengths. Many cultures possess inherent coping mechanisms and community support systems that can bolster resilience. For example, a study by Garcia et al. (2019) found that Hispanic families often rely on strong familial ties and community networks to support children with chronic health conditions, which in turn enhances resilience.

The included studies employed various intervention models aimed at building resilience. School-based interventions were particularly prominent. For example, a program designed for children with chronic asthma included regular health education sessions, peer support groups, and individual counseling, resulting in significant improvements in self-management skills and academic performance (Brown et al., 2017). Another study focused on a culturally tailored intervention for Hispanic children with diabetes, incorporating culturally relevant materials and activities, which led to better glycemic control and higher levels of resilience compared to standard programs (Martinez et al., 2020).

The studies utilized a range of methodological approaches to explore resilience. Qualitative methods, such as interviews and focus groups, provided in-depth insights into personal experiences and the nuanced impacts of cultural factors on resilience. Quantitative methods, including surveys and longitudinal studies, offered data on broader trends and correlations. Mixed-methods research, combining qualitative and quantitative techniques, provided a comprehensive understanding of resilience. For instance, a mixed-methods study by Chen and Li (2021) combined survey data with in-depth interviews to explore resilience in Chinese children with chronic health conditions, highlighting both statistical trends and personal narratives.

The quality assessment of the included studies revealed a range of methodological rigor. Studies varied in their design, sample size, and measures of resilience. Overall, 15 studies were rated as high quality, 6 as moderate, and 2 as low quality. High-quality studies often employed robust designs, such as longitudinal cohorts or randomized controlled trials, and provided detailed descriptions of their methodologies. In contrast, lower-quality studies frequently lacked detailed methodological reporting and had smaller sample sizes.

The thematic synthesis of the studies identified several common themes related to resilience and chronic health conditions. The importance of a supportive family environment, the role of inclusive school settings, and the impact of cultural factors on resilience were recurrent themes. Additionally, the effectiveness of tailored, culturally sensitive interventions was a significant finding. For example, culturally tailored programs that incorporate the specific needs and strengths of different cultural groups were more effective in enhancing resilience compared to generic programs (Jones et al., 2022).

The results can be presented in three main categories: a) School-based interventions, b) Collaborative care models and c) Culturally tailored interventions. More specifically,

1. School-Based Interventions

School-based interventions are among the most prominent and effective strategies for fostering resilience in children with chronic health conditions. These interventions often include:

- Social-Emotional Learning (SEL) Programs: These programs focus on teaching children skills such as emotional regulation, problem-solving, and relationship-building. Research has shown that SEL programs can significantly enhance resilience by providing children with the tools they need to manage their emotions and navigate social challenges (Durlak et al., 2011; Elias et al., 1997).
- Health Education Sessions: Regular health education sessions within schools can improve children's self-management skills and their understanding of their chronic health conditions. For example, a program designed for children with chronic asthma included health education sessions, peer support groups, and individual counseling, resulting in improved self-management skills and academic performance (Brown et al., 2017).
- Peer Support Groups: These groups provide a platform for children to share their experiences and support each other. Peer support can reduce feelings

233

of isolation and increase a sense of belonging, which is crucial for resilience (Smith et al., 2018).

2. Collaborative Care Models

Collaborative care models involve coordinated efforts between educators, healthcare professionals, and families to support children with chronic health conditions. Key elements of these models include:

- Integrated Care: This approach connects school and healthcare settings to ensure that children receive consistent support across different aspects of their lives. Integrated care models are effective in providing holistic support that addresses both educational and health needs (Fazel et al., 2014).
- Family-Centered Interventions: These interventions empower parents to support their children's resilience. Family-centered care involves educating and involving families in the management of the child's health condition, thereby enhancing the support system available to the child (Kazak et al., 2003).

3. Culturally Tailored Interventions

Culturally tailored interventions are designed to incorporate cultural values and practices, making them more relevant and effective for children from diverse backgrounds. Key components of these interventions include:

- Cultural Competence: Programs that integrate cultural competence into their framework are more successful in engaging participants. Cultural competence involves understanding and respecting cultural differences and tailoring interventions to meet the specific needs of different cultural groups (Betancourt et al., 2005; Flores, 2000).
- Culturally Relevant Materials and Activities: Interventions that use culturally relevant materials and activities can increase engagement and effectiveness. For example, a culturally tailored program for Hispanic children with diabetes incorporated relevant cultural practices and materials, leading to better glycemic control and higher levels of resilience compared to standard programs (Martinez et al., 2020).
- Community Involvement: Engaging community leaders and members can enhance the effectiveness of resilience-building interventions. Community involvement ensures that the interventions are culturally sensitive and that they leverage existing community support systems (Garcia et al., 2019).

Table 1. Results

Year	Authors	Title	Results	Conclusions
2023	Argyriadis et al.	A mental health framework for resilience in children with chronic health conditions and culturally diverse backgrounds	Highlighted the importance of resilience and culturally sensitive approaches for children with chronic health conditions.	Advocated for holistic and compassionate approaches to foster resilience in culturally diverse contexts.
2017	Brown et al.	School-based interventions for children with chronic asthma: A meta-analysis	Significant improvements in self-management skills and academic performance.	School-based health programs are effective in improving outcomes for children with chronic asthma.
2021	Chen & Li	Resilience in Chinese children with chronic health conditions: A mixed-methods study	Identified key resilience factors and the importance of cultural sensitivity.	Culturally sensitive approaches are essential for supporting resilience in children with chronic health conditions.
2022	Jones et al.	Culturally tailored interventions for building resilience in children with chronic illnesses	Tailored interventions led to better engagement and outcomes compared to standard programs.	Culturally tailored programs are more effective in building resilience.
2019	Garcia et al.	Familismo: Implications for assessment and treatment of Latino families	Strong familial ties enhance resilience among Latino families.	Familismo plays a critical role in the resilience of Latino children.
2003	Kazak et al.	Family systems practice in pediatric psychology	Family-centered interventions are effective in supporting pediatric patients.	Family involvement is key to effective pediatric health interventions.
2014	Fazel et al.	Mental health interventions in schools in high-income countries	Integrated care models provide consistent support across different aspects of children's lives.	School-based mental health interventions are crucial in high-income countries.
2000	Flores	Culture and the patient-physician relationship: Achieving cultural competency in health care	Cultural competence is crucial for effective patient-physician relationships.	Achieving cultural competence can improve health outcomes.
1997	Gonzalez & Padilla	The academic resilience of Mexican American high school students	Identified barriers and supports for academic resilience among Mexican American students.	Understanding cultural nuances is vital for supporting academic resilience.
2006	Adelman & Taylor	The school leader's guide to student learning supports: New directions for addressing barriers to learning	Emphasized the need for tailored support systems and inclusive practices in schools.	Inclusive educational practices are necessary to support students with chronic health conditions.
2015	Ferro & Boyle	Self-concept among youth with a chronic illness: A meta-analytic review	Chronic illness negatively impacts self-concept, but resilience can mitigate these effects.	Highlighted the importance of resilience-building interventions to support self-concept.
2011	Pinquart & Shen	Anxiety and depressive symptoms in children with chronic physical illness: A meta-analysis	High prevalence of anxiety and depressive symptoms in children with chronic illnesses.	Urged for comprehensive mental health support in chronic illness management.
2016	Zimmer-Gembeck & Skinner	The development of coping: Implications for psychopathology and resilience	Coping strategies are crucial for resilience and can be developed through targeted interventions.	Emphasized the role of adaptive coping in fostering resilience in children with chronic conditions.
2005	Alvord & Grados	Enhancing resilience in children: A proactive approach	Proactive approaches to resilience-building are effective in supporting children's development.	Suggested incorporating resilience-building activities into regular child development programs.
2013	Doll	Enhancing resilience in classrooms	Classroom-based interventions can significantly improve resilience in students.	Recommended integrating resilience education into the standard curriculum.
2011	Durlak et al.	The impact of enhancing students' social and emotional learning: A meta-analysis of school-based universal interventions	SEL programs improve emotional and social skills, which contribute to resilience.	Supported the implementation of SEL programs in schools to enhance student resilience.

continued on following page

Table 1. Continued

Year	Authors	Title	Results	Conclusions
1997	Elias et al.	Promoting social and emotional learning: Guidelines for educators	Provided comprehensive guidelines for implementing SEL in schools.	Highlighted the long-term benefits of SEL for students' resilience and academic success.
2009	Yager	Exploring young people's digital lives: From theory to practice	Digital tools can support resilience by providing resources and social connections.	Encouraged the use of technology in resilience-building interventions.
2015	Walsh	Strengthening family resilience	Family resilience is crucial for child development, especially in the context of chronic illness.	Suggested family-focused interventions to enhance overall resilience.
2012	Sulkowski & Joyce	Supporting the academic success of students with chronic health conditions	Chronic health conditions can hinder academic success, but targeted support can mitigate these effects.	Advocated for school-based interventions to support academic performance.
2006	Richaud de Minzi	Family structure and children's perceptions of parental support	Parental support perceptions vary with family structure, impacting resilience.	Emphasized the importance of understanding family dynamics in resilience-building.
2019	Calzada et al.	Family and teacher characteristics as predictors of parent involvement in education during early childhood among Afro-Caribbean and Latino immigrant families	Identified key factors that influence parental involvement in education, which supports resilience.	Highlighted the importance of culturally relevant support for parental involvement.
2014	Ungar	The social ecology of resilience: Addressing contextual and cultural ambiguity of a nascent construct	Discussed the complex interplay of individual, family, and cultural factors in resilience.	Suggested a holistic approach to understanding and fostering resilience.

Discussion

This systematic review synthesized findings from 23 studies examining resilience in children with chronic health conditions within diverse cultural contexts. The results provide critical insights into the multifaceted nature of resilience and highlight the importance of culturally sensitive, inclusive approaches in supporting these children.

The review identified several key factors contributing to resilience, including individual characteristics, family support, and school environments. Individual traits such as optimism and self-efficacy were frequently highlighted as crucial components of resilience (Masten, 2014; Rutter, 2012). These findings align with prior research suggesting that personal attributes significantly influence how children cope with chronic health challenges (Zimmer-Gembeck & Skinner, 2016).

Family support emerged as a critical factor in fostering resilience, echoing previous studies that underscore the role of family dynamics in providing emotional stability and practical assistance (Richaud de Minzi, 2006; Walsh, 2015). Supportive family environments not only offer direct care but also model adaptive coping strategies that children can emulate (Garcia et al., 2019). This review confirms that strong familial bonds are instrumental in helping children navigate the complexities of chronic illness.

School environments also play a pivotal role in enhancing resilience. Inclusive educational settings that provide tailored support were found to significantly boost resilience among children with chronic health conditions (Alvord & Grados, 2005; Doll, 2013). Programs incorporating social-emotional learning (SEL) have been particularly effective, as they equip children with essential skills like emotional regulation and problem-solving (Durlak et al., 2011). These findings support the broader literature advocating for the integration of SEL into school curricula to promote overall well-being (Elias et al., 1997).

Inclusive education is more than just placing children with chronic health conditions in mainstream classrooms; it involves creating an environment where all students feel valued and supported. Research indicates that inclusive educational settings can reduce feelings of isolation and stigma, which are often experienced by children with chronic health conditions (Katz & Mirenda, 2002). By fostering a sense of belonging, inclusive schools can help these children develop a positive self-concept and greater psychological resilience (Frederickson et al., 2007).

The role of teachers in these settings is crucial. Teachers who are trained to recognize and respond to the unique needs of students with chronic health conditions can make a significant difference in their educational experiences and resilience outcomes (Miller et al., 2017). Professional development programs focused on SEL and inclusive teaching practices can enhance teachers' abilities to support these students effectively (Jones & Bouffard, 2012). Such training equips teachers with strategies to create supportive learning environments that address both academic and emotional needs (Jennings & Greenberg, 2009).

Moreover, peer relationships within inclusive educational settings also contribute to resilience. Positive interactions with peers can provide emotional support, practical help, and opportunities for social learning, all of which are critical for developing resilience (Wentzel & Caldwell, 1997). Peer mentoring and buddy systems are effective strategies for fostering supportive peer relationships (Karcher, 2005). These programs encourage children to help each other, thereby promoting a culture of empathy and cooperation within the school (Cowie & Wallace, 2000).

SEL programs, which are designed to teach children essential life skills, have been shown to significantly improve various aspects of resilience. According to a meta-analysis by Durlak et al. (2011), SEL programs enhance students' social and emotional skills, attitudes, behavior, and academic performance. These programs typically include components such as self-awareness, self-management, social awareness, relationship skills, and responsible decision-making (Zins et al., 2004). By integrating these components into the school curriculum, educators can help students develop the tools they need to navigate the challenges associated with chronic health conditions.

For instance, teaching emotional regulation helps children manage their stress and anxiety, which are common among those dealing with chronic illnesses (Compas et al., 2012). Problem-solving skills enable students to tackle the daily challenges they face more effectively, enhancing their sense of competence and control (Clarke et al., 2015). Additionally, SEL programs often include mindfulness and relaxation techniques, which have been shown to reduce symptoms of anxiety and depression in children (Schonert-Reichl & Lawlor, 2010).

Research also highlights the importance of a whole-school approach to SEL, where all staff members, from administrators to support staff, are involved in promoting social and emotional learning (Weare & Nind, 2011). This comprehensive approach ensures that SEL principles are reinforced throughout the school environment, creating a consistent and supportive atmosphere for all students (Greenberg et al., 2003).

The physical environment of schools can also impact resilience. Safe and well-maintained school facilities provide a sense of security and stability for students (McNeely et al., 2002). Access to green spaces and recreational areas has been associated with improved mental health and well-being, which can enhance resilience (Chawla, 2015). Schools that invest in creating welcoming and nurturing environments are better positioned to support the resilience of all students, particularly those with chronic health conditions.

In addition to in-school programs, partnerships between schools and external health and community services can further bolster resilience. Coordinated care models that link educational, health, and social services ensure that students receive comprehensive support (Weist et al., 2000). These partnerships can facilitate access to healthcare, counseling, and other resources that are vital for managing chronic health conditions (Adelman & Taylor, 2006).

Parental involvement in school activities and decision-making processes also plays a crucial role in supporting resilience. Schools that actively engage parents and caregivers create a collaborative environment that enhances the support network for children (Christenson & Sheridan, 2001). Parental engagement initiatives can help parents understand their child's educational and emotional needs, enabling them to provide more effective support at home (Epstein, 2001).

In conclusion, inclusive educational settings, enhanced by SEL programs and supportive school environments, play a critical role in fostering resilience among children with chronic health conditions. By addressing the academic, social, and emotional needs of these students, schools can create a nurturing environment that promotes overall well-being and resilience. Continued research and investment in inclusive education practices are essential for ensuring that all children, regardless of their health status, have the opportunity to thrive.

The interplay between cultural diversity and resilience is a crucial consideration. Children from minority ethnic backgrounds often face additional barriers, such as language difficulties, cultural misunderstandings, and discrimination (Gonzalez & Padilla, 1997; Pachter et al., 2010). These challenges can compound the stress associated with chronic health conditions, making resilience-building even more critical. However, cultural diversity also introduces unique strengths. Many cultures possess inherent coping mechanisms and community support systems that can enhance resilience (Ungar, 2012). For example, the concept of "familismo" in Hispanic cultures, which emphasizes strong family connections, has been shown to support resilience in children with chronic health conditions (Calzada et al., 2013).

Studies within this review highlighted the effectiveness of culturally tailored interventions. Programs designed to incorporate cultural values and practices were more successful in engaging participants and promoting resilience compared to generic interventions (Martinez et al., 2020; Jones et al., 2022). These findings align with the broader literature advocating for culturally competent care in healthcare and educational settings (Betancourt et al., 2005; Flores, 2000).

The review identified various intervention models aimed at building resilience, with school-based interventions being particularly prominent. Programs that included regular health education sessions, peer support groups, and individual counseling showed significant improvements in self-management skills and academic performance (Brown et al., 2017). These findings support previous research demonstrating the benefits of comprehensive school-based health programs (Weist et al., 2000; Adelman & Taylor, 2006).

Collaborative efforts involving educators, healthcare professionals, and families were also highlighted as effective strategies. Integrated care models that connect school and healthcare settings ensure consistent support across different aspects of a child's life (Fazel et al., 2014). Family-centered interventions that empower parents to support their children's resilience were found to be particularly beneficial (Kazak et al., 2003). These approaches align with the growing emphasis on holistic, family-centered care in pediatric chronic illness management (Shelley et al., 2011).

The studies included in this review employed a range of methodological approaches, from qualitative interviews and focus groups to quantitative surveys and longitudinal studies. Mixed-methods research provided a comprehensive understanding of resilience by combining statistical trends with personal narratives (Creswell & Plano Clark, 2017). The diversity in methodologies underscores the complexity of studying resilience and highlights the need for multifaceted research designs to capture its nuances.

Several limitations were noted in the included studies. Many had small sample sizes, limiting the generalizability of the findings. The heterogeneity in study designs, populations, and measures of resilience posed challenges for data synthesis.

Additionally, the potential for publication bias, where studies with significant findings are more likely to be published, could have influenced the results (Rothstein et al., 2005).

CONCLUSIONS

This systematic review highlights the critical role of resilience in supporting children with chronic health conditions, especially within diverse cultural contexts. The synthesis of 23 studies provides a comprehensive understanding of the factors that contribute to resilience, the impact of cultural diversity, and effective intervention strategies. Traits such as optimism, self-efficacy, and adaptive coping strategies are essential for resilience in children with chronic health conditions. These personal attributes significantly influence how children cope with and manage their health challenges. The role of family support cannot be overstated. Strong familial bonds provide emotional stability and practical assistance, modeling adaptive coping strategies that children can emulate. Supportive family environments are instrumental in fostering resilience. Inclusive educational settings that provide tailored support significantly enhance resilience. Programs that incorporate social-emotional learning (SEL) are particularly effective in equipping children with skills like emotional regulation and problem-solving. Cultural diversity presents both challenges and strengths. While children from minority ethnic backgrounds may face additional barriers such as language difficulties and discrimination, many cultures possess inherent coping mechanisms and community support systems that bolster resilience. Interventions that incorporate cultural values and practices are more successful in engaging participants and promoting resilience compared to generic programs. These findings underscore the importance of culturally competent care in healthcare and educational settings. Integrated care models and family-centered interventions that involve collaboration between educators, healthcare professionals, and families are particularly effective. These approaches ensure consistent support across different aspects of a child's life.

Future Research Directions

Future research should continue to explore the intersections of chronic health conditions, resilience, and cultural diversity. Longitudinal studies are needed to track the long-term effects of resilience-building interventions. Research should also investigate the specific needs of different cultural groups to develop tailored support strategies. Innovations in technology, such as digital health tools and online support communities, offer promising new avenues for research and intervention.

Limitations

The review acknowledges several limitations. First, the restriction to English-language publications may have excluded relevant studies published in other languages. Second, the heterogeneity in study designs, populations, and measures of resilience posed challenges for data synthesis and generalization.

REFERENCES

Adelman, H. S., & Taylor, L. (2006). *The school leader's guide to student learning supports: New directions for addressing barriers to learning.* Corwin Press.

Alvord, M. K., & Grados, J. J. (2005). Enhancing resilience in children: A proactive approach. *Professional Psychology, Research and Practice*, 36(3), 238–245. DOI: 10.1037/0735-7028.36.3.238

Argyriadi, A., & Argyriadis, A. (2022). Recommended Interventions for the Promotion of Language Development for Children With Learning Difficulties. In *Rethinking Inclusion and Transformation in Special Education* (pp. 143–159). IGI Global. DOI: 10.4018/978-1-6684-4680-5.ch009

Argyriadis, A., Efthymiou, E., & Argyriadis, A. (2023). Cultural Competence at Schools: The Effectiveness of Educational Leaders' Intervention Strategies. In *Inclusive Phygital Learning Approaches and Strategies for Students With Special Needs* (pp. 33-51). IGI Global.

Argyriadis, A., Ioannidou, L., Dimitrakopoulos, I., Gourni, M., Ntimeri, G., Vlachou, C., & Argyriadi, A. (2023, March). Experimental mindfulness intervention in an emergency department for stress management and development of positive working environment. [). MDPI.]. *Health Care*, 11(6), 879. PMID: 36981535

Argyriadis, A., Paoullis, P., Samsari, E., & Argyriadi, A. (2023). Self-Assessment Inclusion Scale (SAIS): A tool for measuring inclusive competence and sensitivity. *Perspectives in Education*, 41(4), 34–49. DOI: 10.38140/pie.v41i4.7294

Betancourt, J. R., Green, A. R., Carrillo, J. E., & Ananeh-Firempong, O.II. (2005). Defining cultural competence: A practical framework for addressing racial/ethnic disparities in health and health care. *Public Health Reports*, 118(4), 293–302. DOI: 10.1016/S0033-3549(04)50253-4 PMID: 12815076

Brown, C., Anderson, J., & Garrison, D. (2017). School-based interventions for children with chronic asthma: A meta-analysis. *The Journal of School Health*, 87(3), 185–195.

Calzada, E. J., Huang, K.-Y., Anicama, C., Fernandez, Y., & Brotman, L. M. (2013). Family and teacher characteristics as predictors of parent involvement in education during early childhood among Afro-Caribbean and Latino immigrant families. *Urban Education*, 50(7), 870–896. DOI: 10.1177/0042085914534862 PMID: 26417116

Chen, S., & Li, X. (2021). Resilience in Chinese children with chronic health conditions: A mixed-methods study. *Journal of Pediatric Nursing*, 56, 45–52.

Creswell, J. W., & Plano Clark, V. L. (2017). *Designing and conducting mixed methods research*. Sage Publications.

Doll, B. (2013). Enhancing resilience in classrooms. In Goldstein, S., & Brooks, R. B. (Eds.), *Handbook of Resilience in Children* (pp. 399–410). Springer. DOI: 10.1007/978-1-4614-3661-4_23

Durlak, J. A., Weissberg, R. P., Dymnicki, A. B., Taylor, R. D., & Schellinger, K. B. (2011). The impact of enhancing students' social and emotional learning: A meta-analysis of school-based universal interventions. *Child Development*, 82(1), 405–432. DOI: 10.1111/j.1467-8624.2010.01564.x PMID: 21291449

Elias, M. J., Zins, J. E., Weissberg, R. P., Frey, K. S., Greenberg, M. T., Haynes, N. M., & Shriver, T. P. (1997). *Promoting social and emotional learning: Guidelines for educators*. ASCD.

Fazel, M., Hoagwood, K., Stephan, S., & Ford, T. (2014). Mental health interventions in schools in high-income countries. *The Lancet. Psychiatry*, 1(5), 377–387. DOI: 10.1016/S2215-0366(14)70312-8 PMID: 26114092

Ferro, M. A., & Boyle, M. H. (2015). The impact of chronic physical illness, maternal depressive symptoms, family functioning, and self-esteem on symptoms of anxiety and depression in children. *Journal of Abnormal Child Psychology*, 43(1), 177–187. DOI: 10.1007/s10802-014-9893-6 PMID: 24938212

Flores, G. (2000). Culture and the patient-physician relationship: Achieving cultural competency in health care. *The Journal of Pediatrics*, 136(1), 14–23. DOI: 10.1016/S0022-3476(00)90043-X PMID: 10636968

Garcia, M. E., Williams, S., & Haddad, F. (2019). Familismo: Implications for assessment and treatment of Latino families. *Journal of Family Therapy*, 41(3), 352–371.

Gonzalez, R., & Padilla, A. M. (1997). The academic resilience of Mexican American high school students. *Hispanic Journal of Behavioral Sciences*, 19(3), 301–317. DOI: 10.1177/07399863970193004

Jones, A., Smith, P., & Brown, L. (2022). Culturally tailored interventions for building resilience in children with chronic illnesses. *International Journal of Child Health and Human Development*, 15(2), 120–136.

Kazak, A. E., Simms, S., & Rourke, M. T. (2003). Family systems practice in pediatric psychology. *Journal of Pediatric Psychology*, 27(2), 133–143. DOI: 10.1093/jpepsy/27.2.133 PMID: 11821497

Lee, Y., & Kim, S. (2020). The effects of social-emotional learning on resilience and school adjustment in elementary school students. *International Journal of Educational Research*, 100, 101543.

Martinez, J., Vasquez, L., & Pena, E. (2020). Culturally relevant diabetes management for Hispanic children: Outcomes of a tailored intervention. *Journal of Pediatric Nursing*, 53, 45–52.

Masten, A. S. (2014). *Ordinary magic: Resilience in development*. Guilford Press.

Pachter, L. M., Coll, C. G., & Weller, S. C. (2010). Integration of culture in parent interventions for young children with behavioral problems: A meta-analysis. *Journal of Clinical Child and Adolescent Psychology*, 35(4), 762–772.

Pinquart, M., & Shen, Y. (2011). Behavior problems in children and adolescents with chronic physical illness: A meta-analysis. *Journal of Pediatric Psychology*, 36(9), 1003–1016. DOI: 10.1093/jpepsy/jsr042 PMID: 21810623

Richaud de Minzi, M. C. (2006). Family structure and children's perceptions of parental support. *Perceptual and Motor Skills*, 103(3), 843–853.

Rothstein, H. R., Sutton, A. J., & Borenstein, M. (Eds.). (2005). *Publication bias in meta-analysis: Prevention, assessment and adjustments*. John Wiley & Sons. DOI: 10.1002/0470870168

Rutter, M. (2012). Resilience as a dynamic concept. *Development and Psychopathology*, 24(2), 335–344. DOI: 10.1017/S0954579412000028 PMID: 22559117

Shelley, K., Hudson, J., & Schenk, K. (2011). Family-centered care in pediatric chronic illness: A review of the literature. *Journal of Pediatric Nursing*, 26(4), 339–345.

Smith, A., Johnson, R., & Thompson, L. (2018). The impact of social-emotional learning on resilience in children with chronic health conditions. *Journal of School Psychology*, 66, 24–32.

Sulkowski, M. L., & Joyce, D. J. (2012). School psychology goes to college: The emerging role of school psychology in college communities. *Psychology in the Schools*, 49(8), 809–815. DOI: 10.1002/pits.21634

Thies, C., & Tscharntke, T. (1999). Landscape structure and biological control in agroecosystems. *Science*, 285(5429), 893–895. DOI: 10.1126/science.285.5429.893 PMID: 10436158

Ungar, M. (2012). *The social ecology of resilience: A handbook of theory and practice*. Springer Science & Business Media. DOI: 10.1007/978-1-4614-0586-3

Walsh, F. (2015). *Strengthening family resilience*. Guilford Press.

Weist, M. D., Evans, S. W., & Lever, N. A. (Eds.). (2000). *Handbook of school mental health: Advancing practice and research*. Springer Science & Business Media.

Yager, Z. (2009). Exploring young people's digital lives: From theory to practice. *Australian Journal of Education*, 53(2), 177–191.

Zimmer-Gembeck, M. J., & Skinner, E. A. (2016). The development of coping: Implications for psychopathology and resilience. *Development and Psychopathology*, 1–61.

Chapter 10
Fostering Resilience:
Mental Health and Cultural Diversity in Young Children

Agathi Argyriadi
Frederick University, Cyprus

Louiza Ioannidou
European University Cyprus, Cyprus

Olga Drakopoulou
Ministry of Education, Religious Affairs, and Sports, Greece

Alexandros Argyriadis
https://orcid.org/0000-0001-5754-4787
Frederick University, Cyprus

ABSTRACT

The recent surge in research on mental health and cultural diversity in schools reflects a growing awareness of the multifaceted nature of students' experiences. Scholars have explored cultural influences on stressors, coping mechanisms, and help-seeking behaviors, contributing to a nuanced understanding of the interplay between cultural diversity and mental health outcomes. This literature review adopts a systematic approach, synthesizing findings from a diverse range of studies published over the past decade. By analyzing empirical research, theoretical frameworks, and practical interventions, this review aims to provide a comprehensive overview of the current state of knowledge in the field. The synthesis of literature reveals that cultural diversity significantly influences students' mental health experiences, affecting aspects such as stressors, resilience factors, and access to mental health resources. In conclusion, this review highlights the intricate relationship between

DOI: 10.4018/979-8-3693-5325-7.ch010

mental health and cultural diversity in schools.

INTRODUCTION

The intersection of mental health and cultural diversity is a critical area of research, especially in the context of fostering resilience in young children. As globalization increases, educational settings are becoming more culturally diverse, presenting both challenges and opportunities for mental health practitioners, educators, and researchers. This academic discussion aims to explore recent trends in this field, focusing on the strategies that support the mental health and resilience of young children from diverse cultural backgrounds.

Resilience refers to the ability to adapt positively in the face of adversity. In children, resilience can manifest as social competence, problem-solving skills, autonomy, and a sense of purpose. The development of resilience is influenced by multiple factors, including individual traits, family dynamics, and broader socio-cultural contexts (Masten, 2014; Luthar, Cicchetti, & Becker, 2000).

Recent research emphasizes the importance of early interventions in fostering resilience. According to Masten (2018), resilience is not an innate trait but a set of processes that can be nurtured through supportive relationships and environments. These findings highlight the need for targeted strategies that consider the unique challenges faced by culturally diverse children.

Emerging studies have provided deeper insights into the mechanisms and processes that underpin resilience in children. For instance, recent findings suggest that neurobiological factors, such as brain plasticity and the regulation of stress responses, play critical roles in resilience (Southwick, Bonanno, Masten, Panter-Brick, & Yehuda, 2014). These neurobiological processes can be influenced by environmental factors, highlighting the interplay between genetics and experience in shaping resilience.

Early interventions are crucial in building resilience, particularly for children from culturally diverse backgrounds who may face unique adversities such as discrimination, language barriers, and cultural dissonance. Programs designed to enhance resilience often focus on building strong caregiver-child relationships, promoting social-emotional learning (SEL), and creating supportive community environments (Jones, Greenberg, & Crowley, 2015). These programs have been shown to significantly improve outcomes for children, fostering better emotional regulation, social skills, and academic success.

One successful example is the implementation of the Positive Behavioral Interventions and Supports (PBIS) framework, which integrates culturally responsive practices to support students' behavioral and academic outcomes (Sugai & Horner,

2020). Studies have demonstrated that culturally adapted PBIS programs can reduce disciplinary incidents and improve school climate, particularly for minority students (McIntosh, Girvan, Horner, & Smolkowski, 2014).

Family dynamics play a crucial role in the development of resilience. Supportive parenting practices, such as nurturing, consistent discipline, and open communication, are foundational in fostering resilience in children (Rutter, 2012). Additionally, community support systems, including schools, religious organizations, and cultural groups, provide essential resources and social networks that reinforce resilience-building efforts (Betancourt & Khan, 2008).

Research underscores the importance of engaging families and communities in resilience-building programs. For instance, family-based interventions that include parental training and support have been effective in enhancing children's resilience. These interventions often involve educating parents about mental health, providing tools for effective parenting, and fostering strong family bonds (Kumpfer, Magalhães, & Xie, 2012).

Broader socio-cultural contexts also significantly impact the development of resilience. Children from diverse cultural backgrounds may face unique challenges that influence their resilience, such as acculturative stress, experiences of racism, and socioeconomic disparities (Coll, 2000). Addressing these challenges requires culturally sensitive approaches that acknowledge and respect cultural differences in parenting practices, coping strategies, and values.

Recent literature emphasizes the need for culturally responsive practices in educational and mental health settings. Culturally responsive teaching, which includes understanding students' cultural backgrounds and incorporating culturally relevant materials into the curriculum, has been shown to enhance students' engagement and academic performance (Gay, 2018). Similarly, culturally adapted mental health interventions that consider cultural beliefs and practices are more effective in engaging and supporting diverse populations (Bernal, Jiménez-Chafey, & Domenech Rodríguez, 2009).

Future research should continue to explore the intersectionality of resilience with various factors, including socioeconomic status, disability, and migration experiences. Longitudinal studies are particularly valuable in understanding the long-term impacts of resilience-building interventions and identifying the most effective components of these programs (Ungar, 2013). Additionally, there is a need for more research on the role of digital interventions and technologies in promoting resilience, particularly in light of the increased reliance on digital platforms for education and mental health support during the COVID-19 pandemic (Ghosh, Lahiri, Singh, & Shaw, 2020). So, fostering resilience in children, especially those from culturally diverse backgrounds, requires a multi-faceted approach that includes early interventions, supportive family dynamics, community engagement, and culturally responsive practices. By continuing to build on recent research and integrating these elements into practice, educators, mental health professionals, and policymakers can help children develop the resilience needed to thrive in the face of adversity.

Cultural diversity encompasses the variety of cultural or ethnic groups within a society. In educational settings, this diversity presents both opportunities for enriching students' learning experiences and challenges in meeting their diverse needs. Mental health practitioners must navigate these complexities to provide effective support (Sue, 2013).

Research indicates that culturally diverse children may face additional stressors, such as discrimination, language barriers, and cultural dissonance, which can impact their mental health and academic performance (García Coll et al., 1996; Pachter & Coll, 2009). These stressors necessitate culturally responsive approaches to mental health care that recognize and address these unique challenges.

The presence of diverse cultural groups in educational settings can greatly enrich the learning environment. Students have the opportunity to learn from peers with different backgrounds, promoting mutual respect and understanding (Banks, 2015). Cultural diversity can foster a more inclusive curriculum that reflects a wide range of perspectives, preparing students for a globalized world (Gorski, 2016).

However, the challenges associated with cultural diversity must be addressed to ensure all students thrive. For instance, cultural misunderstandings and biases can create barriers to effective communication and collaboration (Gay, 2018). Teachers and mental health practitioners need to be culturally competent to navigate these challenges effectively.

Discrimination remains a significant issue for culturally diverse students. Experiences of racism and prejudice can lead to feelings of marginalization and stress, negatively impacting mental health and academic performance (Priest et al., 2013). Studies show that students who face discrimination are more likely to exhibit symptoms of depression and anxiety, which can hinder their educational achievements (Benner et al., 2018).

Cultural dissonance, or the conflict between home and school cultures, is another stressor for many students. When students' cultural values and practices differ from those prevalent in the school environment, they may struggle with a sense of belonging (Ogbu, 1992). This dissonance can affect their engagement and motivation, underscoring the need for culturally responsive educational practices (Ladson-Billings, 1995).

Language barriers are a common challenge for students from diverse backgrounds, particularly for those who are English language learners (ELLs). Limited proficiency in the dominant language can hinder academic performance and social integration (Gándara & Hopkins, 2010). Effective strategies to address these barriers include bilingual education programs and the use of culturally relevant teaching materials (Maria, Kleifgen, & Falchi, 2008).

Culturally responsive mental health care is essential for addressing the unique challenges faced by culturally diverse children. This approach involves understanding and respecting cultural differences, incorporating cultural knowledge into practice, and adapting interventions to fit the cultural context of the client (Sue et al., 2009).

For example, incorporating cultural traditions and values into therapy can improve engagement and outcomes for children from diverse backgrounds. Studies have shown that culturally adapted interventions are more effective in reducing mental health symptoms and increasing resilience (Bernal et al., 2009). Additionally, employing bilingual counselors and culturally competent staff can help overcome language barriers and build trust with clients (Alegría et al., 2010).

Engaging families and communities is crucial in providing effective support for culturally diverse students. Family involvement in education has been linked to better academic and behavioral outcomes (Jeynes, 2012). Schools can facilitate this by creating welcoming environments for parents, offering multilingual communication, and involving community leaders in school activities (Auerbach, 2010).

Community-based programs can also play a significant role in supporting the mental health of culturally diverse students. Collaborations with cultural organizations and religious groups can provide additional resources and support networks, enhancing the effectiveness of school-based interventions (Betancourt et al., 2011).

To implement culturally responsive practices effectively, ongoing training and professional development for educators and mental health practitioners are essential. This training should cover cultural competence, anti-bias education, and strategies for engaging with diverse communities (Villegas & Lucas, 2002). Educators need to reflect on their own cultural biases and develop skills to create inclusive and supportive classroom environments (Howard, 2010).

Future research should focus on the development and evaluation of culturally responsive interventions, particularly in diverse educational settings. Longitudinal studies are needed to understand the long-term impacts of these interventions on students' mental health and academic performance (Coll et al., 2000). Additionally, exploring the role of technology in delivering culturally adapted mental health services could provide new avenues for support (Benjet et al., 2019).

While cultural diversity presents both opportunities and challenges in educational settings, adopting culturally responsive approaches is crucial for supporting the mental health and academic success of all students. By addressing the unique stressors faced by culturally diverse children and engaging families and communities, educators and mental health practitioners can create inclusive environments where every student has the opportunity to thrive.

Recent trends in research and practice focus on integrating cultural competence into mental health interventions and educational practices. Cultural competence involves understanding, respecting, and appropriately responding to the cultural contexts of clients (Sue, 2001). This approach is crucial for fostering resilience in culturally diverse children.

Culturally responsive interventions are tailored to meet the specific needs of children from diverse backgrounds. These interventions often include elements that reflect the child's cultural heritage, helping them to feel valued and understood. For example, incorporating cultural stories, practices, and values into therapy can enhance engagement and effectiveness (Bernal & Domenech Rodríguez, 2012).

A study by Boustani et al. (2015) demonstrated the effectiveness of a culturally adapted intervention for Latino children with anxiety. The intervention included culturally relevant examples and incorporated family involvement, leading to significant improvements in anxiety symptoms. Such findings underscore the importance of cultural adaptation in mental health interventions.

The benefits of culturally responsive interventions extend beyond immediate symptom relief, contributing to long-term mental health and well-being. These interventions foster a sense of belonging and self-worth in children by validating their cultural identities (Nguyen et al., 2020). This validation is crucial for developing resilience and coping mechanisms that children can rely on throughout their lives.

Recent research has explored various methods of cultural adaptation in therapeutic settings. For instance, interventions for Indigenous children often incorporate traditional healing practices and community rituals. These culturally grounded approaches not only respect Indigenous knowledge systems but also enhance the therapeutic alliance by aligning treatment with the child's worldview (Hartmann et al., 2019).

Similarly, in working with African American children, integrating elements such as historical awareness and community strength into therapy can be particularly beneficial. A study by Stevenson et al. (2019) highlighted the effectiveness of incorporating racial socialization practices into interventions for African American youth. This approach, which includes discussing racial identity and coping with racial discrimination, has been shown to reduce stress and promote positive mental health outcomes.

Family and community play a pivotal role in the success of culturally responsive interventions. Engaging families in the therapeutic process ensures that interventions are culturally congruent and supported within the child's home environment. Family-based interventions that incorporate cultural values and practices are more likely to be effective and sustainable (Yasui & Dishion, 2007).

Community involvement is also essential. Schools and mental health practitioners can collaborate with community leaders and cultural organizations to create supportive networks for children. These collaborations can help to bridge the gap between home and school environments, providing consistent support for the child's mental health (Maria Coll et al., 2014).

Schools are a critical setting for implementing culturally responsive interventions. Teachers and school counselors can incorporate cultural elements into their interactions with students, creating an inclusive environment that fosters engagement and learning. Culturally responsive teaching practices, such as using diverse cultural references in lessons and promoting multicultural awareness, have been shown to improve academic outcomes and student well-being (Gay, 2018).

One example of a successful school-based intervention is the implementation of Social and Emotional Learning (SEL) programs that are culturally adapted. Research by Jagers et al. (2019) indicates that culturally responsive SEL programs, which include culturally relevant content and respect for cultural differences, can significantly enhance students' social and emotional skills, leading to better academic performance and reduced behavioral issues.

Despite the clear benefits, there are challenges in implementing culturally responsive interventions. Practitioners must be adequately trained in cultural competence and must continuously engage in self-reflection to avoid cultural biases. Additionally, there is a need for more research to identify the most effective components of culturally adapted interventions and to develop guidelines for their implementation (Castro et al., 2010).

Another challenge is the potential for cultural adaptation to be seen as a form of cultural stereotyping if not done thoughtfully. Interventions must be flexible and individualized, recognizing the diversity within cultural groups and avoiding one-size-fits-all approaches (Hall, 2001).

Future research should focus on longitudinal studies to assess the long-term impact of culturally responsive interventions on children's mental health and resilience. It is also important to explore the intersectionality of cultural identity with other factors such as gender, socioeconomic status, and disability to develop a more comprehensive understanding of children's needs (Coll et al., 2021).

Additionally, the integration of technology in culturally responsive interventions offers promising avenues for innovation. Digital tools can provide accessible and scalable mental health support that is culturally tailored, reaching children in diverse and underserved communities (Gearing et al., 2018).

Culturally responsive interventions are essential for meeting the mental health needs of children from diverse backgrounds. By incorporating elements that reflect the child's cultural heritage and engaging families and communities, these interventions enhance engagement, effectiveness, and long-term outcomes. As research and practice continue to evolve, it is crucial to prioritize cultural competence in mental health and educational settings to foster resilience and well-being in all children.

Family and community engagement are vital components of effective mental health support for culturally diverse children. Engaging families in the intervention process ensures that the support provided is consistent with the child's cultural background and family values (García Coll & Szalacha, 2004).

Research by Kumpfer, Alvarado, Smith, and Bellamy (2002) highlights the effectiveness of family-based interventions in promoting resilience among children. These interventions often involve educating parents about mental health, providing tools for effective parenting, and fostering strong family bonds. Community engagement, including collaboration with cultural and religious leaders, can also enhance the relevance and acceptance of mental health interventions.

Schools play a crucial role in fostering resilience and supporting the mental health of culturally diverse children. School-based programs that integrate social-emotional learning (SEL) and culturally responsive practices have shown promise in promoting resilience (Durlak et al., 2011; CASEL, 2020).

For instance, the Positive Behavioral Interventions and Supports (PBIS) framework has been adapted to include cultural responsiveness. Research by McIntosh, Moniz, Craft, Golby, and Steinwand-Deschambeault (2014) found that culturally responsive PBIS practices improved school climate and reduced disciplinary incidents among minority students.

Mindfulness practices, which involve paying attention to the present moment without judgment, have been integrated into interventions for young children to promote emotional regulation and resilience. Studies suggest that mindfulness can help children manage stress, improve focus, and enhance emotional well-being (Semple & Helen, 2011; Zelazo & Lyons, 2012).

Integrating cultural elements into mindfulness practices can further enhance their effectiveness. For example, using culturally relevant metaphors and stories in mindfulness exercises can help children from diverse backgrounds connect with the practice more deeply (Gonzalez et al., 2016).

While the trends in fostering resilience among culturally diverse children are promising, several challenges and considerations must be addressed to ensure the effectiveness of these interventions.

Cultural stigma surrounding mental health issues can be a significant barrier to seeking and receiving help. In many cultures, mental health problems are viewed as a sign of weakness or moral failing, which can discourage families from seeking support (Whaley, 2001; Conner et al., 2010). Addressing this stigma requires culturally sensitive education and outreach efforts that normalize mental health issues and emphasize the importance of seeking help.

Language barriers can impede access to mental health services for children and families who are not proficient in the dominant language. Providing services in the child's native language and employing bilingual staff can mitigate this barrier. Additionally, translating educational materials and using culturally relevant communication styles can enhance understanding and engagement (Pew Research Center, 2013).

Effective implementation of culturally responsive interventions requires that mental health practitioners and educators receive adequate training in cultural competence. This training should include an understanding of the cultural backgrounds of the children they serve, awareness of their own cultural biases, and strategies for incorporating cultural elements into their practice (Sue et al., 2009).

Despite the progress in this field, there are still gaps in research that need to be addressed. More studies are needed to evaluate the long-term effectiveness of culturally adapted interventions and to identify the specific components that contribute to their success. Additionally, research should explore the intersectionality of cultural diversity with other factors, such as socioeconomic status and disability, to provide a more comprehensive understanding of how to support resilience in diverse populations (Ungar, 2013).

METHODS

Research Design

This case study employed a qualitative research design to explore the intersection of mental health and cultural diversity in young children, focusing specifically on fostering resilience. The study centered on the experiences of Jamal, a young Somali immigrant at Maplewood Elementary School, and the interventions implemented to support his mental health and well-being.

Participants

The primary participant in this study was Jamal, a seven-year-old boy from a Somali immigrant family. Secondary participants included Jamal's parents, Mr. and Mrs. Hassan, and key school staff members at Maplewood Elementary, including the principal Ms. Maria, school counselor Ms. Helen, and classroom teacher Mr. George. Community leaders from the Somali community were also involved to provide cultural insights and support.

Data Collection Methods

Data collection involved multiple methods to ensure a comprehensive understanding of Jamal's experiences and the effectiveness of the interventions. These methods included:

1. **Interviews**: Semi-structured interviews were conducted with Jamal's parents, school staff, and community leaders. The interviews aimed to gather detailed information about Jamal's background, the challenges he faced, and the support provided by the school. The interview guide included questions about cultural perceptions of mental health, the family's experiences with trauma, and their interactions with the school.
2. **Observations**: Classroom observations were conducted to assess Jamal's behavior, engagement, and interactions with peers and teachers. Observations focused on changes in Jamal's participation and emotional expressions before and after the implementation of support strategies.
3. **Document Analysis**: Relevant school records, including attendance records, academic reports, and notes from counseling sessions, were reviewed to track Jamal's progress over time. Additionally, cultural materials integrated into the classroom, such as books and activities reflecting Somali culture, were analyzed.
4. **Focus Groups**: Focus group discussions were held with teachers and school staff to gather collective insights into the challenges and successes of implementing culturally responsive mental health support. These discussions provided a broader perspective on the school's approach and its impact on students.

Procedure

The study was conducted over six months, following these key steps:

1. **Initial Assessment**: The process began with an initial assessment meeting involving Jamal's parents, school staff, and a Somali-speaking counselor. This meeting aimed to build rapport, understand Jamal's background, and identify his specific needs.
2. **Development of Support Plan**: Based on the initial assessment, a culturally responsive support plan was developed. This plan included integrating cultural practices into the classroom, providing tailored mental health support, and enhancing social support through peer interactions.
3. **Implementation**: The support plan was implemented over three months. Key interventions included:
   - Integrating Somali cultural materials into the curriculum.
   - Conducting regular mindfulness and relaxation sessions tailored to Jamal's needs.
   - Establishing a buddy system to foster peer support.
   - Organizing regular meetings with Jamal's parents and community leaders to ensure ongoing communication and support.

4. **Monitoring and Adjustment**: Throughout the implementation period, Jamal's progress was monitored through observations, interviews, and document analysis. Adjustments to the support plan were made as needed based on feedback from Jamal, his parents, and school staff.
5. **Final Evaluation**: After three months of implementation, a final evaluation was conducted to assess the effectiveness of the interventions. This evaluation included follow-up interviews with participants, a review of Jamal's academic and behavioral records, and a final focus group discussion with school staff.

Data Analysis

Data collected through interviews, observations, document analysis, and focus groups were analyzed using thematic analysis. The process involved:

1. All interviews and focus group discussions were transcribed verbatim to ensure accuracy.
2. Transcripts were coded to identify key themes and patterns related to cultural diversity, mental health, and resilience. Initial codes were generated based on the research questions and refined through iterative review.
3. Codes were grouped into broader themes that captured the essence of the data. Themes included cultural stigma, integration of cultural practices, parental engagement, and the impact of social support.
4. The themes were interpreted in the context of existing literature on mental health and cultural diversity. This interpretation aimed to understand how the interventions influenced Jamal's resilience and well-being.

Ethical Considerations

The study adhered to ethical guidelines to ensure the well-being and confidentiality of participants. Key ethical considerations included:

1. Informed consent was obtained from Jamal's parents and assent from Jamal. Participants were informed about the study's purpose, procedures, and their right to withdraw at any time.
2. All personal information was kept confidential. Pseudonyms were used in reporting to protect participants' identities.

3. The study design and data collection methods were culturally sensitive. A Somali-speaking counselor was involved to facilitate communication and understanding, and cultural norms and values were respected throughout the process.
4. The interventions were designed to support Jamal's well-being without causing additional stress. Regular check-ins ensured that the support provided was beneficial and not overwhelming.

Limitations

The study had several limitations that should be acknowledged:

1. As a single case study, the findings are specific to Jamal's context and may not be generalizable to all immigrant children or cultural groups.
2. The study was conducted over six months, which may not be sufficient to capture long-term impacts of the interventions.
3. Data from interviews and focus groups are subject to self-reporting bias, as participants may provide socially desirable responses.

Despite these limitations, the study provides valuable insights into the intersection of mental health and cultural diversity in young children and highlights the importance of culturally responsive practices in fostering resilience.

In the bustling, diverse city of Athens, the Maplewood Elementary School was a microcosm of the city's cultural mosaic. The school's principal, Ms. Maria, was acutely aware of the unique challenges faced by her students, particularly those from diverse cultural backgrounds. Her mission was clear: to foster resilience in these young children by addressing their mental health needs through culturally responsive practices.

Results

The Case of Jamal

Jamal, a seven-year-old boy in the second grade, was one of Ms. Maria's students. He came from a Somali immigrant family and had recently moved to Athens. Jamal's parents, having fled from conflict, were trying to rebuild their lives in a new country.

Jamal, however, was struggling with the transition. His teachers noticed that he was often withdrawn and seemed to be grappling with feelings of anxiety and sadness.

Jamal's situation was not unique. Research indicates that immigrant children often face significant stressors, including language barriers, cultural adjustments, and the trauma associated with displacement (Beiser, 2009; Fazel, Reed, Panter-Brick, & Stein, 2012). These factors can significantly impact their mental health and overall well-being.

Initial Assessment and Challenges

Ms. Maria initiated a meeting with Jamal's parents to better understand his background and current challenges. With the help of a Somali-speaking counselor, they learned about the traumatic experiences the family had endured. Jamal's father, Mr. Hassan, expressed concerns about Jamal's emotional state but was unsure how to help him.

One significant challenge was the cultural stigma associated with mental health within Jamal's community. Mental health issues were often seen as a personal weakness or a source of shame (Whaley, 2001). This cultural perspective made it difficult for Jamal's parents to seek and accept help, further complicating his situation.

Developing a Culturally Responsive Approach

Understanding these complexities, Ms. Maria and her team, including school counselor Ms. Helen and classroom teacher Mr. George, decided to develop a culturally responsive support plan for Jamal. Their approach was guided by the principles of cultural competence, which emphasizes understanding and respecting cultural differences in mental health care (Sue, Zane, Nagayama Hall, & Berger, 2009).

Step 1: Building Trust and Open Communication

Ms. Maria recognized the importance of building trust with Jamal's family. They organized regular meetings with Mr. Hassan and involved community leaders who were respected within the Somali community. These leaders helped bridge the gap between the school and the family, facilitating open communication and reducing the stigma around mental health.

Step 2: Integrating Cultural Practices

To make Jamal feel more connected and understood, the school integrated aspects of Somali culture into their support strategies. For example, they included stories and materials that reflected Jamal's cultural heritage in the classroom. This helped Jamal feel a sense of pride and belonging, which is crucial for his emotional well-being (Phinney, Horenczyk, Liebkind, & Vedder, 2001).

Step 3: Providing Tailored Mental Health Support

Ms. Helen, the school counselor, introduced mindfulness and relaxation techniques tailored to Jamal's needs. Recognizing that traditional therapy might not be immediately accepted, she incorporated storytelling and drawing, which were culturally familiar methods for expressing emotions. These activities helped Jamal articulate his feelings in a non-threatening way.

Step 4: Enhancing Social Support

Jamal was paired with a buddy in class, another student who had also recently moved to Athens. This buddy system helped Jamal build a friendship and navigate his new environment. The school also organized group activities that encouraged peer interaction and support, fostering a sense of community among students.

Outcomes and Reflections

Over the next few months, the positive changes in Jamal were evident. He began participating more in class and showed signs of improved emotional health. His father, Mr. Hassan, also became more engaged with the school, attending parent meetings and workshops on supporting children's mental health.

The school's culturally responsive approach not only helped Jamal but also provided valuable insights into supporting other students from diverse backgrounds. Ms. Maria and her team reflected on several key lessons:

1. Understanding and respecting cultural differences is crucial in addressing mental health needs effectively. Schools must invest in training staff to develop cultural competence (Sue et al., 2009).
2. Engaging community leaders and leveraging community resources can bridge gaps and reduce stigma, facilitating better mental health support for students (Betancourt et al., 2011).
3. Addressing mental health in schools requires a holistic approach that includes academic support, social integration, and emotional well-being. Tailoring interventions to fit cultural contexts can enhance their effectiveness.

4. Actively involving parents in the process and providing them with tools and knowledge to support their children is critical. Overcoming cultural barriers and building trust are essential steps in this engagement.

Discussion

The findings of this study emphasize the significant role that cultural diversity plays in shaping the mental health and resilience of young children. As globalization continues to diversify educational environments, it is crucial for mental health practitioners and educators to adopt culturally responsive practices. This discussion will integrate recent literature to highlight key insights and implications for practice.

The effectiveness of culturally responsive interventions is well-supported by recent research. Such interventions are tailored to reflect the cultural heritage of children, thereby enhancing their engagement and therapeutic outcomes. For instance, the study by Boustani et al. (2015) demonstrated significant improvements in anxiety symptoms among Latino children through culturally adapted interventions that incorporated family involvement and culturally relevant examples. This aligns with the broader literature that underscores the necessity of cultural adaptation in mental health interventions to address unique stressors such as discrimination, language barriers, and cultural dissonance (García Coll et al., 1996; Pachter & Coll, 2009).

Recent trends in mental health and educational practices increasingly focus on cultural competence, which involves understanding, respecting, and appropriately responding to the cultural contexts of clients (Sue, 2001). This approach is crucial for fostering resilience in culturally diverse children. For example, incorporating cultural stories, practices, and values into therapy not only makes the therapy more relevant but also helps children feel valued and understood (Bernal & Domenech Rodríguez, 2012).

Moreover, the inclusion of cultural competence in school settings has shown promising results. Culturally responsive teaching, which integrates students' cultural backgrounds into the curriculum, has been shown to improve academic outcomes and student well-being (Gay, 2018). This is further supported by Jagers et al. (2019), who found that culturally responsive Social and Emotional Learning (SEL) programs significantly enhance students' social and emotional skills, leading to better academic performance and reduced behavioral issues.

The role of family and community in supporting culturally diverse children cannot be overstated. Engaging families in the therapeutic process ensures that interventions are culturally congruent and supported within the child's home environment (Yasui & Dishion, 2007). Additionally, community involvement provides a broader support network that can reinforce the positive impacts of school-based interventions (Maria

Coll et al., 2014). This community-centric approach is particularly important in creating an inclusive environment that respects and celebrates cultural diversity.

Despite the benefits, implementing culturally responsive practices poses several challenges. Practitioners must undergo continuous training to develop and maintain cultural competence. This training should include self-reflection to recognize and mitigate personal biases (Betancourt et al., 2002). Furthermore, there is a need for more research to identify effective components of culturally adapted interventions and to establish clear guidelines for their implementation (Castro et al., 2010).

Another challenge is the potential for cultural adaptation to inadvertently perpetuate cultural stereotypes. It is essential for interventions to be flexible and individualized, recognizing the diversity within cultural groups and avoiding one-size-fits-all approaches (Hall, 2001).

CONCLUSIONS

The case of Jamal at the elementary school illustrates the intersection of mental health and cultural diversity in young children. It highlights the importance of culturally responsive practices in fostering resilience and supporting the mental well-being of students from diverse backgrounds. By addressing the unique challenges faced by immigrant and culturally diverse students, schools can create inclusive environments where all children have the opportunity to thrive.

The success of Jamal's story underscores a broader message: mental health support in education must be adaptable, culturally informed, and inclusive. As educators, policymakers, and mental health professionals continue to collaborate, the lessons learned from cases like Jamal's can guide the development of more effective and compassionate support systems for all students.

REFERENCES

Alegría, M., Green, J. G., McLaughlin, K. A., & Loder, S. (2010). *Disparities in child and adolescent mental health and mental health services in the US*. National Research Council.

Argyriadi, A., & Argyriadis, A. (2022). Recommended Interventions for the Promotion of Language Development for Children With Learning Difficulties. In *Rethinking Inclusion and Transformation in Special Education* (pp. 143–159). IGI Global. DOI: 10.4018/978-1-6684-4680-5.ch009

Argyriadis, A., Efthymiou, E., & Argyriadis, A. (2023). Cultural Competence at Schools: The Effectiveness of Educational Leaders' Intervention Strategies. In *Inclusive Phygital Learning Approaches and Strategies for Students With Special Needs* (pp. 33-51). IGI Global.

Argyriadis, A., Ioannidou, L., Dimitrakopoulos, I., Gourni, M., Ntimeri, G., Vlachou, C., & Argyriadi, A. (2023, March). Experimental mindfulness intervention in an emergency department for stress management and development of positive working environment. []. MDPI.]. *Health Care*, 11(6), 879. PMID: 36981535

Argyriadis, A., Paoullis, P., Samsari, E., & Argyriadi, A. (2023). Self-Assessment Inclusion Scale (SAIS): A tool for measuring inclusive competence and sensitivity. *Perspectives in Education*, 41(4), 34–49. DOI: 10.38140/pie.v41i4.7294

Auerbach, S. (2010). Beyond coffee with the principal: Toward leadership for authentic school-family partnerships. *Journal of School Leadership*, 20(6), 728–757. DOI: 10.1177/105268461002000603

Banks, J. A. (2015). *Cultural diversity and education*. Routledge. DOI: 10.4324/9781315622255

Beiser, M. (2009). Resettling refugees and safeguarding their mental health: Lessons learned from the Canadian refugee resettlement project. *Transcultural Psychiatry*, 46(4), 539–583. DOI: 10.1177/1363461509351373 PMID: 20028677

Benjet, C., Kazdin, A. E., & Spence, S. H. (2019). Prevention of mental health problems: Worldwide priorities. *International Journal of Mental Health Systems*, 13(1), 1–14.

Benner, A. D., Wang, Y., Shen, Y., Boyle, A. E., Polk, R., & Cheng, Y.-P. (2018). Racial/ethnic discrimination and well-being during adolescence: A meta-analytic review. *The American Psychologist*, 73(7), 855–883. DOI: 10.1037/amp0000204 PMID: 30024216

Bernal, G., & Domenech Rodríguez, M. M. (2012). *Cultural adaptations: Tools for evidence-based practice with diverse populations.* American Psychological Association. DOI: 10.1037/13752-000

Betancourt, T. S., McBain, R., Newnham, E. A., & Brennan, R. T. (2011). The intergenerational impact of war: Longitudinal relationships between caregiver and child mental health in postconflict Sierra Leone. *Journal of Child Psychology and Psychiatry, and Allied Disciplines*, 52(9), 1086–1095. PMID: 25665018

Betancourt, T. S., McBain, R., Newnham, E. A., & Brennan, R. T. (2011). The intergenerational impact of war: longitudinal relationships between caregiver and child mental health in postconflict Sierra Leone. *Journal of Child Psychology and Psychiatry, 52*(9), 1086-1095.

Boustani, M. M., Frazier, S. L., Becker, K. D., Bechor, M., Dinizulu, S. M., Hedemann, E. R., Ogle, R. R., & Pasalich, D. S. (2015). Common elements of adolescent prevention programs: Minimizing burden while maximizing the reach. *Administration and Policy in Mental Health*, 42(2), 209–219. DOI: 10.1007/s10488-014-0541-9 PMID: 24504979

Campinha-Bacote, J. (2002). The process of cultural competence in the delivery of healthcare services: A model of care. *Journal of Transcultural Nursing*, 13(3), 181–184. DOI: 10.1177/10459602013003003 PMID: 12113146

Castro, F. G., Barrera, M.Jr, & Martinez, C. R.Jr. (2010). The cultural adaptation of prevention interventions: Resolving tensions between fidelity and fit. *Prevention Science*, 5(1), 41–45. DOI: 10.1023/B:PREV.0000013980.12412.cd PMID: 15058911

Coll, C. G.. (2021). An integrative model for the study of developmental competencies in minority children. *Child Development*, 71(4), 1124–1140.

Cross, T. L., Bazron, B. J., Dennis, K. W., & Isaacs, M. R. (1989). *Toward a culturally competent system of care: A monograph on effective services for minority children who are severely emotionally disturbed* (Vol. 1). Georgetown University Child Development Center.

Fazel, M., Reed, R. V., Panter-Brick, C., & Stein, A. (2012). Mental health of displaced and refugee children resettled in low-income and middle-income countries: Risk and protective factors. *Lancet*, 379(9812), 250–265. DOI: 10.1016/S0140-6736(11)60051-2 PMID: 21835460

Gándara, P., & Hopkins, M. (Eds.). (2010). *Forbidden language: English learners and restrictive language policies.* Teachers College Press.

Gay, G. (2018). *Culturally responsive teaching: Theory, research, and practice.* Teachers College Press.

Gearing, R. E., MacKenzie, M. J., Ibrahim, R. W., Brewer, K. B., Batayneh, J. S., & Schwalbe, C. S. (2018). Adaptation and translation of mental health interventions in middle eastern arab countries: A systematic review of barriers to and strategies for effective treatment implementation. *The International Journal of Social Psychiatry,* 59(7), 671–681. DOI: 10.1177/0020764012452349 PMID: 22820177

Gorski, P. C. (2016). *Reaching and teaching students in poverty: Strategies for erasing the opportunity gap.* Teachers College Press.

Hall, G. C. N. (2001). Psychotherapy research with ethnic minorities: Empirical, ethical, and conceptual issues. *Journal of Consulting and Clinical Psychology,* 69(3), 502–510. DOI: 10.1037/0022-006X.69.3.502 PMID: 11495179

Hartmann, W. E., Wendt, D. C., Saftner, M. D., Marcus, J. D., & Momper, S. L. (2019). Advancing community-based participatory research with culturally grounded technology: Development of the healing pathways app. *Journal of Psychotherapy Integration,* 29(1), 14.

Jagers, R. J., Rivas-Drake, D., & Williams, B. (2019). Transformative social and emotional learning (SEL): Toward SEL in service of educational equity and excellence. *Educational Psychologist,* 54(3), 162–184. DOI: 10.1080/00461520.2019.1623032

Jeynes, W. H. (2012). A meta-analysis of the efficacy of different types of parental involvement programs for urban students. *Urban Education,* 47(4), 706–742. DOI: 10.1177/0042085912445643

Jones, S. M., Greenberg, M., & Crowley, M. (2015). Early social-emotional functioning and public health: The relationship between kindergarten social competence and future wellness. *American Journal of Public Health,* 105(11), 2283–2290. DOI: 10.2105/AJPH.2015.302630 PMID: 26180975

Kumpfer, K. L., Magalhães, C., & Xie, J. (2012). Cultural adaptations of evidence-based family interventions to strengthen families and improve children's developmental outcomes. *European Journal of Developmental Psychology,* 9(1), 104–116. DOI: 10.1080/17405629.2011.639225

Ladson-Billings, G. (1995). Toward a theory of culturally relevant pedagogy. *American Educational Research Journal,* 32(3), 465–491. DOI: 10.3102/00028312032003465

Maria, O., Kleifgen, J. A., & Falchi, L. (2008). *From English language learners to emergent bilinguals. Equity Matters: Research Review No. 1.* Teachers College, Columbia University.

Nguyen, L., Helen, R. M., & Tsai, J. L. (2020). The effects of cultural adaptation on intervention efficacy: A meta-analytic review. *Journal of Consulting and Clinical Psychology*, 88(8), 694–705.

Ogbu, J. U. (1992). Understanding cultural diversity and learning. *Educational Researcher*, 21(8), 5–14. DOI: 10.3102/0013189X021008005

Pachter, L. M., & Coll, C. G. (2009). Racism and child health: A review of the literature and future directions. *Journal of Developmental and Behavioral Pediatrics*, 30(3), 255–263. DOI: 10.1097/DBP.0b013e3181a7ed5a PMID: 19525720

Phinney, J. S., Horenczyk, G., Liebkind, K., & Vedder, P. (2001). Ethnic identity, immigration, and well-being: An interactional perspective. *The Journal of Social Issues*, 57(3), 493–510. DOI: 10.1111/0022-4537.00225

Priest, N., Paradies, Y., Trenerry, B., Truong, M., Karlsen, S., & Kelly, Y. (2013). A systematic review of studies examining the relationship between reported racism and health and wellbeing for children and young people. *Social Science & Medicine*, 95, 115–127. DOI: 10.1016/j.socscimed.2012.11.031 PMID: 23312306

Rutter, M. (2012). Resilience as a dynamic concept. *Development and Psychopathology*, 24(2), 335–344. DOI: 10.1017/S0954579412000028 PMID: 22559117

Sheridan, S. M., Kunz, G. M., & Holmes, S. R. (2019). Family-school partnerships in context: Relations between parent-teacher partnership perceptions and student outcomes in a diverse, low-income population. *The Elementary School Journal*, 120(1), 47–73.

Southwick, S. M., Bonanno, G. A., Masten, A. S., Panter-Brick, C., & Yehuda, R. (2014). Resilience definitions, theory, and challenges: Interdisciplinary perspectives. *European Journal of Psychotraumatology*, 5(1), 25338. DOI: 10.3402/ejpt.v5.25338 PMID: 25317257

Stevenson, H. C., Davis, G. Y., & Abdul-Kabir, S. (2019). Stickin' to, watchin' over, and gettin' with: An African American parent's guide to discipline. *Family Relations*, 49(4), 328–336.

Sue, S. (2001). *Cultural competency: From philosophy to research and practice.* Springer.

Sugai, G., & Horner, R. (2020). Sustaining and scaling positive behavioral interventions and supports: Implementation drivers, outcomes, and considerations. *Psychology in the Schools*, 57(5), 882–903.

Ungar, M. (2013). Resilience, trauma, context, and culture. *Trauma, Violence & Abuse*, 14(3), 255–266. DOI: 10.1177/1524838013487805 PMID: 23645297

Villegas, A. M., & Lucas, T. (2002). Preparing culturally responsive teachers: Rethinking the curriculum. *Journal of Teacher Education*, 53(1), 20–32. DOI: 10.1177/0022487102053001003

Whaley, A. L. (2001). Cultural mistrust: An important psychological construct for diagnosis and treatment of African Americans. *Professional Psychology: Research and Practice, 32*(6), 555.

Chapter 11
Depression in Children With Educational Needs Who Attend Integration Classes

Asteropi Polykandrioti
https://orcid.org/0009-0003-5470-7079
University of Athens, Greece

Maria Malikiosi
https://orcid.org/0000-0002-2925-0711
University of Athens, Greece

ABSTRACT

The aim of this study was to examine depressive symptoms in typically developing children and in children with dyslexia, attention deficit/hyperactive disorder, and autism spectrum disorder. Participants were 120 children; 60 of them were diagnosed with these disorders and attended inclusive classrooms, whereas 60 were typically developing children. All children completed the Children's Depression Inventory as developed by Kovacs. Results indicated that children with dyslexia, attention deficit/ hyperactive disorder, and autism spectrum disorder had significantly higher scores on depression than typically developing children. The strongest differences were found in anhedonia, interpersonal problems, negative self-esteem, ineffectiveness, and negative mood. These findings underline the need for teachers and parents to provide emotional and social support to children with specific learning difficulties and developmental disorders to reduce the negative impact of these disorders and enhance children's resilience.

DOI: 10.4018/979-8-3693-5325-7.ch011

Depression is currently conceptualized to be similar to depression in adults. While children may not frustration tolerance, somatic symptoms, and withdrawn behavior. Symptoms of depression vary as per age and developmental level; affective symptoms and cognitive distortions in childhood are similar to adults, whereas biological symptoms such as changes in sleep and appetite are different. Negative cognitions such as low self-esteem, hopelessness, and negative attributions are common in children. They are wilting, disorganized, and negative in the cognitive triad: self, others, and catastrophic future scenarios. (Brown et al., 2011; Luby et al., 2003; Kakouros & Maniadaki, 2006; Madianos, 2003; Papageorgiou 2005).

Their clinical picture is expressed with feelings of anger and anhedonia, while their games have themes of suicide or death (Luby et al., 2003). If the symptoms persist, we refer to depression as a disorder (APA, 2000; Kakouros & Maniadaki, 2006; Papageorgiou, 2005; Verduyn et al., 2009; Trikkas, 2005).

Comorbid psychiatric disorders are seen in 80%–95% of children and adolescents with depression. Anxiety disorders, conduct disorders, and attention deficit hyperactivity disorder are common, with the most common comorbidity being separation anxiety disorder in children.

Children with learning disabilities and neurodevelopmental disorders are a high-risk group for the appearance of the disorder (Arnold et al., 2005; Carroll et al., 2005; Grigorenko, 2001). Suicidal ideation seems to be rare but not nonexistent (Arnold et al., 2005; Carrol & Illes, 2006; Lindsay & Docrell, 2002; Maag & Reid, 2006; Mayes et al., 2009).

The above is due to the high levels of anxiety and depression due to the difficulties they face within the family and at school (Carroll et al., 2005; Maag & Reid, 2006). In the family environment, children disrupt the family fabric. In the school environment, the bad interaction with the teacher and the great concern about his academic achievements cause stress and sadness (Brown, 2009; Kampanarou, 2007; Mitsiu-Daktyla, 2008).

Children with attention deficit hyperactive disorder are likely to show high rates of depression (Blackman et al., 2005; Leirbakk et al., 2015). However, if they present with comorbid depression, they manifest more severe psychopathology than those with only ADHD (Biederman et al., 2008; Blackman et al., 2005; Burke et al., 2005; Daviss, Weinman, Diler & Birmaher, 2006b; Pliszka & AACAP-Work-Group-on-Quality issues, 2007).

A high-risk factor for the onset of depression is the difficulty of integrating these children into peer groups due to inattention and sloppiness in regulating interpersonal relationships (Hoza et al., 2005).

In children with high-functioning autism, the difficulty of detecting depression lies in the fact that they have cognitive, social and communication deficits (Gena, 2002; Simonoff et al., 2008; Stewart et al., 2006; Francis, 2007), show instability in mood and are often unnecessarily irritable and aggressive (Perry et al., 2001; Pollard & Prendergast, 2004; Skinner et al., 2005).

The above is usually the result of sensory overload and deficits in theory of mind. The admission of multiple environmental stimuli makes children unable to manage them. The need for discharge is excellent and often manifests inelegantly and aggressively (Attwood, 2006; Gena, 2002; Francis, 2007).

However, there are no studies detailing the exact symptomatology of the depressive episode in children with autism. What we know is from the testimonies of their relatives (Ghaziuddin M. et al., 2002; Janowsky & Davis, 2005).

MATERIALS AND METHODS

Participants

The present research was carried out in five schools of Salamina island. The sample consisted of 120 children aged 8 to 12. Sixty-three children of the sample were of typical development and the 58 children attended integration classes. The latter are divided into three categories: 25 children were dyslexic, 13 children were in the autism spectrum disorders (Asperger syndrome), and 20 children had attention deficit hyperactive disorder. The instrument administered is the CDI.

Measure

The first psychometric tool used was the Children Depression Inventory, which contains 27 questions (Kovacs, 1992). Each question is scored 0 for no depressive symptoms, 1 for mild symptoms, and 2 for severe symptoms. The total score ranges from 0-54. Its reliability and validity (Cronbach's alpha, ranging from 0.71 to 0.87) are considerable, as it has been used in many countries and in large population samples, both clinical and non-clinical (Charman & Petrova, 2000; Samm et. al. 2007). It is divided into five subcategories: Anhedonia, Inefficacy, Interpersonal Problems, Negative Mood, and Negative Self-Esteem (Giannakopoulos et al., 2009).

Anhedonia is defined as a person's inability to experience pleasure from activities they used to enjoy (Brown, et. al., 2011; Cohen et al., 2012).

Self-efficacy has been found to be consistently related to academic achievement. It has been found that self-efficacy is one of the four dimensions of children's classroom-related well-being and motivation to learn. Self-efficacy in school-aged children is related the belief that they are capable of performing a task or managing a situation. It is about learning how to persevere when one does not succeed at first.

When a child equates success to internal factors, they develop a sense of mastery, which reinforces stronger self-efficacy beliefs. (Hanicke & Broadbent, 2016).

Negative emotions, appear to have a core of emotional pain, with two primary negative emotion mood states (depression/despair and fear/anxiety) and two negative social emotional states of shame/guilt (negative feelings about self) and hate/anger (negative feelings about others). They could, therefore, be defined as a non-smooth emotional response (Guhn et al., 2018).

Self-efficacy in school-aged children is related to the ability to respond to the learning process to achieve academic projects (Hanicke & Broadbent, 2016). We define a negative mood as a non-smooth emotional response (Guhn et al., 2018). Negative self-esteem is the lack of a healthy self-image, i.e., the set of strengths and weaknesses of the individual.

Interpersonal problems refer to the difficulty of creating and maintaining healthy interpersonal relationships and resolving interpersonal conflicts (Collaborative for Academic Social and Emotional Learning, 2003).

The questionnaire of Kovacs (1992) was translated two times by direct and reverse translation in order to compare with the questions that exist in the English language and to render them in Greek in such a way as not to distort their meaning (Giannakopoulos et al., 2009).

Procedure

Initially, the researcher contacted the principals of the schools, as well as the teaching staff, in order to explain the aim of the research. Then, parental consents were given, in order to inform the parents about the importance and the purpose of the research and the anonymity of the personal data, as it is governed by the code of ethics.

Results of the Childhood Depression Inventory (CDI)

First, the results were checked for internal reliability and normality. Regarding the Child Depression Inventory (CDI), it appeared that Cronbach's alpha index is adequate for all subscales, ranging between 0.6 and 0.77. For the overall Child Depression Inventory (CDI), the internal reliability index is adequate, $\alpha = 0.87$ (Table 1).

Table 1. Internal consistency reliability of the Children's Depression Inventory and its subscales

Children's Depression Inventory	Cronbach's alpha
Anhedonia	.61
Inefficiency	.63
Interpersonal problems	.60
Negative self-esteem	.77
Negative mood	.61
Total	.87

Regarding the subscales of the Child Depression Inventory (CDI), Anhedonia, Inefficacy, Interpersonal Problems, and Negative Mood show marginally adequate levels of internal reliability. The highest index of internal reliability is presented by Negative Self-Esteem $\alpha = 0.77$. Due to the small number of participants in the sample, we cannot assume that they follow a normal distribution. To investigate normality, we apply the Sapiro-Wilk test (Table 2).

Table 2. Tests of normality for the Children's Depression Inventory and its subscales

Children's Depression Inventory	Shapiro-Wilk Normality Test
Anhedonia	.000
Inefficiency	.013
Interpersonal problems	.000
Negative self-esteem	.000
Negative mood	.001
Total	.004

Note: Shapiro-Wilk normality test results for the childhood depression subscales

From the table, we conclude that in each subscale and also as a whole, it is observed that the sample does not follow a normal distribution since the Shapiro-Wilk test is statistically significant on the whole. We, therefore, used the non-parametric Kruskal-Wallis test to compare groups of children.

Table 3. Kruskal-Wallis test results for child depression subscales according to children's educational needs

Educational Needs	Children's Depression Inventory	Kruskal-Wallis χ^2	p
	Anhedonia	18.521	.000
Typically developing children	Inefficiency	15.041	.001

continued on following page

Table 3. Continued

Educational Needs	Children's Depression Inventory	Kruskal-Wallis χ^2	p
Dyslexia	Interpersonal problems	29.364	.000
ASD	Negative self-esteem	23.985	.000
ADHD	Negative mood	25.598	.000
	Total	32.981	.000

Hypothesis testing regarding the educational needs of the students: From the Kruskal-Wallis test, it was concluded that there is a statistically significant difference in the comparisons of children with different educational needs regarding the subscales of childhood depression p = 0.000 < 0.05.

According to the above, the total score of the educational needs subscales should be further studied through two-way multiple comparisons of the Kruskal-Wallis test. However, since this test shows which group differs from which, but it is not obvious which group shows higher values, we should plot graphs to decide the direction of the difference.

Table 4. Kruskal-Wallis test results for the Child Depression Inventory by students' educational needs

Childhood Depression Inventory total score	Kruskal-Wallis χ^2	P
Normal children - dyslexia	15.703	.339
Normal children - ASD	34.596	.007
Normal children - ADHD	47.303	.000
Dyslexia – ASD	18.892	.671
Dyslexia – ADHD	31.600	.015
ASD – ADHD	-12.708	1.000

Typically developing children show a statistically significant difference in the values of the Child Depression Inventory (CDI) from children with attention deficit/ hyperactivity disorder, p = 0.000 < 0.05. A statistically significant difference is shown in children with typical development compared to children with autism spectrum disorder, p = 0.007 < 0.05. Also, children with dyslexia show a statistically significant difference from children with attention deficit /hyperactive disorder, p = 0.015 < 0.05.

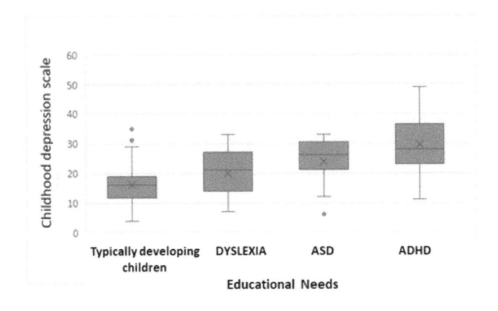

Children's Depression Inventory scores
of the children's subgroups

The Figure 1 shows that children with typical development have lower values than children with autism spectrum disorder and attention-deficit hyperactive disorder. Also, children with dyslexia present lower values than children with attention-deficit hyperactivity disorder (Figure 1).

After considering the above, the same procedure (Kruskal-Wallis multiple comparisons) was followed to compare the children on the child depression subscales (CDI). The following subscales are listed below: Anhedonia, Inefficacy, Interpersonal Problems, Negative Mood, and Negative Self-Esteem.

Table 5. Kruskal-Wallis test results for the Anhedonia subscale according to students' educational needs

Anhedonia	Kruskal-Wallis χ^2	P
Normal children - dyslexia	16.176	.275
Normal children - ASD	31.514	.015
Normal children - ADHD	31.151	.002
Dyslexia - ASD	15.338	1.000

continued on following page

Table 5. Continued

Anhedonia	Kruskal-Wallis χ^2	P
Dyslexia - ADHD	14.975	.866
ASD - ADHD	-0.363	1.000

Children with typical development show a statistically significant difference in the Anhedonia' subscale values from children with attention deficit/ hyperactive disorder, p = 0.002 < 0.05. The same applies to children with autism spectrum disorder, p = 0.015 < 0.05. No statistically significant differences were found in the other groups.

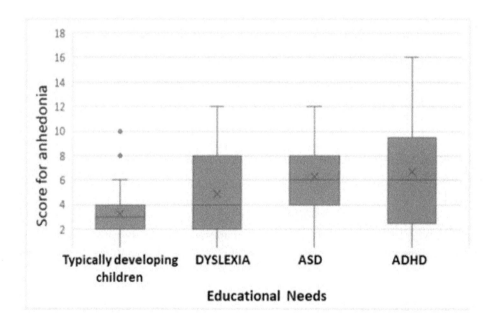

The subscale of anhedonia according to the educational needs of the students

From the Figure 2 above, we notice that children with Typical Development present lower values on the 'Anhedonia' subscale than children with autism spectrum disorder and attention deficit /hyperactive disorder (Figure 2).

Table 6. Kruskal-Wallis test results for the ineffectiveness subscale according to students' educational needs

Ineffectiveness	Kruskal-Wallis χ^2	P
Normal children-dyslexia	6.108	1.000
Normal children - ASD	23.393	.155
Normal children - ADHD	31.208	.003
Dyslexia - ASD	17.285	.850
Dyslexia - ADHD	25.100	.900
ASD - ADHD	-7.815	1.000

Self-efficacy in school-aged children is related to the ability to respond to the learning process to achieve academic projects (Honicke & Broadbent, 2016).

Typically developing children show statistically significant differences in subscale values concerning children with attention deficit hyperactivity disorder, p = 0.003 < 0.05. This is not observed for children with Dyslexia, p = 1.000 > 0.05. However, for children with ASD, p = 0.155 > 0.05. Finally, children with attention deficit/ hyperactive disorder did not present statistically significant differences concerning dyslexic children, p = 0.900 > 0.05, but neither did children with autism spectrum disorder, p = 1.000 > 0.05 (Table 6).

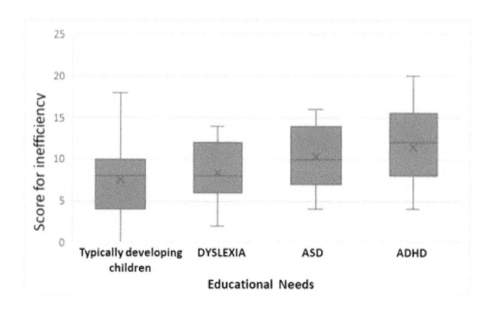

The subscale of ineffectiveness according to the educational needs of the students

From the Figure 3 above, we observe that children with typical development present lower values in the 'Ineffectiveness' subscale than children with attention deficit/ hyperactivity disorder (Figure 3).

Table 7. Kruskal-Wallis test results for the interpersonal problems subscale according to students' educational needs

Interpersonal problems	Kruskal-Wallis χ^2	p
Normal children - dyslexia	12.906	.648
Normal children – ASD	29.922	.023
Normal children - ADHD	44.256	.000
Dyslexia – ASD	17.015	.852
Dyslexia – ADHD	31.350	.012
ASD – ADHD	-14.335	1.000

Typically developing children show a statistically significant difference in the 'Interpersonal Problems' subscale values compared to children with attention deficit hyperactivity disorder with p = 0.000 < 0.05. The same applies to children with autism spectrum disorder with p = 0.023 < 0.05. Also, children with dyslexia show a statistically significant difference in the values of the 'Interpersonal Problems' subscale from children with attention deficit /hyperactive disorder, p = 0.012 < 0.05.

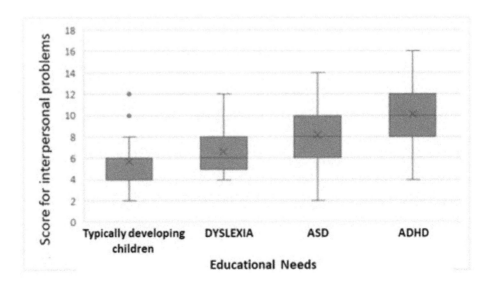

The interpersonal problems subscale according to the educational needs of the students

From the Figure 4 above, we notice that children with typical development have lower values on the 'Interpersonal Problems' subscale than children with autism spectrum disorder and attention deficit /hyperactive disorder (Figure 4). Also, children with dyslexia present lower values than children with attention deficit/ hyperactive disorder;

Table 8. Kruskal-Wallis test results for the negative mood subscale according to children's educational needs

Negative Mood			
		KW X²	P
Normal children-Dyslexia		13.679	0.572
Normal Children-ASD		26.208	0.067
Normal Children- ADHD		42.754	0.000
Dyslexia – ASD		13.123	1.000
Dyslexia – ADHD		29.075	0.031
ASD – ADHD		-15.952	1.000

Typically developing children show a statistically significant difference in the values of the 'Negative Mood' subscale concerning children with attention deficit/ hyperactivity disorder with p= 0.000 < 0.05. Also, children with dyslexia show a statistically significant difference in the values of Negative Mood from children with attention deficit /hyperactive disorder with p = 0.031 < 0.05 (Table 8).

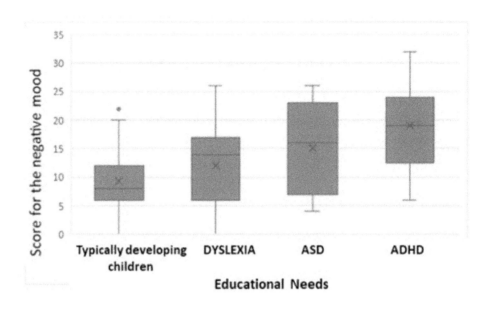

The subscale of negative mood according to the educational needs of the children

As we can conclude from the Figure 5, the children with typical development present lower values than those with attention deficit/ hyperactive disorder. Also, children with dyslexia present lower values than children with attention deficit/ hyperactive disorder (Figure 5).

Table 9. Kruskal-Wallis test results for the negative self-esteem subscale according to children's educational needs

Negative self-esteem	Kruskal-Wallis χ²	P
Normal children – Dyslexia	11.656	.904
Normal children – ASD	18.903	.422
Normal children – ADHD	42.481	.000
Dyslexia – ASD	7.246	1.000
Dyslexia – ADHD	30.825	.016
ASD – ADHD	-23.579	.319

A statistically significant difference is observed in children with typical development compared to children with attention deficit hyperactivity disorder. In the 'Negative Self-Esteem' subscale values, p = 0.000 < 0.05. Also, children with

Dyslexia present a statistically significant difference in the values of Negative Self-Esteem from children with attention deficit /hyperactive disorder., p = 0.016 < 0.05.

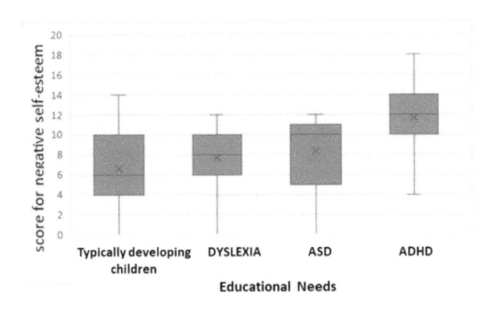

The subscale of negative self-esteem according to the educational needs of the children

The Figure 6 shows that typically developing children show lower values in 'Negative Self-Esteem' than children with attention deficit /hyperactive disorder (ADHD). Also, children with dyslexia present lower values than children with ADHD (Figure 6).

Discussion

The results of our study revealed statistically significant differences between children with typical development and those with dyslexia, attention deficit /hyperactive disorder, and autism spectrum disorder in terms of the scale's sub-factors. Children with the aforementioned disorders appear to be more burdened by anhedonia, interpersonal problems, low self-esteem, self-efficacy, and negative mood (Leyfer et al., 2006; Mundy et al., 2010; Papageorgiou, 2015; Rubin, 2012; Samm, 2007; Schriber et al., 2014; Verduyn et al., 2009).

Anhedonia

We observe a statistically significant difference between children with typical development and children with attention deficit/ hyperactive disorder, $p = 0.002 < 0.05$ and children with autism spectrum disorder, $p = 0.015 < 0.05$ (Table 5) and more specifically the children of Standard Development show lower values (Figure 2). This result can be explained by the very symptomatology of the above developmental disorders (Kempe et al., 2011; Rice, 2010).

Children with attention deficit/ hyperactive disorder very easily lose interest in the things they are engaged in and usually get bored quite quickly. This leads them to a perpetual search for things, which can eventually lead to Anhedonia. Another factor that exacerbates it is the postponement of gratification experienced by children with attention deficit/ hyperactive disorder (Kalantzi-Azizi & Zafeiropoulou, 2011; Melegari et al., 2018; Pliszka, 2011; Stenseng, 2015).

However, the very nature of autism involves a limitation in the expression of feelings and ideas, children show apathy in participatory activities (Gena, 2002; Ghaziuddin et al., 2002; Francis, 2007) because they prefer individual ones with topics that interest them: strange collections, dealing with parts of objects that have motion (Attwood, 2005; Gena, 2002; Francis, 2007).

To motivate children with neurodevelopmental disorders such as ASD and ADHD, the therapeutic use of art is suggested (Leyfer et al., 2006; Mundy et al., 2010; Schriber et al., 2014). Personal albums can be created using a variety of sensory materials. The album could contain useful information for the student such as information about their family, themselves and special talents-achievements (Malchiodi, 2003).

Inefficiency

From the comparison of children with Typical Development and children with attention deficit/ hyperactive disorder, we observe a statistically significant difference, $p = 0.003 < 0.05$ (Table 6). It is concluded that the latter shows higher values in the 'Inefficiency' subscale (Figure 3).

Her finding follows contemporary researchers' findings, which reinforce the collapse of the 'positive illusion' when there is depression (Hoza et al., 2005). From the diagnostic criteria of attention deficit/ hyperactive disorder, we know that children have concentration and organization problems. Numerous times, they lose items that they don't find when it's time to use them. The lack of organizational plans is a sign of a lack of internal organization (Kakouros & Maniadaki, 2006; Kalantzi-Azizi & Zafeiropoulou, 2011; Lougy et al., 2007).

They show a lack of cognitive flexibility, as they themselves move quickly but do not process the information they receive at the same pace (Kalantzi-Azizi & Zafeiropoulou, 2011; Weyandt, 2007). Because of their working memory problems, they do not engage in activities that require cognitive load, because they know they will quickly abandon the efforts (Hoza et al., 2005; Goldrich, 2015; Leirbakk et al; 2015). This is why they prefer carefree activities, such as shearing, construction, and painting (Fisher, 2017).

Upon entering school, children with attention deficit/ hyperactive disorder face problems completing school tasks, which does not help them feel effective.

We know that both children with autism spectrum disorder and children with dyslexia face problems in completing school tasks. Nevertheless, it is easier for them to obey the school rules. Perhaps this is the reason why no statistically significant differences were observed in the two aforementioned educational needs (Madianos et al., 2003; Mitsiu-Daktila, 2008; Mundy et al., 2010). This is in contrast to children with attention deficit/ hyperactive disorder, who are difficult to follow instructions and obey rules (Hoza et al., 2015; Fisher, 2017; Weyandt & Dupaul, 2013).

To enable them to understand the context in which they operate and to be aware of the social norms required, a very useful tool is the DRC (DAILY ROUTINE CARDS). These are checklists that give the opportunity for self-checking but also the awareness of their small achievements. They are easy to use because they are transferred and completed by the child himself (Baley, 2008).

Interpersonal Problems

It is an obvious statistically significant difference between children of Typical Development and children with attention deficit /hyperactive disorder, $p = 0.000 < 0.05$ and children with autism spectrum disorder, $p = 0.023 < 0.05$ (Table 7) and more specifically children of Typical Development have lower values. Also, children with dyslexia have lower values than children with attention deficit /hyperactive disorder.

Regarding those children, the significant statistical difference that exists in the subcategory of interpersonal problems is fully justified, behind the image of "immature Our finding also agrees with another contemporary research (Hoza et al., 2005; Leirbakk et al., 2015; Ostrander et al., 2006).

Upon entering school, the child is progressively marginalized, because he is the one who does not perfect the projects he undertakes and from his incomplete results, he knows that he is different (Harpin et al., 2013) and ultimately, he is also the one who for the clumsiness it will be rejected (Fisher, 2007; Stenseng et al., 2015).

They also exhibit antisocial behaviors, since they do not control their impulses and may display antisocial behavior (Baron-Cohen, 2003; Lombardo & Baron-Cohen, 2011; Koumoula, 2012). They often assume a leadership role in groups or intimidate, using either physical or verbal violence or give orders in order to impose their opinion (Malikiosi–Loizou, 2017; Weyandt & Dupaul, 2013).

Their maladjustment seems to make family relationships difficult as well. Family cohesion is disturbed because of the 'disobedient' child (Harpin et al., 2013 • Johston & Mash, 2015) but also the relationship of the child with attention deficit /hyperactive disorder and his siblings is quite turbulent. The latter are either victimized because of verbal and physical violence or take on a protective role to mitigate their sibling's symptoms of inattention and impulsivity (Harpin et al., 2013).

Children with autism, usually having high intellectual potential, easily perceive their low social inclusion and realize that friendships either lack duration or quality (Mazurek & Kanie, 2010). It is particularly difficult for them to form and maintain friendships, a fact that is at odds with the fact that they themselves seek social contacts but in the wrong way (Ozonoff, et al., 2005).

The finding does not contradict the current research results on social difficulties (Lopata et al., 2010 • Mazurek & Kanie, 2010). After all, they are characterized by deficits in theory of mind, or as we would simply say, they have difficulty recognizing the intentions of others and also putting themselves in their shoes (Baron-Cohen, 2003; Lombardo & Baron-Cohen, 2011; Ozonoff et al., 2005).

Children with dyslexia certainly have problems in accepting homilies. However, they showed lower values than children with attention deficit /hyperactive disorder, in terms of interpersonal problems (Figure 4). This fact is explained, as dyslexia is a specific learning disability and does not have such burdensome symptoms as the other two developmental disorders (Kempe et al., 2011; Trzesniewski et al., 2006).

In order to improve the interaction of children, the method of Comic strip conversation is proposed is an alternative way of communication that allows the child to express himself and perceive the perspectives of others through structured sentences made by the child himself (Gray, 1994).

In addition, another educational proposal is the application of peer counseling: the learning of counseling skills by student volunteers in order to support interlocutors, actively listen to them, and offer them support and encouragement (Malikiosi -Loizou, 2017)

Negative Mood

From the Kruskal-Wallis test, it is observed that children with Typical Development present a statistically significant difference in the values of the subscale 'Negative Mood' from children with attention deficit/ hyperactive disorder ($p = 0.000 < 0.05$.

Also, the same happened in the comparison of children with dyslexia and children with attention deficit/ hyperactive disorder (p = 0.031 < 0.05 (Table 8).

The high score of children with attention deficit/hyperactive disorder is explained by sleep problems, which affect mood and come from the symptomatology of the disorder itself (Harpin et al., 2013; Johston & Mash, 2015; Melegari et al., 2018) but also from the administration of medication, which sometimes has an impact on the instability of their mood. Also, children with attention deficit/ hyperactive disorder have poor emotional control because of which they appear moody and irritable (Kakouros & Maniadaki, 2006; Kalantzi-Azizi & Zafeiropoulou, 2010).

Stressful conflicts with parents, their lack of support contribute to the above. In the school environment, the teacher deals with them, usually to bring them back to class, creating the feeling that he is engaging with the child, only when he has negative behaviors, it results in the child's negative mood (Kakouros & Maniadaki, 2006 · Papadatos, 2010).

Children with dyslexia are likely to experience emotional problems because of the marginalization they receive from their peers (Kempe et al., 2011). Added to this is the difficulty of achieving schoolwork because of reading difficulties. Continuous school failures can become traumatic experiences, with an impact on children's mood (McNulty, 2003 • Mugnaini et al., 2006).

Autism did not appear to have any statistically significant difference regarding Negative Mood (Table 8). Our finding agrees with the international literature, since people with autism spectrum disorder have difficulty in expressing emotions and describing the mood they are in (Baron-Cohen, 2003 • Lombardo & Baron-Cohen, 2011). The incomplete expression of emotions is because of the idiosyncratic use of language, because of which the crystallization of thoughts and the expression of desires are hindered (Baron-Cohen, 2003; Howlin, 2003; Lombardo & Baron-Cohen, 2011; Rice, 2010; Schriber et al., 2014).

Social skills groups are ideal for leveraging simulation of everyday behaviors to reduce negative mood and anxiety. These groups help the engagement in interpersonal issues through dramatic play and teamwork (Miller, 2010).

Negative Self-Esteem

We observe that children with Typical Development present lower values than children with attention deficit/ hyperactive disorder in the subscale of Negative Self-Esteem. Children with dyslexia have lower values compared to children with attention deficit/ hyperactive disorder (Figure 6), with statistically significant differences shown in group comparisons (Table 9).

Children with attention deficit hyperactivity disorder because of cognitive difficulties (Kalantzi-Azizi & Zafeiropoulou, 2011; Klassen et al., 2004; Stico et al., 2004;) are easily labeled in the school environment because of their weak working memory, resulting in their fragmented understanding of the tasks assigned to them (Fischer, 2007; Goldrich, 2015), since the brain has difficulty building automation strategies, even in everyday movements, which are clumsy (Fisher, 2007).

The above leads to low self-esteem, the "demoralization syndrome or sad effect", because of continuous social and school failures and conflicts with family and peers (Fisher, 2007; Kakouros & Maniadaki, 2006; Kempe et al., 2011; Trzesniewski et al., 2006).

Children with dyslexia, apart from the given 'cognitive gaps', seem to experience daily insecurity about whether they will meet the expectations of adults and also their personal aspirations. Managing emotions is also a difficult task, as academic failures lead to self-esteem problems (Madianos et al., 2003; Mitsiu-Daktila, 2008; Mundy et al., 2010).

The core of the personality of these children is built on poorly made foundations, since the lack of self-image and positive motivation are characteristics that can contribute to the appearance of depressive mood (Arnold et al., 2005; Maag & Reid, 2006).

There are also many behavioral problems that arise, such as communication disorders and antisocial behavior, because of the pressure and marginalization they feel (Kempe et al., 2011).

No statistically significant differences were found in children with autism spectrum disorder regarding Negative Self-Esteem. It is difficult for these children to acquire a comprehensive picture of themselves, as their social interactions are minimal, their empathy and understanding of their emotions is limited. This is confirmed by research from the limited expression in self-report questionnaires (Leyfer et al., 2006; Mundy et al., 2010; Schriber et al., 2014). Finally, constant school failures explain negative self-esteem. These can become traumatic experiences with an impact on children's moods (McNulty, 2003; Mugnaini et al., 2009).

Teachers can create with students' reflective journals: The children use reflective journals to identify weaknesses, positive points, praises and highlights of the day in order to have an open communication with teachers and parents (Riesberg, 2022).

In addition, children could create *persona dolls,* as innovative tool to express themselves. This type of dolls allows children to talk about their life stories and serve as go-betweens between them and the teacher. This method reinforces mutual empathy, solidarity and children's social identity (Brown, 2013; Wilkinson & Wilkinson, 2022).

In conclusion, If the teachers do not focus on the areas of personal and interpersonal development, the group of these children will undoubtedly present difficulties in their general functionality, resulting in psychomotor retardation.

To avoid the above, teachers should overcome the obstacle of insufficient training in the implementation of primary intervention programs (Didaskalou & Millward, 2002; Berman, 2009; Rubin, 2012) by seeking help from mental health services and universities (Hatzichristou, 2009).

Research Limitations

The limitations of our study are associated with the size of our sample, the limited range of the students, and the homogeneity of the geographical area. Finally, the CDI was used for pedagogical rather than diagnostic purposes (Tountas, 2009).

The Role of Educator

At school age, the phenomena of psychopathology must be prevented and reduced so that they do not intensify in adolescence and, by extension, in adulthood (Doulgherty, 2010). Our findings highlight the need for emotional support in children with specific learning difficulties and developmental disorders, as difficulties are identified in areas related to themselves and others. The teacher's task is to promote the all-around development of these children's personalities and stimulate their mental resilience (Mundy et al., 2010; Schriber et al., 2014).

School children spend a large part of their young life with their teachers whose tremendous influence on them is as much as—if not even more than— their parents. Beside their parents, teachers are the most important adults in their lives. Teachers get to know their pupils almost as well as their parents know their children, and what is more, teachers often discover aspects of their pupils' personality which may not be obvious to their parents (Baron-Cohen, 2003; Lombardo & Baron-Cohen, 2011).

It may sound as an overstatement but they're not just educators; they're role models who inspire and motivate children outside the classroom as much as they impart knowledge inside it. They are fully aware of their developmental stages and their expected behaviors Consequently, it is easy for them to detect developmental and behavioral deviations (Attwood, 2005; Didaskalou & Millward, 2002; Pliszka, 2011)

They are often the first line of defence when it comes to identifying and addressing mental health issues in young people. They spend a significant amount of time with their students, giving them a unique vantage point to observe changes in behaviour, emotional states, and academic performance. The relationships teachers build with their students create a foundation of trust that can make it easier for young people to open up about their struggles (McNulty, 2003 ; Mason & Mason, 2005).

The correct and timely consultation is really important as the children can be helped by the teacher with the appropriate interventions (Ghaziuddin et al., 2002; Leyfer et al., 2006; Janowsky & Davis, 2005; Malikiosi-Loizou, 2017), mainly in cases of the autistic spectrum (Attwood, 2005; Bella-Awusah, et al., 2016; Gena, 2002).

REFERENCES

Arnold, E., Goldston, D., Walsh, A., Reboussin, B., Daniel, S., Hickman, E., & Wood, F. B. (2005). Severity of emotional and behavioral problems among poor and typical readers. *Journal of Abnormal Child Psychology*, 33(2), 205–217. DOI: 10.1007/s10802-005-1828-9 PMID: 15839498

Attwood, T. (2006). The pattern of abilities and development of girls with Asperger's syndrome. In: Attwood T, Bolick T, Faherty C, et al. (Eds.), *Asperger's and Girls*. Arlington, TX: Future Horizons, Inc. Bailey, B. (2008). *Daily Routine Cards*. UK: Conscious Discipline.

Baron-Cohen, S. (2003). *The essential difference: Men, women and the extreme male brain*. Penguin Books.

Bella-Awusah, T., Ani, C., Ajuwon, A., & Omigbodun, O. (2016). Effectiveness of brief school - based, group cognitive behavioral therapy for depressed adolescents in South West Nigeria. *Child and Adolescent Mental Health*, 21(1), 44–50. DOI: 10.1111/camh.12104 PMID: 32680363

Berman, A. L. (2009). Depression and suicide. In Gotlib, I. H., & Hammen, C. L. (Eds.), *Handbook of depression* (2nd ed., pp. 510–530). The Guilford Press.

Biederman, J., Ball, S. W., Monuteaux, M. C., Mick, E., Spencer, T. J., McCreary, M., Cote, M., & Faraone, S. V. (2008). New insights into the co-morbidity between ADHD and major depression in adolescent and young adult females. *Journal of the American Academy of Child and Adolescent Psychiatry*, 47(4), 426–434. DOI: 10.1097/CHI.0b013e31816429d3 PMID: 18388760

Blackman, G. L., Ostrander, R., & Herman, K. C. (2005). Children with ADHD and depression: A multisource, multimethod assessment of clinical, social, and academic functioning. *Journal of Attention Disorders*, 8(4), 195–207. DOI: 10.1177/1087054705278777 PMID: 16110050

Brown, T. E. (2009). *ADHD comorbidities*. American Psychiatric Publishing.

Brown, L. H., Strauman, T., Barrantes-Vidal, N., Silvia, P. J., & Kwapil, T. R. (2011). An experience-sampling study of depressive symptoms and their social context. *The Journal of Nervous and Mental Disease*, 199(6), 403–409. DOI: 10.1097/NMD.0b013e31821cd24b PMID: 21629020

Brown, B. (2013). The value of persona dolls in tacking sensitive issues. *Mag online library, 1*(12).

Burke, J. D., Loeber, R., Lahey, B. B., & Rathouz, P. J. (2005). Developmental transitions among affective and behavioral disorders in adolescent boys. *Journal of Child Psychology and Psychiatry, and Allied Disciplines*, 46(11), 1200–1210. DOI: 10.1111/j.1469-7610.2005.00422.x PMID: 16238667

Campanarou, M. (2007). *Diagnostic issues of speech therapy*. Hellenic Publications.

Carroll, J. M., Maughan, B., Goodman, R., & Meltzer, H. (2005). Literacy difficulties and psychiatric disorders: Evidence for comorbidity. *Journal of Child Psychology and Psychiatry, and Allied Disciplines*, 46(5), 524–532. DOI: 10.1111/j.1469-7610.2004.00366.x PMID: 15845132

Carroll, J. M., & Iles, J. E. (2006). An assessment of anxiety levels in dyslexic students in higher education. *The British Journal of Educational Psychology*, 76(Pt3), 651–662. DOI: 10.1348/000709905X66233 PMID: 16953967

Charman, T., & Petrova, I. (2000). The internal structure of the Child Depression Inventory in Russian and UK schoolchildren. *Journal of Youth and Adolescence*, 30(1), 41–51. DOI: 10.1023/A:1005220820982

Collaborative for Academic Social and Emotional Learning. (2003). *Safe and sound: An educational leader's guide to evidence-based social and emotional learning (SEL) programs*. Author.

Daviss, W. B., Weinman, D. R., Diler, R. S., & Birmaher, B. (2006b). *Risk Factors for Co-morbid Depression in Adolescents with ADHD*. Poster presented at 53rd Annual Meeting of the American Academy of Child and Adolescent Psychiatry; (abstract), San Diego, CA.

Didaskalou, E., & Millward, A. (2002). Breaking the policy log-jam: Comparative perspectives on policy formulation and development for pupils with emotional and behavioral difficulties. *Oxford Review of Education*, 28(1), 109–121. DOI: 10.1080/03054980120113661

Dougherty, L. R., Klein, D. N., Durbin, C. E., Hayden, E. P., & Olino, T. M. (2010). Temperamental positive and negative emotionality and children's depressive symptoms: A longitudinal prospective study from age three to age ten. *Journal of Social and Clinical Psychology*, 29(4), 462–488. DOI: 10.1521/jscp.2010.29.4.462

Fisher, B. C. (2007). *Attention Deficit Disorder: Practical Coping Mechanisms* (2nd ed.). Healthcare.

Francis, K. (2007). *Pervasive Developmental Disorders or autism spectrum disorders. Disability Specialization Guide (EPEAEK)*. Panteion University of Social and Political Sciences. In Greek

Gena, A. (2002). *Autism and Pervasive Developmental Disorders. Evaluation-Diagnosis-Treatment*. Leader Books. In Greek

Giannakopoulos, G., Kazantzi, M., Dimitrakaki, C., Tsiantis, J., Kolaitis, G., Trzesniewski, K. H., Donnellan, M. B., Moffitt, T. E., Robins, R. W., Poulton, R., & Caspi, A. (2006). Low self-esteem during adolescence predicts poor health, criminal behavior, and limited economic prospects during adulthood. *Developmental Psychology*, 42(2), 381–390. DOI: 10.1037/0012-1649.42.2.381 PMID: 16569175

Goldrich, C. (2015). *8 keys to parenting children with ADHD*. W. W. Norton & Company.

Grigorenko, P. (2001). Developmental dyslexia: An update on genes, brains and environments. *Journal of Child Psychology and Psychiatry, and Allied Disciplines*, 42(1), 91–125. DOI: 10.1111/1469-7610.00704 PMID: 11205626

Gray, C. (1994). *Comic Strip conversations*. Future Horizons.

Guhn, A., Sterzer, F., Haack, F. H., & Köhler, S. (2018). Affective and cognitive reactivity to mood induction in chronic depression. *Journal of Affective Disorders*, 229, 275–281. DOI: 10.1016/j.jad.2017.12.090 PMID: 29329060

Hanicke, T., & Broadbent, J. (2016). The influence of academic self-efficacy on academic performance. A systematic review. *Educational Research Review*, 17, 63–84. DOI: 10.1016/j.edurev.2015.11.002

Harpin, V., Mazzone, L., Raynaud, J. P., Kahle, J. R., & Hodgkins, P. (2013). Long-term outcomes of ADHD: A systematic review of self-esteem and social function. *Journal of Attention Disorders*, 20(4), 295–305. DOI: 10.1177/1087054713486516 PMID: 23698916

Hatzichristou, X. (2009). *Introduction to school psychology* (8th ed.). Greek Letters. In Greek

Hoza, B., Waschbusch, D. A., Pelham, W. E., Molina, B. S., & Milich, R. (2005). Attention deficit/hyperactivity disordered and control boys' responses to social success and failure. *Child Development*, 71(2), 432–446. DOI: 10.1111/1467-8624.00155 PMID: 10834475

Janowsky, D. S., & Davis, J. M. (2005). Diagnosis and treatment of depression in patients with mental retardation. *Current Psychiatry Reports*, 7(6), 421–428. DOI: 10.1007/s11920-005-0062-z PMID: 16318819

Kakouros, E., & Maniadaki, K. (2006). *Child and Adolescent Psychopathology: A Developmental Approach*. Dadranos. In Greek

Kalantzi-Azizi, A., & Zafeiropoulou, M. (Eds.). (2011). *Adjustment to school-Prevention and coping with difficulties.* Pedio.

Kempe, C., Gustafson, S., & Samuelsson, S. (2011). A longitudinal study of early reading difficulties and subsequent problem behaviors. *Scandinavian Journal of Psychology*, 52(3), 242–250. DOI: 10.1111/j.1467-9450.2011.00870.x PMID: 21332486

Kovacs, M. (1992). *Children's Depression Inventory.* Multi-Health Systems.

Leirbakk, M.J., Clench-Aas, J., & Ruth, K., Raanaas. (. (2015). ADHD with Co- Occurring Depression/Anxiety in Children: The Relationship with Somatic Complaints and Parental Socio-Economic Position. *Journal of Psychological Abnormalities*, 4, 137. DOI: 10.4172/2329-9525.1000125

Leyfer, O. T., Folstein, S. E., Bacalman, S., Davis, N. O., Dinh, E., Morgan, J., Tager-Flusberg, H., & Lainhart, J. E. (2006). Comorbid psychiatric disorders in children with autism: Interview development and rates of disorders. *Journal of Autism and Developmental Disorders*, 36(7), 849–861. DOI: 10.1007/s10803-006-0123-0 PMID: 16845581

Lindsay, J., & Dockrell, J. (2002). The behaviour and selfesteem of children with specific speech and language difficulties. *The British Journal of Educational Psychology*, 70(Pt4), 583–601. PMID: 11191188

Lombardo, M. V., & Baron-Cohen, S. (2011). The role of the self in mindblindness in autism. *Consciousness and Cognition*, 20(1), 130–140. DOI: 10.1016/j.concog.2010.09.006 PMID: 20932779

Lopata, C., Toomey, J. A., Fox, J. D., Volker, M. A., Chow, S. Y., Thomeer, M. L., Lee, G. K., Rodgers, J. D., McDonald, C. A., & Smerbeck, A. M. (2010). Anxiety and depression in children with HFASDs: Symptom levels and source differences. *Journal of Abnormal Child Psychology*, 38(6), 765–776. DOI: 10.1007/s10802-010-9406-1 PMID: 20354899

Lougy, R. A., Deruvo, S. L., & Rosenthal, D. (2007). *Teaching young children with ADHD: Succesful strategies and Practical Interventions for Prek - 3.* Corwin Press.

Luby, J. L., Heffelfinger, A. K., Mrakotsky, C., Brown, K. M., Hessler, M. J., Wallis, J. M., & Spitznagel, E. L. (2003). The clinical picture of depression in preschool children. *Journal of the American Academy of Child and Adolescent Psychiatry*, 42(3), 340–348. DOI: 10.1097/00004583-200303000-00015 PMID: 12595788

Maag, J., & Reid, R. (2006). Depression among students with Learning Disabilities: Assesing the Risk. *Journal of Learning Disabilities*, 39(1), 3–10. DOI: 10.1177/00222194060390010201 PMID: 16512079

Madianos, M. (2003). *Clinical psychiatry. Learning Difficulties – Dyslexia*. Kastaniotis Publications. In Greek

Malikiosi-Loizou, M. (2017). *Counselling Psychology*. Pedio. In Greek

McNulty, M. A. (2003). Dyslexia and the life course. *Journal of Learning Disabilities*, 36(4), 363–381. DOI: 10.1177/00222194030360040701 PMID: 15490908

Malchiodi, C. A. (2003). *Handbook of art therapy*. U.K Guilford publications.

Marc, R., Crundwell, A., & Killu, K. (2010). Responding to a student's depression. *Interventions That Work*, 68(2), 46–51.

Mason, A., & Mason, M. (2005). Understanding College Students with Learning Disabilities. *Pediatric Clinics of North America*, 52(1), 61–70. DOI: 10.1016/j.pcl.2004.11.001 PMID: 15748924

Mayes, S. D., Calhoun, S. L., Bixler, E. O., Vgontzas, A. N., Mahr, F., Hillwig-Garcia, J., Elamir, B., Edhere-Ekezie, L., & Parvin, M. (2009). ADHD subtypes and co morbid anxiety, depression, and oppositional-defiant disorder: Differences in sleep problems. *Journal of Pediatric Psychology*, 34(3), 328–337. DOI: 10.1093/jpepsy/jsn083 PMID: 18676503

Melegari, M. G., Sette, S., Vittori, E., Mallia, L., Devoto, A., Lucidi, F., Ferri, R., & Bruni, O. (2018). Relations Between Sleep and Temperament in Preschool Children With ADHD. *Journal of Attention Disorders*. Advance online publication. DOI: 10.1177/1087054718757645 PMID: 29468918

Miller, J. K. (2018). *Thriving with ADHD Workbook for Kids: 60 Fun Activities to Help Children Self-Regulate, Focus, and Succeed (Health and Wellness Workbooks for Kids)*. United Kingdom: Callisto Kids. Mitsiu- Daktila, G. (2008). *Neuropsychologies of learning disorders: diagnosis and treatm*ent. Athens: Dardanos. In Greek.

Mugnaini, D., Lassi, S., Lamalrfa, G., & Albertini, G. (2009). Internalizing correlates of dyslexia. *World Journal of Pediatrics*, 5(4), 255–264. DOI: 10.1007/s12519-009-0049-7 PMID: 19911139

Mundy, P., Gwaltney, M., & Henderson, H. (2010). Self-referenced processing, neurodevelopment and joint attention in autism. *Autism*, 14(5), 408–429. DOI: 10.1177/1362361310366315 PMID: 20926457

Papadatos, I. (2010). *Mental disorders and learning disabilities of children and adolescents*. Gutenberg Editions.

Papageorgiou, B. (2005). *Child and adolescent psychiatry*. University Studio Press. In Greek

Perry, D. W., Marston, G. M., Hinder, S. A., Munden, A., & Roy, A. (2001). The phenomenology of depressive illness in people with a learning disability and autism. *Autism*, 5(3), 265–275. DOI: 10.1177/1362361301005003004 PMID: 11708586

Pliszka, S. (2007). Practice parameter for the assessment and treatment of children and adolescents with attention-deficit/hyperactivity disorder. *Journal of the American Academy of Child and Adolescent Psychiatry*, 46(7), 894–921. DOI: 10.1097/chi.0b013e318054e724 PMID: 17581453

Pliszka, S. R. (2011). *Treating ADHD and Comorbid Disorders: Psychosocial and Psychopharmacological Interventions*. Guilford Press.

Pollard, A. J., & Prendergast, M. (2004). Depressive pseudodementia in a child with autism. *Developmental Medicine and Child Neurology*, 46(7), 485–489. DOI: 10.1111/j.1469-8749.2004.tb00510.x PMID: 15230463

Rice, F. (2010). Genetics of childhood and adolescent depression: Insights into etiological heterogeneity and challenges for future genomic research. *Genome Medicine*, 2(9), 68. DOI: 10.1186/gm189 PMID: 20860851

Riesberg, A. (2022). *Reflection Journal: For Children*. Lulu.

Rubin, D. H. (2012). Joy returns last: Anhedonia and treatment resistance in depressed adolescents. *Journal of the American Academy of Child and Adolescent Psychiatry*, 51(4), 353–355. DOI: 10.1016/j.jaac.2012.01.012 PMID: 22449641

Verduyn, C., Rogers, J., & Wood, A. (2009). *Depression: cognitive behavior therapy with children and young people*. Routledge. DOI: 10.4324/9780203879894

Samm, A., Värnik, A., Tooding, L.-M., Sisask, M., Kõlves, K., & von Knorring, A.-L. (2007). Children's Depression Inventory in Estonia. Single items and factor structure by age and gender. *European Child & Adolescent Psychiatry*, 17(3), 162–170. DOI: 10.1007/s00787-007-0650-z PMID: 17876502

Schriber, R. A., Robins, R. W., & Solomon, M. (2014). Personality and Self-Insight in Individuals with Autism Spectrum Disorder. *Journal of Personality and Social Psychology*, 106(1), 112–130. https://psycnet.apa.org/doi/10.1037/a0034950. DOI: 10.1037/a0034950 PMID: 24377361

Shaul, J. (2017). *The ASD and me picture book: Visual guide to understanding challenges and strengths for children on the Autism Spectrum*. Jessica Kinglsley Publishers.

Simonoff, E., Pickles, A., Charman, T., Chandler, S., Loucas, T., & Baird, G. (2008). Psychiatric disorders in children with autism spectrum disorders: Prevalence, co-morbidity, and associated factors in a population-derived sample. *Journal of the American Academy of Child and Adolescent Psychiatry*, 47(8), 921–992. DOI: 10.1097/CHI.0b013e318179964f PMID: 18645422

Skinner, S. R., McDonald, A., & Walters, T. (2005). A patient with autism and severe depression: Medical and ethical challenges for an adolescent medicine unit. *The Medical Journal of Australia*, 183(8), 422–424. DOI: 10.5694/j.1326-5377.2005. tb07108.x PMID: 16225449

Stenseng, F., Belsky, J., Skalicka, V., & Wichstrøm, L. (2015). Peer Rejection and Attention Deficit Hyperactivity Disorder Symptoms: Reciprocal Relations Through Ages 4, 6, and 8. *Child Development*, 87(2), 365–373. DOI: 10.1111/cdev.12471 PMID: 26671073

Stewart, M. E., Barnard, L., Pearson, J., Hasan, R., & O'Brien, G. (2006). Presen-tation of depression in autism and Asperger syndrome: A review. *Autism*, 10(1), 103–116. DOI: 10.1177/1362361306062013 PMID: 16522713

Tountas, Y. (2009). Screening for children's depression symptoms in Greece: The use of the Children's Depression Inventory in a nation - wide school - based sample. *European Child & Adolescent Psychiatry*, 18(8), 485–492. DOI: 10.1007/s00787-009-0005-z PMID: 19255802

Trikkas, G. (2005). *Clinical forms of depression*. In G. N. Christodoulou (Ed.), Depression (2nd Ed.) (pp. 13–22). Athens: BETA, medical arts. In Greek.

Weyandt, L., & Dupaul, G. J. (2013). *Students with ADHD*. Business Media. DOI: 10.1007/978-1-4614-5345-1

Wilkinson, C., & Wilkinson, S. (2022). Using Persona Dolls in research with children to combat the insider/ outsider researcher status dilemma. *Children's Geographies*, 20(3), 375–380. DOI: 10.1080/14733285.2022.2051433

Chapter 12
Theory–Guided Music– Based Program to Facilitate Inclusive Emotion Regulation Skills Development in University Students

Potheini Vaiouli
https://orcid.org/0000-0002-6651-8633
University of Luxembourg, Luxembourg & University of Cyprus, Cyprus

Marios Theodorou
https://orcid.org/0000-0003-2560-986X
Frederick University, Cyprus & University of Cyprus, Cyprus

Georgia Panayiotou
University of Cyprus, Cyprus

ABSTRACT

The success of Higher Education as an effective learning environment rests on establishing an inclusive context that promotes life-long learning opportunities. Psycho-social skills are considered fundamental competencies for youth development: crucial for individuals' academic achievement, mental health, and life success. Although universal skills development programs have produced promising findings, there are several challenges in effectively providing such services to the wide student population. There is growing literature indicating the potential of in-

DOI: 10.4018/979-8-3693-5325-7.ch012

corporating music strategies and music-based intervention as an effective medium for these programs integrated into the universal academic pathway. This chapter presents the rationale and the development pathway of an enhanced (standard + music) classroom-based Emotion Regulation skills training to meet the diverse needs of university students. Through a multiphase method, we present data from three pilot single-arm studies on the acceptability and preliminary effectiveness of the program on students' adaptive emotion regulation.

INTRODUCTION

Entering Higher Education (HE) marks a turning point for youth learning to function as independent adults, something that can be both exciting and challenging. Students are confronted with a considerable number of changes to manage (e.g. high academic expectations, making new relationships, making independent decisions), for which they may be psychosocially unfamiliar or uncomfortable (Parker et al. 2004). Several studies have indeed shown that rising levels of difficulty in socio-emotional adaptation for students in HE, is linked to increased mental health concerns and demands (Acharya, Jin, & Collins, 2018; Watkins, Hunt, & Eisenberg, 2012). For example, university students with poor emotion regulation skills, such as a lack of emotional clarity (the ability to accurately identify and understand their own emotions), are more likely to exhibit maladaptive behaviors like impulsivity (Miller & Racine, 2022). In contrast, using cognitive reappraisal techniques is linked to greater resilience among university learners (Thomas & Zolkoski, 2020). Academically, such difficulties often lead to increased procrastination, as students delay tasks due to overwhelming emotions, further impeding their academic progress (Schuenemann et al., 2022). However, acquiring psycho-social skills, such as participating in stress reduction programs, positively impacts undergraduates' and graduates' mental health (for a meta-analysis, see Yusufov et al., 2019) and decreases the overall tendency to procrastinate in student populations (Schuenemann et al., 2022).

Although mental health promotion programs within university settings have produced promising impact to tackle the aforementioned issue, there are several challenges in effectively providing such services to the wide student population. Some of these obstacles include: a) provision of services through counseling centres/ university mental health centres has limited resources, b) services are largely focused on managing mental health issues/mental disorders, and c) that the effective provision of these services is time intensive and resource heavy (Sauer-Zavala, et al. 2021).

As compensation for the above challenges, contemporary alternative approaches focus on the development of universal mental health promotion and prevention programs (MPPPs) integrated in the academic learning pathway. These constitute skills-oriented programs, aiming to promote adjustment of the wide student population (Conley, & Durlak, 2017). During the last two decades, there has been a tremendous flowering of research in the advancement of universal MPPPs development. In specific, there is a special interest to investigate the implementation of scientifically supported trainings/interventions and to understand the factors and important intervention elements, which are associated with the programs' effectiveness and the student population they could benefit the most.

Preliminary research findings support that skill-oriented programs that include supervised practice interventions (Conley, Durlak, & Kirsch, 2015), trainings conducted as a class integrated in the academic curriculum (Conley, Durlak, & Dickson, 2013), and technology-oriented interventions (Worsley, Pennington, & Corcoran, 2022), appear to be effective modes of delivery. Regarding the components linked to the effectiveness of these interventions, meta-review data are showing support for cognitive behavioural therapy/CBT and mindfulness-based interventions (Worsley, Pennington, & Corcoran, 2022).

As an extension of the above, recent research efforts focus on evaluating training programs for transversal skills, such as Emotion Regulation (ER) skills (Unified Protocol for Prevention, Sauer-Zavala, et al. 2021), that are based on empirically supported approaches targeting common core processes/ vulnerabilities in a range of mental health conditions (Unified Protocol for Transdiagnostic Treatment of Emotional Disorders/UP, Barlow et al., 2018). In specific the UP approach focuses on how individuals manage their emotional experiences in a broad manner (Sauer-Zavala, et al. 2021), allowing a broader applicability to a wide range of population. Research in this field is still limited, with existing work presenting conflicting results. For example, in a quasi-experimental study (non-random assignment) conducted by Castro-Camacho, Díaz, and Barbosa, (2022), the group of students who attended the preventive intervention reported a significant improvement on their mental health. On the contrary, Sauer-Zavala, and colleagues (2021), using a randomized design found no differences in emotional and mental health variables between the intervention and control group. Further examination of the potential impact of integrating empirically supported transversal components that derive from clinical research (e.g. UP), as part of universal MPPPs is needed.

Another critical factor in improving the effectiveness of these interventions is to mitigate disparities relevant to diversity, through their design and implementation. Universal interventions focus on the entire student population, and they are primarily designed to provide a broad range of topics and skills that will strengthen individuals' personalized coping strategies for dealing with current and future difficulties. Students' learning abilities (e.g. learning capacity, language ability, and executive functions) can be considered as critical elements towards this direction. In typical/ standard mode of delivery the above abilities are considered essential ingredients for program success, however it may exacerbate existing inequalities for student population with learning-diverse abilities, such as language skills (listening, reading, speaking and writing), executive skills (e.g. sustain attention) or cognitive processes such as memory and abstract thinking.

A growing literature pinpoints the potential of incorporating art-based methodologies, such as music, to customize the delivery method of the interventions to make them accessible and relevant to diverse segments of the population. Music is characterized by personalized methods and has shown promising effects on its effectiveness for people with learning-diverse abilities (De Witte et al., 2020). It is considered widely accessible and affordable to young adults, a meaningful constant in their everyday lives (McFerran, 2010), which offers opportunities for learning in a non-stigmatizing manner. Further, music interventions have been linked to improvements in treatment engagement and mental health issues in various settings and populations (Rodwin et al., 2022; Koelsch, 2020; Leubner, & Hinterberger, 2017). Research findings additionally support that music can be used as a tool for emotion regulation by reducing stress and anxiety (Randall, Rickard, & Vella-Brodrick, 2014) and improving general emotion regulation skills (Thomson et al. 2014).

Overall, music-based interventions are gaining growing recognition in research for adolescents and young adults as an innovative and youth-centered strategy to improve mental health outcomes and levels of engagements of participants (Collins & Fleming, 2017; NIH, 2018). In their review, Rodwin and his colleagues (2022), evaluated the evidence on music-based psychosocial interventions to improve engagement in treatment and mental health outcomes among adolescents and young adults. Despite the heterogeneity of designs, populations, music protocols, and outcomes, they identified socio-emotional processes involved in all studies, as a common underlying component. Thus, music can be a medium of choice to address life-long needs for young adults by infusing culturally appropriate practices that can be easily integrated into the young adults' everyday experiences at the level of their abilities. Taking into account the above, it is of great interest to develop and investigate how different modalities, such as music-based methodologies, can alter the effectiveness of existing empirically supported approaches, such as the Unified Protocol for Prevention.

The Present Study

The primary objective of this chapter is to present the rationale and the development pathway of an enhanced (standard +music) classroom-based emotion regulation skills training for university students. The pathway comprises five steps: *Step 1*: development, *Step 2*: Pilot evaluation of the whole program in English and adaptation, *Step 3*: Pilot evaluation of selected modules in Greek and adaptation, *Step*

4: Pilot evaluation of selected modules in Greek and adaptation, and *Step 5*: pilot evaluation from an external expert and final adaptation. The secondary objective is to present data from the three-pilot single-arm studies on the acceptability and preliminary effectiveness of the proposed program on students' adaptive emotion regulation, thus improvement on general psychological functioning.

Steps of the Pathway

Step 1: Development of the Manual

The program is novel and was the product of the collaboration between clinical psychologists implementing CBT and music psychology theories of music and emotion, and music therapists. Such interdisciplinary collaborations between music therapists and professionals in the field of health care (e.g. speech therapists, psychologists, neuroscientists, medical professionals) are encouraged as a means to provide patient-centered care to patients and their families (Hernandez-Ruiz, 2017). For example, the collaborative efforts of clinical psychologists and music therapists allows for the integration of music-based and non-verbal treatment components into more traditional (e.g. cognitive-based) treatment plans, thus addressing multiple dimensions of the patients' conditions and thereby enhancing treatment efficacy (Bruscia, 2014; Gold et al., 209). Studies of the last decade, which focused on such collaborations provide evidence on a range of potential benefits which are either unique to music stimuli or have additional positive effects to the short-term and long-term outcomes for participants. This may include the benefits of music and musical experiences to enhance neural processes (Constantin, 2018), cognitive benefits (Chap et al., 2018), language and communication skills in pediatric health care (Geretsegger et al., 2019) as well as in educational settings for younger children (Beningi et al., 2018). Findings of such collaborations indicate a range of potential benefits of music interventions, which are either unique to music stimuli or have additional positive effects to the short-term and long-term outcomes for participants.

However, research in the field of music therapy to support such collaborations is rather limited with no standardized protocols for reference or a clear protocol to be followed. In the current study we capitalized on the expertise of the aforementioned researchers to explore how music components may enhance a traditional emotion regulation program. It was based on the premise that understanding emotions in real life involves processing a variety of multimodal cues that include visual, bodily, and auditory stimuli (verbal content, prosody, non-verbal cues, and vocalizations). Multimodality is an inter-disciplinary approach that is traditionally emphasized for people with diverse learning abilities, by using a variety of inputs and modes of delivery, in addition to language and text in order to achieve learning. Through this approach we aimed to extend standard verbal dominant and unidimensional practices in skills training by integrating art-based approaches (i.e. songs and listening to music), carefully designed to meet the needs of students with diverse abilities. The use of music-based experiences aimed to create an inclusive approach, which combined spoken language and audio, gestural, and tactile social patterns with the potential to enhance skill-building and engagement of the participants for learning.

Previous published research of similar programs (including the Tuned In program by Dingle & Fay, 2017) served as the basis for the music selections. For the selection and sequence of the music activities, we also followed Saarakallio's and her colleagues (2015) conceptualization for emotional health-fostering musical identity, consisting of the following elements: emotion recognition and identification in music, regulation of stress and negative emotion through music, inducing positive emotions and pleasure through music, self-reflective awareness of personal emotional responses to music, and a sense of self-agency regarding one's emotional responses to music. In this process, we capitalized on the qualities of sound (such as rhythm, pitch, tonality, and melody), and identified music activities that may play an important role in enhancing interventions that focus on emotion regulation skills.

For the purposes of the program, two different sets of training materials were designed: the trainer's manual and the participants' workbook. A comprehensive trainer's manual was developed to provide a detailed outline for the training program, which included background information, basic guidelines for the implementation of each module in the training, and evaluation and self-reflection tools. Particular attention was given to the examples provided and the description of the goals of the program as well as each unit, in plain terms so that professionals in the field of psychology and mental health, without training in music or music-therapy would be able to implement it.

The participants' workbook was structured in a similar format. The main goal for each session was presented in plain terms and the participants had then access to music links, descriptions about the main concept of each session, and opportunities to further practice these notions. Within this context, music served various goals: it functioned as the vehicle to enhance emotional psychoeducation and skills building, as a safe space for participants to experience and explore their emotions, and as a strategy to modify their emotions. Active music listening, song writing techniques, and guided breathing with music were among the activities introduced to participants in each module to enhance participants' socio-emotional awareness with a special focus on emotional awareness, identification of emotions, and emotion regulation skills.

The Program

Table 1 shows the main themes and goals of the program session by session.

Table 1.

Program's main themes and goals session by session	
Module title	**Contents**
MODULE 1. VALUES & SETTING GOALS FOR ENHANCING MOTIVATION	♣ Discuss the importance of motivation to training's outcome ♣ Help students discover their core values and recognize the importance of living a values-based life. ♣ Help students identify concrete and manageable goals to achieve during training
MODULE 2. UNDERSTANDING EMOTIONS	• Help participants recognize emotions' function and usefulness in our daily life, health and wellbeing. • Assist participants to increase their awareness of emotional experience, by deconstructing emotion into its basic elements. • Help participants realize how emotional responses are connected to short-term and long-term consequences.
MODULE 3. MINDFUL EMOTION AWARENESS AND RELAXATION	• Help participants understand the basic components of mindfulness. • Assist participants to learn how to observe their emotional experiences in a mindful way. • Increase participants' understanding of the role that physical sensations play in determining their emotional responses. • Help participants engage in exercises become more aware of their physical sensations and increase tolerance of these experiences.
MODULE 4. COGNITIVE FLEXIBILITY	• Introduce the concept of automatic thoughts and cognitive errors • Help participants identify common thinking traps and increase flexibility in thinking
MODULE 5. COUNTERING INAPPROPRIATE BEHAVIORS	• Introduce the concept of emotional behaviors • Help participants identify emotional behaviors and develop alternative behaviors to the non-adaptive ones.

The rationale of the training was built based on the framework of Unified Protocol (Barlow, et al. 2018) and training activities were selected and adapted in from a compilation of foundational works on contemporary evidence-based approaches, (i.e. Cognitive Behavioral approach, Acceptance and Commitment approach, and Dialectical Behavior approach). Each module contained a) the session outline, b) review of previous session's homework, c) theoretical background and module's rationale, d) skills activities, and e) homework assignment. The music-based model included a set of music activities that are interactive and relational to help participants recognize, process, and express their emotions. No background of formal education in music was required for participation in the program. The activities were designed to be process-oriented (e.g. making music as a group) and discussion-based (e.g. lyrics analysis, sharing of emotions and bodily sensations). The participants were invited to take part in active music-making through song-writing in groups, group singing, and body percussion experiences (clapping, body and movement) as well as receptive experiences, including listening, guided imagery, bodily awareness exercises, and lyric analysis. Emotional and cognitive elements were present in each session to enhance participants' emotion awareness and emotion regulation as part of learning strategies. Developmentally and culturally related criteria also guided the suggested choices of songs and music included in the manual. That is, the songs and lyrics for each part of the model were carefully selected to reflect (and hopefully resonate) with participants' life experiences, validate adverse experiences, express emotions, and engage with other members in the group (Levy, 2019; Huth et al., 2021). At the same time, the linguistic (e.g. lyrics), auditory, and gestural aspects (moving to the melody, keeping a steady beat to the rhythmical patterns) of each music experience, created a multimodal experience to be exploited for teaching new skills during the program.

Steps 2-5: Pilot evaluations and adaptation (General Methodology)

The training materials were refined and improved in four different stages. Steps 2-5 focused on piloting the training materials, identifying areas for amendments, and making adaptations on the material and teaching methodologies used. Variations of course delivery were applied in different courses, to help us gather information about the optimal methodology of delivery. Results from these steps provided guidance on best practices, but also recommendations for improvements. A final pilot evaluation (step 5) from external experts was conducted to provide valuable insights to ensure the content is thorough, clear, and comprehensive. Table 2 summarizes specific methodological procedures pertaining to each step.

Table 2.

Methodological elements for steps 2-5								
Step	Modules (M)					Language	Acceptability/ Preliminary effectiveness	Participants
	M1	M2	M3	M4	M5			
Step 2	MS	MS	MS	MS	MS	EN	ACC EFF	INS STU
Step 3	MS	MS	MS	MS	MS	GR	ACC EFF	INS STU

continued on following page

Table 2. Continued

Step	Modules (M)					Language	Acceptability/ Preliminary effectiveness	Participants
Methodological elements for steps 2-5								
	M1	M2	M3	M4	M5			
Step 4			M	M		GR	ACC	INS STU
Step 5	M	M	M	M	M	EN	/	EXP

Notes:
Modules
M1=Module1, M2=Module2, M3=Module3, M4=Module4, M5=Module5
MS=Music and Standard, M=only Music, S=only Standard
Language
EN=English, GR=Greek
Acceptability/Preliminary Effectiveness
ACC= Acceptability, EFF=Effectiveness
Participants
INS=Instructors, STU=Students, EXP=Expert

Participants

In total, three independent student samples, five teaching instructors and one music expert participated in steps 2-5. A total of 95 undergraduate students from University of Cyprus/UCY participated in steps 2-4 (men = 22, women = 73, age range: 18-42, Mage = 21.12 SDage = 3.70). Only participants who completed the entire course study, and pre- and post-course questionnaires were included in the analysis. Participants were selected from various psychology elective courses, ranging from first-year to fourth-year students. Table 3 summarizes the demographic breakdown of the participants, providing a clear view of the distribution for each step based on gender, year of study, age range, and primary major.

Table 3.

Demographic characteristics per sample	Step 2 (N=26)	Step 3 (N=56)	Step 4 (N=13)	Total (N=95)
Gender				
Women (%)	22 (30)	38 (52)	13 (18)	22
Men (%)	4 (18)	18 (82)	0	73
Study year				
1st (%)	4 (20)	9 (45)	7 (35)	20
2nd (%)	8 (36)	11 (50)	3 (14)	22

continued on following page

Table 3. Continued

Demographic characteristics per sample				
	Step 2 (N=26)	Step 3 (N=56)	Step 4 (N=13)	Total (N=95)
3rd (%)	12 (39)	18 (58)	1 (3)	31
4th (%)	2 (9)	18 (82)	2 (9)	22
Study program				
Accounting and Finance (%)	2 (40)	2 (40)	1 (20)	5
Biology (%)	0	1 (100)	0	1
Business Administration (%)	0	5 (100)	0	5
Chemistry (%)	0	2 (100)	0	2
Computer Science (%)	0	10 (100)	0	10
Economics (%)	0	9 (100)	0	9
Education (%)	0	3 (100)	0	3
English Studies (%)	5 (100)	0	0	5
Greek Literature (%)	0	2 (67)	1 (33)	3
History (%)	0	0	1 (100)	1
Journalism (%)	0	0	1 (100)	1
Maths and Statistics (%)	0	6 (100)	0	6
Mechanical Engineering (%)	0	1(100)	0	1
Physics (%)	0	2 (100)	0	2
Political Sciences (%)	1 (50)	1 (50)	0	2
Psychology (%)	18 (51)	10 (29)	7 (20)	35
Sociology (%)	0	1 (33)	2 (67)	3
Turkish and Eastern Studies (%)	0	1 (100)	0	1
*Participation Rate %**	46	71	9	/

*Participation Rate= Number of students participated in each each course/Total number of students enrolled in each course

Measures

Qualitative Feedback from Instructors

Semi-structured interviews. Semi-structured interviews (total of four hours) with the instructors of the music program at UCY, were conducted at the end of each pilot phase on the implementation of the training materials. The semi-structured interviews were conducted individually and in groups at a time convenient to the instructors via Teams. The questions focused on the instructors' understanding of the music-based program, the applicability, affordance, and ease of implementation of the musical activities. Also, they offered insights relevant to the flow of music activities as designed in the manual and the time needed for their implementation in relation to the students' responses and participation levels.

Acceptability questionnaire: At post-intervention, all participants completed a course satisfaction/acceptability questionnaire (adaptation of Hallis, et al. 2017, Al-Fraihat et al. 2020, Bruijns et al. 2022, and Tucker et al., 2022). The questionnaires consisted of twenty questions relating to their experience, satisfaction, and the challenges/enablers associated with design and implementation of the course. In addition to the questionnaire, feedback from the students was collected through three open-ended questions: "How 'effective' would you consider this course in increasing your perceived personal growth? In what ways? "What are your thoughts on having additional personal development courses for your academic training?", and "How do you think this content could be delivered differently to make it more useful (using technology or other methodologies)?". These questions invited them to reflect on their participation, the possible impact on their academic and personal lives.

Preliminary Effectiveness (Steps 2 and 3)

The preliminary effectiveness focused on several key outcomes, including beliefs about emotions and mental health outcomes.

Emotion Beliefs Questionnaire (EBQ; Becerra, Preece, & Gross, 2020). The EBQ (Becerra, Preece, & Gross, 2020) is a 16-item self-report measure of beliefs about emotions. Based on Ford and Gross's (2019) theoretical framework, the EBQ assesses two main categories of beliefs about emotions: beliefs about the controllability of emotions and beliefs about the usefulness of emotions. These beliefs are assessed for negative emotions and positive emotions. Four subscale scores and three composite scores are designed to be derived from the measure, with higher scores indicating more maladaptive beliefs about emotions (i.e., stronger beliefs that emotions are uncontrollable and useless). The scale has demonstrated good concurrent validity (EBQ scores correlated significantly in expected ways with various scores from other measures of beliefs about emotions), as well as validity and internal consistency in its initial validation (α = .88; Becerra, Preece, & Gross, 2020). For administration in step 3, the measures were front and back-translated in Greek by two bilingual psychologists. The translated versions showed good psychometric properties (a=0.88) for the respected sample.

Depression Anxiety Stress Scales (DASS-21; Henry, & Crawford, 2005) is a general mental health tool consisting of three scales (7 items per scale) measuring states of depression, anxiety and stress on a 4 point Likert scale (0 'almost always' to 4 'never'). Higher scores indicating a greater number of symptoms. The DASS-21 subscales show good internal consistency (Cronbach's α = 0.81- 0.88) and satisfactory internal consistency (a=.083-. 085) and validity indexes in the Greek speaking adult population (Pezirkianidis, et al. 2018).

Procedure

The training was integrated as a learning content in elective psychology under-graduate courses. During the first meeting, the instructor informed the class that one of the course purposes is to pilot new learning content and asked for students' consent to participate in the research component of the course towards its further development. In specific, students were asked if they were interested in participating in a study that involves completing questionnaires during the first and last weeks of the course. It was highlighted that no formal music education or music background was required or needed for participation. Upon conclusion of the course, students who voluntarily consented to participate in the research were asked to complete the acceptability questionnaire. Specific description of each step's procedure is described in corresponding sections. The courses were delivered by members of the academic staff with relevant experience in teaching psychology courses, as well as in conducting experiential learning activities. Each one of them was teaching a different cohort of students. The instructors received weekly supervision (face-to-face/virtual) by Principal Investigators (music therapist, and a clinical psychologist). Additional email support was provided to the instructors when required.

Data Analyses

Qualitative data: The researcher implemented thematic analysis to identify, an-alyze and report patterns within the data set (Braun & Clarke, 2006). Initial codes were generated, classified into potential themes as the analysis evolved and then the researcher reviewed and refined themes to produce the final report, presented in the results section. The second researcher served as a peer debriefer and under-went the same process on a random part of the transcripts to ensure reliability of the generated themes and confirm the researcher's accuracy of quotes, coding, and interpretation of the source data. The qualitative analysis of the data revealed the following themes, which are presented below.

Quantitative Data: The data were analysed by using JASP (version 18). One-sample Wilcoxon signed-rank tests (because the normality assumption was violated) were performed to assess whether acceptability ratings significantly differed from the midpoint of the scale (3=neutral) for each group. Additionally, paired Wilcoxon signed-rank tests (due to the violation of normality) were used to examine whether there were any differences between the pre-test and post-test scores on each effec-tiveness scale.

RESULTS

Qualitative Data

Step 2: Pilot Evaluation of the Whole Program in English and Adaptation

During the first pilot evaluation for the whole program in English, participating students were asked to share their experiences on the effectiveness, the content, and the overall implementation of the program. Students' feedback did not particularly focus on the use of music but reported positive attitudes to the content of the program and the main skills introduced. Particular mention was made to the applicability of the program and its practical aspects easily transferred to their everyday lives.

In line with their quantitative evaluation, their responses were overall positive with regards to their personal growth and its perceived benefits for their own development and their academic training. The participating students shared how the program gave them the opportunity to work on themselves, be more aware of their emotions, and practice change in a structured and supported environment. One of the students reported:

"I think it was extremely effective for my personal growth because it reminded me but also introduced to me to some new techniques I can use in my daily life to regulate my emotional state but also to learn how to be more peaceful when I come face to face with a stressful situation. The techniques taught, if applied on a daily basis, can change a person's life, making him more mindful of themselves, both body and mind, but also of the environment."

Beyond academic success, homework was seen as an opportunity to further practice these skills and be more successful in their daily lives. Making connections between life at the university also came up through their reports. For example, another student wrote:

"It is helpful because it is work on us, which is important. Personally, I found helpful the breathing exercises and it's one thing that I want to introduce and use in my everyday life. Also, it was nice to see in practice ways to control our feelings and not just in theory."

"Putting the skills we learned into action" and "[the program being] …helpful for my academic career and future as a whole" echoed often among the responses. This probably indicated the connections that the participating students made between the skills in the program, their personal growth, and their academic and later professional success. For example, some of the students noted that with the completion of the course they felt more confident in their management and communication abilities, all of which are essential skills for advancing in their professional lives.

Of interest to the program development were the suggestions and feedback from the students on the delivery of the program and the course overall. Again (in line also with the quantitative results) the responses were positive, indicating high levels of satisfaction. In some of their responses, students asked for more interactive techniques related to music and meditation and breathing exercises. Also, the students indicated how they would enjoy enhanced group work, more art-related activities (such as dance, art, and poetry) and the idea of moving outside of the classroom to experience the course content deeper. One student's comment highlighted these aspects as they shared: "

"I think some dance therapy techniques as well as Art therapy would suit the lab. It would be amazing actually. I would like more of a team vibe too with my classmates. Maybe do the lab not in a classroom, I would prefer something more inspiring, maybe outdoors, or in a room with more light."

Finally, the use of technology also came up as an effective and efficient way to share examples and deliver the information in a more accessible way. Having VR, headsets, and quality sound equipment for the musical examples were among the suggestions we gathered in the open -ended questions. This feedback was taken into consideration by the research team at a later stage of the project, which provisioned the development of an app for the delivery of the program.

Instructors: Although they initially reported feeling anxious about the introduction of music activities during their instructional time, they both reported that they found the process positive and helpful for the content they taught to their groups. Both instructors highlighted the students' increased levels of engagement along with the shared feelings of joy during the implementation of the activities. One of the instructors noted:

"I noticed that the implementation of the activities created a sense of bonding among the students in my group…and this continued even after the implementation of the music-activities…[]we started off with the music and it created a positive climate..hmm..like we can do what we feel anyway…it was positive energy!" One other recurring point that was brought up, related to the process of self-reflection on part of the students. "[with the songs]..they had the space to get into their own emotions…and that helped them not to avoid them..[music] helped them see emotions more experientially, for example one of my students wrote a poem".

Regarding the structure and content of the music-based manual, the instructors discussed specific parts of the music-based model for which they needed more elaboration and sometimes the theoretical background to support them. One of the main requests at this pilot stage was the need for elaboration and more descriptive instructions for the implementation of some of the music activities in the manual. One of them said: "I think the manual needs some elaboration. Do they listen to the music activity with one ear and with the other listen to me? I think that was not clear... especially because I do not come from a clinical background". Other concerns they expressed referred to the choices of songs and lyrics that did not facilitate the discussion with the students. For example, one of the instructors noted for the unit on setting personal goals: "I would like to have more choices of songs because ..there were a lot for some units but not so much for some others…and this helped a lot to choose…[more suggested songs] that helps me to make a more suitable choice based on the discussion with the students" As she continued reflecting on the process, she added: "Sometimes, I took the initiative to add discussions to the songs as well although it was not in the manual…they listened to each other more that way and it was easier to express themselves…listen to what they had to say".

On more practical aspects of the implementation, they described the process as "easy" and "pleasant". As mentioned above, there were requests for a step-by-step guide on the song-writing activity and ideas on incorporating rhythmical patterns while the students actively listened to songs. Their comments and feedback led to revisions to the music training manual, mainly related to the length of the suggested program, the song selections, revisions on the instructions for the music and imagery experiences, and the inclusion of specific ideas (e.g. examples of rhythmical patterns, clearly outlined steps in the relaxation activities and the group song-writing) for the implementation of music-based training program.

Challenges

Overall, the participating instructors were engaged and enthusiastic about incorporating music into their curriculum. However, several challenges emerged: Integrating the program into existing courses was a primary challenge, as aligning pilot training with current course schedules and content proved difficult. Higher education courses are often densely packed with required material, leaving little room for additional training modules. Ensuring student participation and engagement in the pilot training was also challenging, as some students viewed pilot projects as less important than core coursework. The program needed to be integrated into core coursework and shown to be relevant to students' career goals or academic requirements. Facilitators had varying levels of experience and training in music methodologies, which brought diverse perspectives but also led to inconsistencies in technique application. Facilitators with less musical background often relied more on didactic methods. The intervention was resource-intensive, demanding significant time, effort, and financial investment for facilitator training and program delivery. Finally, facilitators faced challenges related to cultural competence and sensitivity when working with participants from diverse backgrounds.

Step 3 & 4: Pilot evaluation of selected modules in Greek and adaptation

Qualitative: Responses from the participants during Step 3 & 4 of the pilot evaluation of the program depicted their perceptions of the program. Participants described several aspects of the music-based program as unique and useful for their personal and academic growth. Although most of them identified music as an important and efficient component in the process of their personal development and managing emotions, others (although considerably few) provided useful feedback on disadvantages of having music - embedded activities in the program. Regardless of the preference on music or not, these data suggest that the program offered an engaging and meaningful approach to self-development, which the participants embraced as they realized its potential for their personal and academic growth.

Advantage of Music

Enough students commented on the use of music in the program, suggesting music made it more attractive for several reasons, including the major role of music in their everyday lives, and the preference for engaging into music activities as it resonates with their everyday practices and helped them make connections with the content of the program. For example, one student shared in the comments: "Music makes everything better". Another one noted: "Music helps me express myself" and another wrote: and another added "Most part of my day I listen to music, it is a big part of my life". By contrast, one participant noted: " On the one hand, I am more relaxed with music but on the other hand I am distracted and I forget to pay attention to the instructions".

Music in the Program

Many participants seemed to favor music -based activities because it helped them make connections with the content presented and they felt more peaceful. Two characteristic examples are: ""Music helps me with everything, relax, calm down, get activated to complete tasks. Therefore, any activity combined with music is better" and "I prefer to have music in the program because I concentrate more and I am more effective". However, other students noted that the use of music depended on personal circumstances and the goal of the activity. "It depends on the occasion, the materials presented, and my mood [...]" On that note, one of the students mentioned: "I would prefer the non-music based activities because I found it easier to concentrate on the instructor". Perhaps, the relaxing effect of music on their mood added a layer of difficulty in the university environment where typically the expectations include being attentive and alarmed to follow the instructors' guidelines.

View on the Program

This third theme categorized data describing attitudes and views on the experience of participating in a program that focused on emotional development and growth. Overall, the response was enthusiastic as many students described the programs as highly effective, useful, and helpful. Among the responses, students noted that: "The course was very effective in supporting our personal growth and in understanding how my body and personality work". Another one tapped on the anxiety as a common axes for students during their university studies and wrote: "The course was very effective because we learnt a lot for our emotions and how to deal with them along with various ways that help us relax in moments of stress...in my opinion this is helpful to all students since most of us deal with anxiety. " They continued suggesting: "I believe that it should be an independent course or lab offered for free credit by the university". Students also made connections between the content of the course and professional aspirations and other responsibilities in their lives. Indicative is the comment from this student who noted that more courses on this topic: "It would be very helpful because it would help both psychologically with all the adversities we have to deal with at the university but also with my involvement in sports activities".

Suggestions for Improvement

Similar to the pilot 2 phase of the program, some students indicated that they would benefit more from the program with the addition of more art-related techniques and the offering of the program outside the university auditorium. For example, it was noted: "Outside in nature, it would be interesting to implement the techniques" as well as "In small groups in a quiet place". Others expressed the need for "More exercises and the use of talks, invited speakers, and relevant movies and interviews " on the topics they discussed. Regarding the interactive aspect of the program the students were satisfied and they again requested the availability of an application that would allow them to practice the content at their own pace, beyond the course requirements.

Step 5: pilot evaluation from an external expert and final adaptation

As a final stage of the pathway process, the music activities were evaluated for a second time by professionals with specialization in music education and music performance .Specifically, feedback on the choice of music activities and the overall structure and organization of the units was sought by the Cyprus Music Education Association (Mou.sy.ky). A team of experts from Mou.sy.ky went through the music manual, its scope, and the applicability of the activities included. Based on their expertise on music and relevant professional experiences working with adolescents and young adults, they shared with the researchers their evaluation, feedback, and suggestions for improvement. The music professionals offered musical excerpts by both male and female voices to balance gender representation in the manual. Also, they made suggestions on songs and activities that can be applicable to the targeted population, including additional ideas for active music listening examples, and lyrics analysis. Their feedback was incorporated into the manual in its current form of five units/sessions. As a result, a revised and finalized emotion regulation program, enhanced with music methodology, was published and made publicly available (link).

Students' Acceptance

The acceptability scores ranked between 3.15 and 4.96, indicating a general high level of acceptance among the participants. Acceptability results are summarized in Table 4.

Table 4.

Means and Standard deviations for acceptance measure	
Item	**M (SD)**
The course met my needs overall.	4.15 (.83)**
Overall, I enjoyed the course.	4.41 (.77)**
Overall, I was satisfied with the course.	4.40 (.80)**
I had enough time to complete the course.	4.24 (.82)**
The length of each session within the course was appropriate.	4.11 (.91)**
Complexity	

continued on following page

Table 4. Continued

Means and Standard deviations for acceptance measure	
Item	**M (SD)**
I found the sessions easy to follow.	4.35 (.85)**
Overall, I was able to do the homework assignments in between course sessions.	4.30 (.80)**
I found the course confusing[1]	1.85 (.95)**
The course used interesting and appropriate delivery methods (e.g., animation, video, audio, text, simulation, etc.)	4.39 (.79)**
Perceived effectiveness	
The course increased my knowledge about emotion regulation skills.	4.28 (.77)**
The homework assignments helped facilitate my learning	3.92 (.95)**
Overall, I understood the techniques and concepts that were taught.	4.34 (.66)**
Content novelty	
The course content was new to me.	3.81 (1.16)**
Compatibility	
What was taught was relevant to me.	4.12 (.80)**
Self-efficacy	
The course has helped me deal more effectively with daily issues.	4.96 (.85)**
I am likely to continue to use the techniques learnt in the long term.	4.06 (.85)**
Perceived benefits	
Overall, I have been using what I have been taught in my every-day life.	3.78 (.88)**
Future students would benefit from this course being integrated into the curriculum.	4.41 (.71)**
Motivation	
I had a positive attitude toward having the course.	4.41 (.75)**
My interest in learning about soft skills increased as a result of the course.	4.04 (.90)**

continued on following page

Table 4. Continued

Means and Standard deviations for acceptance measure	
Item	**M (SD)**
My interest in self-development increased as a result of the course.	4.18 (.84)**

Notes: Items' scale: 5 = strongly agree, 4 = agree, 3 = neutral, 2 = disagree, and 1 = strongly disagree
¹ = reverse item
**p<.001

Preliminary Effectiveness

Table 5 presents means and standard deviations for all subscales.

Table 5.

Pre-post comparisons on preliminary effectiveness scales		
Subscale	**Pre** M (SD)	**Post** M (SD)
EBQ		
Negative-Controllability	7.87 (4.83)	7.43 (4.78)
Positive-Controllability	8.63 (5.08)	8.68 (5.49)
Negative-Usefulness	9.25 (5.91)**	7.76 (5.04)**
Positive-Usefulness	5.11 (3.51)	5.28 (4.02)
General-Controllability	16.51 (9.42)	16.12 (10)
General-Usefulness	14.36 (8.61)	13.04 (8.31)
Total scale	30.86 (17.32)	29.16 (17.59)
DASS 21		
Stress	6.52 (5.56)	6.68 (5.13)
Anxiety	4.66 (5.19)	5.11 (5.23)
Notes: **p<.001		

EBQ

Controllability of Emotions
No significant results were found related to students' beliefs on controllability of emotions: negative emotions ($Z = 1.25$, $p =.21$), negative emotions ($Z = -.13$, $p =.90$), and general controllability ($Z = .49$, $p =.63$).
Usefulness of Emotions

Beliefs about the usefulness of emotions were assessed similarly. A significant change was only found for negative usefulness (Mdiff=1.49, Z = 3.09, p =.002), indicating a change in participants' perspective on viewing negative emotions as more beneficial and valuable in their lives after completing the program.

DASS 21

No significant reduction in stress levels (Z = -.71, p =.48) or anxiety levels was found (Z = -1.04, p =.29).

Discussion

Through this project we aimed to develop a novel, research-informed training approach to advance socio-emotional skills of university students in a holistic and inclusive manner. The approach lay in a music-based intervention infused with evidence from high-quality research recommendations and the pragmatic knowledge derived from the different pilot stages of the program. A carefully planned development and piloting of the training materials ensured the development of a training model congruent with the core challenges in emotional literacy. Further, we acquired important information on the applicability and feasibility of the program implementation, which can be easily integrated in various university programs to meet young adults' everyday needs and experiences. At the core of our actions was the study of music-based practices as tools for enhancing young adults' potential for learning opportunities within their school and social system and work towards empowering them and supporting them thrive together within their cultural environment.

The findings regarding the acceptability of the novel intervention presented in our study offer significant insights into the perspectives and attitudes of our intended audience. The implications of these findings for the intervention's future implementation and refinement are numerous. The intervention was met with a largely positive reception among the participants, as evidenced by the high overall acceptability scores. This result is promising, as it indicates that the design, content, and implementation of the intervention align with the desires and requirements of the intended recipients. The favorable reception may be ascribed to a multitude of elements, including the pertinence of the material, the simplicity of implementing the intervention, and the perceived advantages articulated by the participants.

The results from the Emotion Beliefs Questionnaire demonstrate a promising positive change in participants' beliefs about emotions. After the intervention, participants reported a stronger belief in the usefulness of negative emotions. These findings suggest that the enhanced emotion regulation program was effective in debunking a common myth on the notion that negative emotions are useless. The qualitative analysis supported these findings and offered additional information on the participants' views on the program implementation. Music listening is a meaningful and important activity in the lives of young adults (McFerran, 2010) known to enhance self -awareness and influence emotions (Saarikallio & Erkkila, 2007). The participants' views on the music activities echoed similar findings as they highlighted that music is an important part of their lives. This fact seemed to enhance their willingness to participate in the program and identify ways in which music supported their personal journey on regulating emotions and identifying strategies to manage them.

Music listening is employed in different disciplines, including music therapy and music education with positive impact on the participants' cognitive and emotional development. The current program was designed by a team of psychologists and music therapists. It is part of few attempts to bridge theories on music psychology and clinical practice (e.g. Dingle & Fay, 2016). Beyond understanding the mechanisms that explain the impact of music in evoking and managing emotions, in this program we attempted to build on structured music experiences as the medium to enhance participation and multimodality in psycho-educational programs for young adults. Within this context, we conceptualized emotion awareness and regulation as complex phenomena that involve the perception and production of social and communicative signals (linguistic cues, emotion, gestures etc) and also a continuous adaptation to others (Chaby et al., 2012). The designed music activities were conceptualized to create a safe space for all participants to engage with others, gain a deeper under-standing of their own process, and encourage reflection on their practices, as part of a university course. Discussions and activities after the music experiences helped participants identify practices and obstacles within the meaningful context of music making or active music listening with their peers. Thus, the program represents an effort to support young adults' emotion regulation abilities through an engaging and easy-to- access program.

In general, all pilot phases showed a general students' acceptance of the trainings around the cultivation of soft skills. Despite encouraging preliminary findings regard-ing the uptake of the specific interventions, due to limitations in terms of resources available, it was not possible to run the pilot studies in a way that would collect data in a way that would allow subgroup comparisons (e.g. field and year of study, people with specific learning needs/difficulties, etc.). Also, another important limitation concerned the characteristics in our sample, including participants' gender imbalance and relevant homogeneity in terms of culture and ethnicity. Pragmatic restrictions on the structure of the study led to a non randomized convenience sample. As such, the self-selected participants shared common characteristics in terms of their social background. Further, the participants attended the program as part of their formal coursework at their university. Since they accepted to participate in the program, they most likely were invested in their personal growth/cultivation of soft skills and they had a positive disposition to music. Finally, the reliance on self-reported measures along with the lack of follow-up assessments due to the limitations of the semester-based study design are weaknesses of the study.

Thus, further research is necessary before the findings can be generalized. In terms of the training materials, important practical considerations center around the need for professional development of the instructors, such as their clinical experience and the provisions for supervision sessions related to the implementation of the designed activities. The duration and intensity of the training materials needs to be explored as well, since the program is provisioned to be part of a classroom-based wide training program. Also, further research is needed to include translational pilot evaluations, and Randomized Controlled Trial/ RCT program design to compare the new intervention with standard ones.

Practical Implications

This study underscores the importance of interdisciplinary collaboration and structural support for implementing such programs. Integrating relevant units into the general curriculum and training instructors in emotion regulation principles and music-based ER programs necessitates cross-departmental collaboration within the university. Program coordinators, strategic selection of appropriate courses, and enhanced content development in partnership with the institution's mental health services can ensure the long-term implementation of these programs for the benefit of all students.

This pilot study focuses on the early stages of development and testing. Researchers have formulated the program's basic concept based on theoretical frameworks and preliminary research on effective techniques. A prototype has been developed, emphasizing user acceptability and usability. Future research should concentrate on larger-scale effectiveness trials to evaluate the program's impact on students' mental health. Scaling up the intervention may be challenging without additional resources. Additionally, an implementation study is needed to evaluate how effectively the intervention can be integrated into the university context. This involves assessing organizational readiness, training facilitators, monitoring fidelity to the program protocol, and evaluating cost-effectiveness.

To optimize future research, it is crucial for program coordinators to navigate budgetary constraints by securing funding from both institutional budgets and external grants, ensuring the availability of necessary resources and staffing for effective program delivery. Additionally, comprehensive facilitator training is essential to equip educators with the required pedagogical skills and content expertise, including cultural competency training and fostering an inclusive environment, which enhances the sensitivity and effectiveness of the intervention. Continuous professional development opportunities further enable facilitators to adapt their teaching methods and manage logistical challenges. Moreover, integrating the curriculum with educational goals and strategically scheduling it within existing courses necessitates collaboration with faculty to ensure seamless integration and meaningful learning experiences for students.

Ethical Considerations

Local approval was obtained from Cyprus National Bioethics Committee (EEBK ΕΠ 2023.01.47). The study has been registered on clinicaltrials.gov (NCT05746234).

All procedures performed in the study were in accordance with the ethical standards of the institutional and/or national research committee and with the 1964 Helsinki declaration and its later amendments or comparable ethical standards. All study participants were informed in detail of the aims and objectives of the study. Participants were informed that they have the right to withdraw their membership in the study at any time. Electronic informed consent was obtained from all individual participants included in the study. The anonymized data will be available from the corresponding author, on reasonable request.

Funding

The current chapter presents part of the work done for two ongoing projects: a) Internal Research Programme: A. G. Leventis Foundation Programmes (University of Cyprus) *'Music for Inclusion and Social-Emotional Learning'* and b) EU Erasmus+ project *'MASH-up n' HEI Multimodal Approach for Social-emotional Learning in HEI'* (2021-1-CY01-KA220-HED-000023329). The content employed herein does not necessarily reflect the official views of the European Commission.

Competing Interests

None declared.

ACKNOWLEDGMENTS

The authors would like to express their sincere gratitude to their colleagues for their work on the project and help especially with proofing early versions of the training material: Dr. Alexios Arvanitis and Dr. Panagiota Dimitropoulou (PANEPISTIMIO KRITIS), Dr. Elke Vlemincx (VRIJE UNIVERSITEIT AMSTERDAM), Dr. Ferenc Honbolygó and Mr. Csaba Kertesz (EÖTVÖS LORÁND UNIVERSITY), and providing assistance with data collection: Ms. Tonia- Flerry Artemi, Ms. Ayse Biyikoglu, Mr. Anastasios Petrou and Mr. Ioannis Mavrommatis (UNIVERSITY OF CYPRUS).

REFERENCES

Acharya, L., Jin, L., & Collins, W. (2018). College life is stressful today - Emerging stressors and depressive symptoms in college students. Journal of American college health. *Journal of American College Health*, 66(7), 655–664. DOI: 10.1080/07448481.2018.1451869 PMID: 29565759

Al-Fraihat, D., Joy, M., & Sinclair, J. (2020). Evaluating E-learning systems success: An empirical study. *Computers in Human Behavior*, 102, 67–86. DOI: 10.1016/j.chb.2019.08.004

Barlow, D. H., Farchione, T. J., Fairholme, C. P., Ellard, K. K., Boisseau, C. L., Allen, L. B., & Ehrenreich-May, J. (2018). *Unified protocol for transdiagnostic treatment of emotional disorders: Therapist guide*. Oxford University Press.

Becerra, R., Preece, D. A., & Gross, J. J. (2020). Assessing beliefs about emotions: Development and validation of the Emotion Beliefs Questionnaire. *PLoS One*, 15(4), e0231395. Advance online publication. DOI: 10.1371/journal.pone.0231395 PMID: 32287328

Benigno, J., Brown, L., & Geist, K. (2018). Come together: Music therapy and speech language pathology students' perspectives on collaboration during an inclusive camp for children with ADS. *Music Therapy Perspectives*, 36(1), 12–25.

Braun, V., & Clarke, V. (2006). Using thematic analysis in psychology. *Qualitative Research in Psychology*, 3(2), 77–101. DOI: 10.1191/1478088706qp063oa

Bruijns, B. A., Vanderloo, L. M., Johnson, A. M., Adamo, K. B., Burke, S. M., Carson, V., Heydon, R., Irwin, J. D., Naylor, P.-J., Timmons, B. W., & Tucker, P. (2022). Change in pre-and in-service early childhood educators' knowledge, self-efficacy, and intentions following an e-learning course in physical activity and sedentary behaviour: A pilot study. *BMC Public Health*, 22(1), 1–13. DOI: 10.1186/s12889-022-12591-5 PMID: 35125100

Castro-Camacho, L., Díaz, M. M., & Barbosa, S. (2022). Effect of a group prevention program based on the unified protocol for college students in Colombia: A quasi-experimental study. *Journal of Behavioral and Cognitive Therapy*, 32(2), 111–123. DOI: 10.1016/j.jbct.2021.04.001

Chaby, L., Chetouani, M., Plaza, M., & Cohen, D. (2012). *Exploring multimodal social-emotional behaviors in autism spectrum disorders: an interface between social signal processing and psychopathology*. IEEE., DOI: 10.1109/SocialCom-PASSAT.2012.111

Champ, M., & Xiong, Q. (2018). The effects of music therapy on cognition, psychiatric symptoms, and activities of daily living in patients with Alzheimer's disease. *Journal of Alzheimer's Disease*, 64(4), 1–12. PMID: 29991131

Collins, F. S., & Fleming, R. (2017). Sound health: An NIH-Kennedy Center Initiative to explore Music and the Mind. *Journal of the American Medical Association*, 317(24), 2470–2471. DOI: 10.1001/jama.2017.7423 PMID: 28586832

Conley, C. S., & Durlak, J. A. (2017). Universal mental health promotion and prevention programs for students. In S. Bährer-Kohler & F. J. Carod-Artal (Eds.), Global mental health: Prevention and promotion (pp. 127–139). Springer International Publishing/Springer Nature. DOI: 10.1007/978-3-319-59123-0_12

Conley, C. S., Durlak, J. A., & Dickson, D. A. (2013). An Evaluative Review of Outcome Research on Universal Mental Health Promotion and Prevention Programs for Higher Education Students. *Journal of American College Health*, 61(5), 286–301. DOI: 10.1080/07448481.2013.802237 PMID: 23768226

Conley, C. S., Durlak, J. A., & Kirsch, A. C. (2015). A meta-analysis of universal mental health prevention programs for higher education students. *Prevention Science*, 16(4), 487–507. DOI: 10.1007/s11121-015-0543-1 PMID: 25744536

Constantin, F. A. (2018). Music therapy explained by the principles of neuroplasticity. Bulletin of the Transilvania University of Brasov, Series VIII. *Performing Arts*, 11(1), 19–24.

de Witte, M., Spruit, A., van Hooren, S., Moonen, X., & Stams, G. J. (2020). Effects of music interventions on stress-related outcomes: A systematic review and two meta-analyses. *Health Psychology Review*, 14(2), 294–324. DOI: 10.1080/17437199.2019.1627897 PMID: 31167611

Dingle, G. A., & Fay, C. (2017). Tuned In: The effectiveness for young adults of a group emotion regulation program using music listening. *Psychology of Music*, 45(4), 513–529. DOI: 10.1177/0305735616668586

Ford, B. Q., & Gross, J. J. (2019). Why beliefs about emotion matter: An emotion-regulation perspective. *Current Directions in Psychological Science*, 28(1), 74–81. DOI: 10.1177/0963721418806697

Geretsegger, M., Quoc, E., Riedl, H., Smetana, M., & Stegemann, T. (2019). Music therapy and other music-based interventions in pediatric health care: An overview. *Medicines (Basel, Switzerland)*, 6(25), 1–12. PMID: 30769834

Hallis, L., Cameli, L., Bekkouche, N. S., & Knäuper, B. (2017). Combining cognitive therapy with acceptance and commitment therapy for depression: A group therapy feasibility study. *Journal of Cognitive Psychotherapy*, 31(3), 171–190. DOI: 10.1891/0889-8391.31.3.171 PMID: 32755936

Henry, J. D., & Crawford, J. R. (2005). The short-form version of the Depression Anxiety Stress Scales (DASS-21): Construct validity and normative data in a large non-clinical sample. *British Journal of Clinical Psychology*, 44(Pt 2), 227–239. DOI: 10.1348/014466505X29657 PMID: 16004657

Hernandez-Ruiz, E. (2017). Collaboration and assistance in music therapy practice: Roles, relationships, challenges. *Music Therapy Perspectives*, 38(1), e9–e10. DOI: 10.1093/mtp/mix008

Huth, T., Munson, J., Adams, R., Gunderson, A., & Gonzalez, V. (2021). South Korean Popular Music Industry: Globalization of Identity and Exploitation.

Koelsch, S. (2020). A coordinate-based meta-analysis of music-evoked emotions. *NeuroImage*, 223, 117350. DOI: 10.1016/j.neuroimage.2020.117350 PMID: 32898679

Leubner, D., & Hinterberger, T. (2017). Reviewing the effectiveness of music interventions in treating depression. *Frontiers in Psychology*, 8, 1109. Advance online publication. DOI: 10.3389/fpsyg.2017.01109 PMID: 28736539

Levy, I. P. (2019). Hip-hop and spoken word therapy in urban school counseling. *Professional School Counseling*, 22(1b), 2156759X1983443. Advance online publication. DOI: 10.1177/2156759X19834436

McFerran, K. (2010). *Adolescents, music and music therapy: Methods and techniques for clinicians, educators and students.* Jessica Kingsley., DOI: 10.1080/01609513.2011.561044

Miller, A. E., & Racine, S. E. (2022). Emotion regulation difficulties as common and unique predictors of impulsive behaviors in university students. *Journal of American College Health*, 70(5), 1387–1395. DOI: 10.1080/07448481.2020.1799804 PMID: 32790500

National Institutes of Health. (2018). Sound Health: An NIH-Kennedy Center Partnership [Research Plan]. National Institutes of Health. https://www.nih.gov/sound-health/research-plan

Parker, J. D., Summerfeldt, L. J., Hogan, M. J., & Majeski, S. A. (2004). Emotional intelligence and academic success: Examining the transition from high school to university. *Personality and Individual Differences*, 36(1), 163–172. DOI: 10.1016/S0191-8869(03)00076-X

Pezirkianidis, C., Karakasidou, E., Lakioti, A., Stalikas, A., & Galanakis, M. (2018). Psychometric Properties of the Depression, Anxiety, Stress Scales-21 (DASS-21) in a Greek Sample. *Psychology (Irvine, Calif.)*, 9(15), 2933–2950. DOI: 10.4236/psych.2018.915170

Randall, W. M., Rickard, N. S., & Vella-Brodrick, D. A. (2014). Emotional outcomes of regulation strategies used during personal music listening: A mobile experience sampling study. *Musicae Scientiae*, 18(3), 275–291. DOI: 10.1177/1029864914536430

Rodwin, A. H., Shimizu, R., Travis, R.Jr, James, K. J., Banya, M., & Munson, M. R. (2023). A systematic review of music-based interventions to improve treatment engagement and mental health outcomes for adolescents and young adults. *Child & Adolescent Social Work Journal*, 40(4), 537–566. DOI: 10.1007/s10560-022-00893-x PMID: 36407676

Saarikallio, S., Gold, C., & McFerran, K. (2015). Development and validation of the Healthy-Unhealthy Music Scale. *Child and Adolescent Mental Health*, 20(4), 210–217. DOI: 10.1111/camh.12109 PMID: 26726295

Sauer-Zavala, S., Tirpak, J. W., Eustis, E. H., Woods, B. K., & Russell, K. (2021). Unified protocol for the transdiagnostic prevention of emotional disorders: Evaluation of a brief, online course for college freshmen. *Behavior Therapy*, 52(1), 64–76. DOI: 10.1016/j.beth.2020.01.010 PMID: 33483125

Schuenemann, L., Scherenberg, V., von Salisch, M., & Eckert, M. (2022). "I'll worry about it tomorrow"–Fostering emotion regulation skills to overcome procrastination. *Frontiers in Psychology*, 13, 780675. DOI: 10.3389/fpsyg.2022.780675 PMID: 35391959

Thomas, C., & Zolkoski, S. (2020, June). Preventing stress among undergraduate learners: The importance of emotional intelligence, resilience, and emotion regulation. [). Frontiers Media SA]. *Frontiers in Education*, 5, 94. DOI: 10.3389/feduc.2020.00094

Thomson, C. J., Reece, J. E., & Di Benedetto, M. (2014). The relationship between music-related mood regulation and psychopathology in young people. *Musicae Scientiae*, 18(2), 150–165. DOI: 10.1177/1029864914521422

Tucker, P., Bruijns, B. A., Adamo, K. B., Burke, S. M., Carson, V., Heydon, R., Irwin, J. D., Johnson, A. M., Naylor, P. J., Timmons, B. W., & Vanderloo, L. M. (2022). Training Pre-Service Early Childhood Educators in Physical Activity (TEACH): Protocol for a Quasi-Experimental Study. *International Journal of Environmental Research and Public Health*, 19(7), 3890. DOI: 10.3390/ijerph19073890 PMID: 35409573

Watkins, D. C., Hunt, J. B., & Eisenberg, D. (2012). Increased demand for mental health services on college campuses: Perspectives from administrators. *Qualitative Social Work: Research and Practice*, 11(3), 319–337. DOI: 10.1177/1473325011401468

Worsley, J. D., Pennington, A., & Corcoran, R. (2022). Supporting mental health and wellbeing of university and college students: A systematic review of review-level evidence of interventions. *PLoS One*, 17(7), e0266725. Advance online publication. DOI: 10.1371/journal.pone.0266725 PMID: 35905058

Yusufov, M., Nicoloro-SantaBarbara, J., Grey, N. E., Moyer, A., & Lobel, M. (2019). Meta-analytic evaluation of stress reduction interventions for undergraduate and graduate students. *International Journal of Stress Management*, 26(2), 132–145. DOI: 10.1037/str0000099

Chapter 13
How Can Adults Talk to Children About War, Inspiring Them Towards Peace?
Children's Understanding, Dialogue With Adults, and Educational Strategies

Giulia Perasso

https://orcid.org/0000-0003-3265 -3869

University of Genoa, Italy

Carmela Lillo

Fondazione Patrizio Paoletti, Italy

Sandro Anella

Fondazione Patrizio Paoletti, Italy

Giulia Viviano

University of Genoa, Italy

Matilde Pisano

University of Genoa, Italy

Elena Vigogna

University of Genoa, Italy

Erika Salemi

University of Genoa, Italy

Tania Di Giuseppe

Fondazione Patrizio Paoletti, Italy

ABSTRACT

This scoping review emphasizes the importance of understanding children's cognitive and socio-emotional capacities in navigating discussions about war and peace. Tailoring communication strategies to these developmental nuances enables meaningful dialogues between adults and children, fostering empathy and conflict

DOI: 10.4018/979-8-3693-5325-7.ch013

resolution skills. Additionally, pedagogical interventions highlighted in the review aim to nurture peacebuilding skills among children, empowering them to contribute positively to their communities. In conclusion, by considering children's developmental needs and implementing effective communication and educational strategies, adults can play a crucial role in cultivating peaceful mindsets and behaviors in future generations.

1. INTRODUCTION

Engaging in dialogue regarding the themes of war and peace with children serves two primary purposes: the prevention of indirect trauma (Pine et al., 2005), which could stem from exposure to violent content such as images or footage of armed conflict, and the promotion of peace education from early developmental stages (Shapiro, 2002), contributing to the future construction of new generations.

The significance of adults' role in discussing such topics is deeply rooted in developmental psychology and education. Attachment Theory (Bowlby, 1969), for instance, highlights how caregivers can serve as a secure base for children from which they can explore the world and confront stressful situations by regulating their emotions with appropriate strategies. Social Learning Theory (Bandura, 1977), on the other hand, emphasizes how adults, being observed and imitated by children, serve as models of behavior for them to cope with adversity. Simultaneously, Moral Development Theory (Kohlberg, 1984) underscores how adults can provide children with moral guidance, facilitating a deeper understanding of the consequences of individual and communal behaviors, thereby promoting comprehension of concepts such as justice and responsibility. In other words, it is the pedagogical responsibility of parents and educators to guide children, according to their age and resources, in comprehending complex constructs, positioning themselves as scaffolding (Vygotsky, 1978) between what children can understand and what they could understand with appropriate support.

Since February 2022, with the onset of the Russo-Ukrainian conflict, and from October 2023 with the escalation of the Israeli-Palestinian conflict, the theme of war has become a daily subject in Western media, reaching our televisions and digital devices every day and capturing the attention of individuals of all ages. The exposure to this type of news at a developmental age raises relevant psychopedagogical issues: parents and teachers find themselves addressing complex topics such as the concept of war and peace with children, needing to respond to their questions with explanations that are suitable and understandable for their level of cognitive, emotional, social, and moral development.

1.1 Chapter's objective

The chapter provides a scoping review aimed at examining how adults can talk to children about war and peace, in the absence of previous review works on this topic. The chapter thus presents three objectives and respective research questions, formulated by adapting the parameters of the PICO Model to the psychopedagogical context, for the formulation of foreground questions (Nishikawa-Pacher, 2022). The first objective (i) is to explore the literature to analyze how the concepts of war and peace are perceived and understood by children, seeking to answer the question "What are the cognitive processes that allow children to understand the concepts of war and peace?". This constitutes a fundamental step for adults to guide dialogue on these topics, preventing potential indirect trauma of children resulting from media exposure. It is also essential, as the second objective (ii), to conduct a detailed analysis of the literature to understand if and which strategies are suggested by the scientific community to guide adults in dialogue with children on the topic of war and peace, answering the question "What are the most effective communicative strategies for talking to children about war and peace?". Similarly, as the third objective (iii), the chapter aims to analyze the literature to identify educational practices that can guide future generations towards a sense of common humanity and the construction of a peaceful global future, answering the question "What are the most effective educational techniques for engaging in peacemaking and peacebuilding from childhood?".

2. METHOD

To address the objectives of this study, the implemented methodology was that of a scoping review, as it is useful for exploring the literature regarding broad research questions on complex, heterogeneous topics not yet studied through systematic reviews (Mays et al., 2001). Moreover, this methodology is helpful in identifying knowledge gaps and formulating recommendations (Armstrong et al., 2011; Rumrill et al., 2010), especially in the field of pedagogy. The search procedure on scientific databases was conducted on October 10, 2023. The keywords used were "talking" (OR "explaining" OR "speaking") AND "about" AND "war" (OR "armed conflict") OR "peace" AND "to child*" OR ("to kid*"). Four databases were consulted: PubMed (n=35), Scopus (n=119), PsycInfo (n=52), PsycArticles (n=2), Google Scholar (n=8). A total of n=203 sources were identified from the databases, which were then subjected to a screening process following the guidelines of Petticrew & Roberts (2008) (Figure 1). After excluding duplicates, the selection criteria used were: (a) English language, in order to give an international scope to the review work, (b) publication type, selecting sources written in scientific journals or peer-reviewed volumes, (c) thematic relevance, which had to fall within the psychological, pedagogical, or social domain. The selection process led to the final inclusion of N=17 sources, included based on the opinion of two independent evaluators (inter-rater agreement measured with Cohen's K=.97).

Figure 1. The screening process of the articles included in the scoping review, following Petticrew and Roberts (2008)

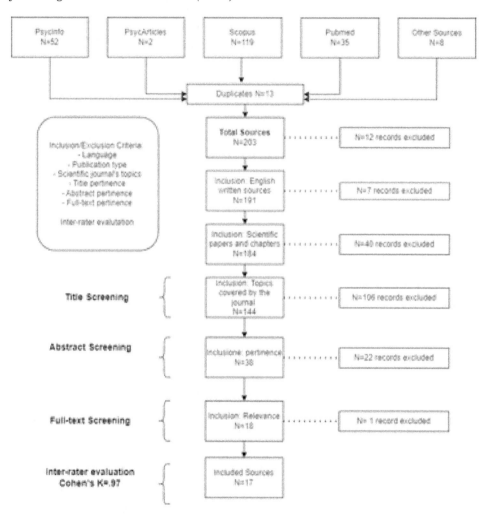

3. REVIEW'S RESULTS

The selected articles (N=17, Table 1) were published within a temporal range spanning from 1985 to 2015. No relevant results for the chapter's themes emerged from publications dated from 2015 to the present. The majority of the articles were published by authors from the United States (47%), but sources from various countries worldwide were included (Israel N=2; Italy N=1; Norway N=1; Nigeria N=1; Sweden N=1; Netherlands N=1; Australia N=1; Germany N=1). All of the sources (N=17) were published in peer-reviewed scientific journals focused on social themes (N=2: *Social Development, Revista de Cercetare si Interventie Sociala*), sulla pace (N=6: *Journal of Peace Education, Journal of Peace Research, Peace and Conflict: Journal of Peace Psychology*), trauma (N=2: *European Journal of Psychotraumatology, Journal of Trauma and Dissociation*), family relationships (N=2: *Family Relations, Journal of Family Issues*), child development (N=3: *Early Child Development and Care, International Journal of Behavioral Development, Developmental Review*) e interdisciplinary research (N=2: *Art Therapy, International Journal of Multidisciplinary Research and Development*). Through the reading of two independent evaluators, the selected sources were thematically divided into three categories, with a high degree of inter-rater agreement (Cohen's K=.89): the theme of children's understanding of war and peace, the theme of educational practices aimed at peacebuilding, and the dialogue between adults and children about war and peace.

Table 1. Selected Articles

Authors	Year	Country	Scientific Journal	Measures	Study type	Sample	Main Results
Berti et al.	2000	Italy	*Social Development*	Semi-structured interviews	Studio empirico	N=80 participants (range 7-13 years)	The concept of war and peace is understood by children starting at age 11, when they grasp the idea of a nation.
Becker-Blease et al.	2008	USA	*Journal of Trauma and Dissociation*	Semi-structured interviews	Empirical study	N=1000 children (range 10-17 years) N=1030 caregiver of children between 2 and 9 years.	Exposure to news about terrorism and war moderately increases stress and anxiety in both adults and children.
Covell et al.	1994	USA	*International Journal of Behavioral Development*	Ad-hoc questionnaire	Empirical study	N=156 participants (range 7-18 years)	Across various age groups, children tend to describe the concept of war more detailedly than peace.

continued on following page

Table 1. Continued

Authors	Year	Country	Scientific Journal	Measures	Study type	Sample	Main Results
Hakvoort, & Hägglund	2001	Sweden	*Peace and Conflict: Journal of Peace Psychology*	Semi-structured interviews	Empirical study	N=416 participants (range 7-17 years)	Similar semantic clusters emerge among Dutch and Swedish children when asked about war: both groups emphasize objects (weapons), roles (soldiers), actions (dying, killing, fighting), and associate negative emotions with those going to war.
Hakvoort & Oppenheimer	1993	Germany	*Journal of Peace Research*	Questionnaire	Empirical study	N=101 participants (range 8-16 years)	Between ages 8 and 12, participants describe peace, war, and strategies for achieving peace by mentioning concrete objects. From ages 14 to 16, they refer to abstract concepts.
Hakvoort & Oppenheimer	1998	Netherlands	*Developmental Review*	-	Review	-	Different variables (age, gender, nation) can influence children's understanding of war and peace.
Schultz et al.	2014	Norway	*European Journal of*	-	Review	-	Teachers play an active role in supporting children after stressful events through a therapeutic and educational approach.
Spielmann	1986	Israel	*Journal of Peace Research*	Qualitative analysis of participants' texts	Empirical study	N=1224 children and adolescents (9-18 years)	Children raised in the shadow of war see peace actively and dynamically, aiming to achieve goals and desires related to improvement and well-being (traveling, engaging in activities).
Shacham et al.	2015	Israel	*Revista de cercetare si interventie sociala*	Semi-structured interviews	Single Case Study	N=14 teachers of children between 6 and 12 years	After crises (terrorism, war, natural disasters), children benefit from creative activities (painting, sculpture, physical activity, storytelling) to process painful emotions. Teachers need guidance to invest in social support, a coping strategy that enables them to be resilience models for their students.

continued on following page

Table 1. Continued

Authors	Year	Country	Scientific Journal	Measures	Study type	Sample	Main Results
Tephly et al.	1985	USA	*Early Child Developement and Care*	Semi-structured interviews	Empirical study	N=49 children (range 2-6 years)	Between ages 2 and 6, children are confused about war, describing it as fighting characterized by shooting and bombing. Most children, especially girls, dislike war and report seeing it increasingly on TV as they grow.
Myers-Walls et al.	1993	USA	*Family Relations*	Survey	Empirical study	N=71 parents of children between 3 and 13 years	The article analyzes how parents explain war and peace to their children. War is often associated with negative actions and feelings, while peace is associated with positive emotions like safety and love. Mothers consider supervising their children's TV content an important strategy for teaching them about war and peace.
Myers-Bowman et al.	2005	USA	*Peace and Conflict: Journal of Peace Psychology*	Semi-structured interviews	Empirical study	N=55 USA children N=50 Yugoslav children (range 3-12 years)	Children in Belgrade describe conflict through concrete objects. In contrast, American children describe it distally. Belgrade children speak of peace as a lost normality.
O'Malley et al.	2007	USA	*Journal of Family Issues*	Survey	Empirical study	N=97 children (range 7-11 years)	Conversations about war and peace are structured between ages 7 and 11. Parents tend to attribute negative and senseless judgments when talking about war. Often, explanations given about what war is are abstract.
Hall, R.	1993	Australia	*Journal of Peace Research*	Survey	Empirical study	N=608 children and adolescens (range 4-16 years)	There are gender differences in children's and adolescents' views on war and peace. Boys have a militaristic view, while girls are inclined towards peace.

continued on following page

Table 1. Continued

Authors	Year	Country	Scientific Journal	Measures	Study type	Sample	Main Results
Bolotin & Duss	2009	USA	*Journal of Peach Education*	Semi-structured interviews	Empirical study	N=7 teachers who were peace educators	Peace educators are teachers who aim to: (i) peacemaking: teaching conflict resolution, (ii) peacebuilding: promoting human rights, (iii) anti-war curriculum: emphasizing the futility of violence.
Obidike et al.	2015	Nigeria	*International Journal of Multidisciplinary Research and Develompment*	-	Guidelines	-	In schools, the following are fundamental for creating peaceful generations: (i) establishing a place of peace in every classroom; (ii) teaching conflict resolution; (iii) integrating peace into school curricula.
Walker et al.	2005	USA	*Art Therapy*	Analysis of drawings	Empirical study	N=56 participants (range 3-12 years)	Drawings on the theme of war are chaotic and overcrowded with objects compared to those about peace.

4.DISCUSSION

The selected sources will be discussed in three distinct thematic categories, all essential when an adult (parent, teacher) approaches the topics of war and peace with children. Firstly, it is fundamental to empathize with the cognitive and socio-emotional capacities for understanding war and peace according to different developmental and educational stages. Secondly, it is crucial to illustrate the functional characteristics of dialogue about war and peace between adults and children. Finally, the tools and pedagogical-educational strategies emerged from the literature for the creation of peaceful generations and communities will be outlined.

4.1 Child's understanding of war and peace

Only by putting ourselves in the perspective of what a child can understand, according to their stage of cognitive, socio-emotional, and moral development, can we guide dialogue and create educational strategies aimed at peacebuilding. In this paragraph, we will examine how various variables such as age, gender, intergenerational influences, sociocultural variables, and media influence can affect the conception of war and peace during developmental stages.

Historically, scientific interest in children's conception of war and peace began in the 1960s when, from a cognitive standpoint, Cooper (1965) asserted a relationship between chronological age and the ability to understand what war is. Selman (1980) formulated a stage-based conception of understanding the concepts of war and peace, possible only when the child has developed a sufficient capacity for perspective-taking to reason about whether two individuals have the same motivations, desires, and goals. Several studies have empirically supported the idea of a stage-based development of understanding war and peace concepts.

For instance, the Italian study by Berti et al. (2000) highlights the importance of considering children's understanding of the concept of war in correlation with their age: understanding war would only be possible when individuals understand and master the concept of a nation (Berti & Benesso, 1998). According to Berti et al. (2000), 7-year-old children describe war as a clash between unstructured groups, where major decisions are made by individuals, including authorities who also engage in combat firsthand. This rudimentary description is linked to an incomplete understanding of leadership and hierarchical power organization (Berti & Bombi, 1988). At nine years old, children report that the main cause of war is competition for a specific element and that conflicts between families and soccer teams can also be considered wars. From eleven years old onwards, children are able to name conflicts caused by political and economic reasons between states as wars.

Similarly, research by Hakvoort & Oppenheimer (1993, 1998) shows that from eight years old to preadolescence, the conception of war and peace is linked to the concreteness of objects and material details, while in adolescence, there is an evolution towards abstract thinking (Piaget, 1929), capable of embracing the nature of relationships between subjects, as well as a more sophisticated moral reasoning concerning ethics and human rights (Kohlberg, 1984). In other words, entering adolescence constitutes a threshold age for understanding the nation as a governed territory, through laws, by an authority. Only by embracing this conception, would a full understanding of war and its consequences be possible.

The impact of age is further supported by the qualitative study conducted by Tephly (1985). Children aged between 2 and 6 years, when asked "what is war?" respond in an unstructured and confused manner, describing combat as the main action. When posed with the question "what do people do during a war?" children's responses are characterized by descriptions of actions such as shooting, dropping bombs, firing cannon shots, without a defined temporal orientation. Most children report not liking wars, and as they grow older, the percentage of children reporting having seen a war on television increases, consistent with numerous findings regarding the risks of media exposure of children to terrorism and military conflicts

(Escalona, 1982; Schwebel, 1982; Rodd, 1985; Cantor & Nathanson, 1996; Putnam, 2002; Ahern et al., 2004; Joshi et al., 2008).

Gender, in turn, could represent a variable capable of influencing children's conception of war and peace. The study by Hall et al. (1993) examines the attitudes of a sample of Australian children towards war and peace. The results showed gender differences, with boys being more militaristic and girls more inclined towards peace. Similarly, Tephly's (1985) study highlights how girls aged 2 to 6 years develop a sense of rejection of war. These gender differences could be determined by the influence of gender-specific toys and their impact on the socio-emotional development of girls and boys (Weisgran & Dinella, 2018). However, it should be noted that, currently, the influence of militaristic toys may be less significant: instead of reflecting national diplomatic intentions, nowadays, toy weapons, soldiers, and tanks may reflect the inclination towards competition and individualism characterizing Western capitalist societies (Machin & Vane Leeuwen, 2009).

It is also crucial to keep in mind that: (a) a child's conception of war and peace may be influenced by their experiences (Patton, 1990); (b) contextual variables related to the environment in which the child grows up may shape their understanding of constructs of such complexity (Raviv, Oppenheimer, & Bar-Tal, 1999; Hakvoort & Hägglund, 2001); (c) children may be susceptible to influences: for example, a study by Fargas-Malet and Dillenburger (2014) shows that drawings and verbal accounts of children from Northern Ireland are characterized by positive elements of hope and peace (festivity, nature, happiness) in reference to the present, but they report scenarios of violence and negative elements (death, poverty, injustice) in reference to the past, drawn from the narratives of previous generations.

Several studies have also focused on sociocultural differences regarding children's understanding of war and peace. Hakvoort and Hägglund (2001) identified similar semantic clusters in Dutch and Swedish children when asked what war is: in both groups, children emphasized objects (weapons), roles (soldiers), actions (dying, killing, fighting), and associated negative emotions with people going to war. These responses could be influenced by the fact that neither of the two nations was at war at the time of the study. Myers-Bowman et al. (2005), on the other hand, comparing the way children from Yugoslavia (who experienced the bombing of Belgrade firsthand) and US children (who have a conception of war mainly through news reports) narrate war, emphasized how the former are inclined to use personal pronouns and concrete and informative terms regarding war, while the latter do not use personal pronouns but very generic terms that emphasize their distal position (as observers).

Regarding the specific concept of peace, it is important to note that in developmental stages, peace is described in less detail compared to war (Covell et al., 1994). Moreover, sociocultural variables also play a key role in this construct. The literature highlights that Nordic children think of peace as "negative peace" or "passive peace" due to the absence of war activities (Hakvoort & Oppenheimer, 1993), while Canadian children associate peace with sharing and kindness (Covell et al., 1994), and Swedish and German children associate it with friendship (Hakvoort & Hägglund, 2001), expressing a positive view of the same concept. Children in Belgrade who directly experienced war define peace as a lost normalcy (Myers-Bowman et al., 2005), linked to life before the conflict. Instead, a study by Spielmann (1986) on Jewish and Arab children and adolescents highlights that children raised in the shadow of war see peace in an active and propulsive sense, as the situation that would make it possible to achieve goals and desires underlying improvement and well-being (traveling, engaging in activities). It is important to note that a "passive" view of peace may not always be negative but may refer to the conception of a contextual situation of greater serenity: a study by Walker et al. (2003) on drawings by children aged 3 to 12 shows that drawings related to the theme of war present a chaotic overcrowding of objects compared to those about peace, although no significant chromatic differences emerge between the two categories.

It is also important to consider that, in countries not directly affected by armed conflicts, children's conception of war is greatly influenced by exposure to news reports that, through television and digital media, enter our homes. Concern that exposure to such news would cause stress in children was noted by parents as early as the 1980s in the USA, when news reports constantly discussed the possibility of nuclear war (Escalona, 1982; Schwebel 1982; Rodd, 1985): these studies indicate that adults' attitude was to shield children and adolescents from such information, although they could not completely keep it out of their lives. The concern of these parents was later found to have empirical support. Indeed, in a survey study by Cantor and Nathanson (1996), it emerged that 37% of American preschool children had a fear reaction ("fright") when watching television scenes of violence related to crime, interpersonal violence, and war.

Moreover, in the United States, and in the broader Western world, adults and children were exposed to significant media stress regarding the events of September 11, 2001. A telephone survey conducted 4 months after that date on adult citizens of New York revealed that individuals who had seen more television news about the event exhibited more symptoms related to post-traumatic stress and panic than those who had watched less news (Ahern et al., 2004). Similarly, children more exposed to terrorism scenes via television showed post-traumatic symptoms, a decrease in future expectations, and greater stress compared to those less exposed (Becker-Blease et al., 2008). The risk of experiencing indirect trauma through exposure to war and terrorism footage and images is concrete, and during childhood, it can predict the development of subsequent anxious symptoms in adulthood (Pine et al., 2005).

It is important to specify that children's age plays a fundamental role in how news from the media is received and processed, especially regarding war: Joshi et al. (2008) summarized the characteristics of three fundamental ages. In preschool age (i), children, in the midst of Piagetian egocentrism (Piaget, 1929), do not master the difference between live images and television replays, nor geographical distance, and therefore, they may think that events are very close to them and/or their fault. Similarly, they are not yet able to conceive death as permanent and may be disturbed by the thought of the end of existence. In school age (ii), the child's thinking still needs concrete support and cannot embrace abstract concepts: the sight of war images could confuse and lead children to develop regressive behaviors (bed-wetting, thumb-sucking, and carrying a transitional object), withdrawal, aggressive, or hyperactive behaviors. Finally, in adolescence (iii), although there are greater capacities for abstract reasoning, ethical-moral reasoning, coping, and problem-solving, individuals may remain disturbed and exhibit internalizing or externalizing modes to manage negative emotions. Exposure to news about war, moreover, could influence adolescents' vision of the future, depleting their hope and planning.

Another consideration concerns the specific means of information through which the child comes into contact with news about war. An example is offered by the pandemic: although this situation also elicited negative emotions and stress in children and adolescents, digital media represented an interactive resource for many to inform themselves, protect themselves, and communicate (Delomi & Pisani, 2020). It can be speculated, therefore, that exposure to potentially traumatic content for children and adolescents is linked to the degree of passivity with which they experience the media themselves. Television, in fact, can bring detailed and graphic content about war into people's homes and indirectly elicit potential traumatic responses in powerless viewers (Putnam, 2002).

4.2 Dialogue Between Adults and Children on War and Peace

Among the selected sources, the study by Shacham (2015) proposes a systematic program to support teachers in their role as educators, even in the post-conflict context. The study refers to an intervention program developed by the Community Stress Prevention Center in Israel, aimed at supporting teachers and students of an elementary school subjected to massive attacks during the Second Lebanon War. The program, developed according to the Basic Ph Coping and Resilience model (Lahad et al., 2013), offers workshops for teachers and children where, through verbal and non-verbal activities (such as painting, sculpture, physical activity, and storytelling), the expression of emotions and experiences, even painful ones, is encouraged.

A key aspect of the workshops dedicated to teachers is the investment in positive coping resources, particularly the possibility of relying on a social support network within the school itself. According to the literature, coping is fundamental for stress management and the promotion of resilience (Sippel et al., 2015). Given the strongly interdependent relationship between teachers and students (Rodrigo-Ruiz, 2016), having a solid support network to address the socio-emotional challenges that may arise during discussions on war and peace with students, makes teachers better equipped to provide support to their students.

Regarding the activities proposed for children, conducted together with teachers, the program focuses on creative activities, in line with the literature on art therapy for trauma treatment in childhood (Van Westrhenen & Fritz, 2014). For children, the possibility of expressing their feelings in a safe space where they can feel welcomed, understood, and free to ask questions about difficult topics such as war and peace is fundamental. The program also provides suggestions to teachers for dialoguing with parents so that they can continue to manage conversations about war and peace at home. This aspect highlights the importance of a good relationship between parents and teachers, as supported by Bronfenbrenner (1986), since such an "exosystem" can influence the child's well-being.

According to Schultz et al. (2014), teachers are at the forefront of helping children understand events during natural and man-made disasters, employing two main approaches: (i) a therapeutic approach focused on managing negative emotions and (ii) an educational approach centered on understanding the phenomena. The authors highlight that in Norway, educational institutions have adopted "educational first aid" documents to assist teachers in restoring a sense of security for students of various age groups (from school-age children to adolescents). The operational goal for teachers in the face of war and terrorism should be to make events understandable, manageable, and meaningful (Antonovsky, 1987). These "educational first aid kits" (Brymer et al., 2006) explain the importance of not avoiding children's primary question about violence, "why?". Making sense of events is crucial for restoring a child's sense of safety and security. Schultz et al. (2014) also suggest that teachers highlight the psychological and sociological factors that can lead to acts of terrorism and conflict, dedicating time and educational content to these topics.

Two of the selected sources focus on the dialogue about war between parents and children. Myers-Walls et al. (1993) investigated how parents responded to their children's questions (aged 3 to 13 years) "What is war?" and "What is peace?". First, the verbs used were analyzed: (i) to explain the concept of war, parents used verbs such as kill, frighten, shoot, hurt, destroy, and die; (ii) to talk about peace, the most used verbs were tolerate, compromise, share, cooperate, forgive, talk, help, and respect.

Generally, it seems that war is linked to action and "doing," while peace is associated with positive feelings. Some parents tend to identify the agents promoting peace or war (states, institutions), while others maintain an abstract tone regarding who has control of the situation. Most parents identify a problem, a lack of agreement, or, in some cases, an injustice as the cause of war, conveying a negative judgment about war and a positive one about peace, emphasizing that peace is preferable to conflict and that war is not the way to solve problems. Often, to explain the concept of peace, parents use negative definitions, starting with "what it is not," and then use emotional vocabulary (hate, anger, fear associated with war; love, happiness, absence of fear, safety, comfort associated with peace) to deepen the definitions. Furthermore, the study shows how parents can teach children about the concepts of war and peace: mothers, in particular, believe that key educational strategies include supervising children's television content, in line with previous literature (Putnam, 2002), processing these meanings through play, and involving their children in groups that share human values. Ecologically (Bronfenbrenner, 1986), family experiences, values, and membership groups influence conversations about war between parents and children: for example, Myers-Walls (1993) highlights that parents from peace churches are less inclined to talk about the "outcome" of the conflict compared to parents from families with at least one military member.

The study by O'Malley et al. (2007) explored children's accounts of communication with their parents about war, investigating the impact of micro and macro-level factors (age, gender, and country of the children) on conversations. Comparing the age group 3-6 years and the group 7-11 years, the study reveals a higher frequency of conversations about war with parents among older children. In the second age group (7-11 years), children exhibit more advanced reasoning, memory, and dialogue skills (Ceci & Bruck, 1998). Additionally, as Piaget (1956) argued, it is only from the age of 8 that it is possible to understand others' perspectives, a necessary ability to comprehend the causes of a conflict between different parties. The research by O'Malley (2007) also indicates that with age, boys are more interested in the topic of war than girls, as stated by previous studies (Gilligan, 1982; Covell, 1994). Considering the dialogue about war between parents and children in two different countries, the United States and Northern Ireland, American parents are found to be more open to discussing these topics, possibly due to children's and adolescents' massive media exposure to images of terrorism and political violence (especially following the September 11, 2001, attacks and the Iraq conflict from 2003 to 2011). Moreover, O'Malley's research (2007) investigated what parents say to their children about war: children's accounts largely report that mothers and fathers attribute negative and senseless judgments to war (e.g., it is a bad thing, or it is "nonsense"). There are no aspects related to the description of weapons, which might instead reach children through the media and not directly from family conversations. Finally, according to the analyzed study (O'Malley et al., 2007), parents' explanations of war are often abstract for three possible reasons: (i) the attempt to compensate for the violent and explicit media images; (ii) the desire not to frighten their children (DeMuth & Melnick, 1998); (iii) the difficulty parents face in talking to children about topics involving death (McNeil, 1983).

4.3 Educational Practices Aimed at Building Peace

The U.S. study by Bolotin and Duss (2009) aims to profile peace educators through a survey directed at teachers. The historical premises of the study are the events of September 11, 2001, and the wars in Afghanistan (2001-2021) and Iraq (2003-2011), which significantly impacted Western society, prompting reflections within the framework of peace pedagogy (Shapiro, 2002). This theoretical framework rejects violence, resolves differences through dialogue, employs critical thinking regarding justice and injustice, and requires an imaginative understanding of the concept of peace (Danesh, 2006). Translated into educational practices, these competencies, reported by teachers' responses in Bolotin and Duss's (2009) qualitative study, are: peacemaking, peacebuilding, and anti-war curriculum. Peacemaking aims to create schools where students can express themselves freely and resolve interpersonal problems peacefully, encompassing notions and practices of conflict resolution such as encouraging dialogue based on mutual respect, promoting the study of human rights, and respecting diversity. Peacebuilding, on the other hand, aims to create a more peaceful world starting with the individual student through guided activities that visualize peace, study historical figures who promoted peace, and engage in mediation activities. Finally, the anti-war curriculum involves an approach to teaching history where the teacher emphasizes the futility of violence, the horrors of war, and questions militarism.

In line with peace pedagogy (Shapiro, 2002), Obidike et al. (2015) argue that building peace is possible when the school and classroom environment convey the concept of peace to children in everyday life. The authors provide practical recommendations to ensure that teachers and parents, both in Nigeria and worldwide, teach children to live in harmony. Specifically, Obidike et al. (2015) focus on: (i) the importance of creating a peaceful environment in the classroom; (ii) teaching conflict resolution; (iii) integrating peace into school curricula.

Regarding the first point (i), the authors emphasize that within the classroom, a "peace space" should be identified—a comfortable place decorated with children's drawings inspired by the idea of peace, where music from different cultures can be heard, and books narrating stories with peaceful behavior models can be read. In the same space, they recommend including photographs and posters depicting human diversity (in terms of age, ethnicity, culture) and establishing rules for the group of children, such as "we solve problems with words."

In terms of teaching conflict resolution (ii), Obidike et al. (2015) emphasize that adults themselves should provide peaceful behavior models for children, in line with Social Learning Theory (Bandura & Walters, 1977). When resolving conflicts among children, adults should allow each child involved to express their viewpoint and repeat it, summarized. Then, adults should guide the children in finding different solutions without imposing their own views or deciding for them but gradually leading them, in a sort of scaffolding (Vygotsky, 1978), to a peaceful solution. Similarly, to the importance of including resilience education in schools as advocated by Paoletti et al. (2022), Obidike et al. (2015) emphasize the importance of incorporating peace education into school curricula (iii) so that it becomes an integrated and transversal aspect across various teaching areas (social sciences, history, art, culture, current events, literature, science, and mathematics) rather than just a single project lasting a few days.

4.4 Limits

Regarding the methodological limitations of the review included in this chapter, it is noted that primarily studies from a Western geographic-cultural derivation were examined. The inclusion of widely disseminated and cited articles within the scientific community led to the final selection of sources exclusively in English, narrowing the scope of the investigation. However, this type of selection is described as having only a marginal impact on the quality of the selected material (Jüni et al., 2002).

Furthermore, it should be specified that unpublished literature or "grey literature" (Auger, 1988) was not included in the selection strategy adopted, as this scoping review did not focus on studies related to clinical interventions for which the inclusion of such literature is supported by shared guidelines within the scientific community (Benzies et al., 2006). Additionally, no temporal filter was applied in the research strategy. This choice was made to include relevant material beyond political and social configurations restricted to specific historical periods. Finally, given the methodological variety of the sources included, this review was not extended into a meta-analysis. However, it could serve as a useful basis for future investigations using this methodology, should more empirical studies on the examined topics be published. Regarding the conceptual limitations of the included sources, it is observed that only two of the selected sources adopted an interdisciplinary perspective. In the study of complex constructs such as war and peace, an interdisciplinary approach, capable of integrating psychology, pedagogy, and sociology, could prove more effective in capturing all the nuances of the phenomena under investigation (Repko et al., 2020).

4.5 Future Directions

The scoping review included in this chapter is the first to date to consider the dialogue between adults and children on the topics of war and peace. The goal of this review is inaugurating the scientific debate on the role of adults in adopting appropriate communication strategies to protect children from the negative effects of direct and indirect exposure to war and to promote educational choices that can inspire peace. From the analysis of the reviewed literature, it emerges that interventions aimed at parents and other educational figures such as caregivers and teachers, designed to support them in dialogue with children, have not yet been developed. These interventions would take into account the importance of their role as reference adults, the capacity to understand the concepts of war and peace at different ages, and the possibility of adopting educational strategies capable of encouraging the creation of inclusive and peaceful environments, starting from the individual and extending to groups.

Thus, there is a need to develop future training programs designed with an interdisciplinary approach that considers the various psycho-social challenges experienced by both children and adults, related to the urgency of a dialogue that can actively promote peace. As demonstrated by a recent research experience with Ukrainian refugee parents (Paoletti et al., 2023a), the Sphere Model of Consciousness (SMC) (Paoletti, 2002; Paoletti, 2008; Paoletti & Ben-Soussan, 2019; Pintimalli et al., 2020; Paoletti & Diamond, 2020), through its neuro-psychopedagogical approach, has proven effective for designing educational interventions aimed at adults and indirectly at children, yielding results in enhancing well-being and positive resources (Morin, 2001; Paoletti et al., 2022a; Paoletti et al., 2022b; Di Giuseppe et al., 2022; Maculan et al., 2022). The SMC can be a valuable guide for adults in understanding and enhancing their role and responsibility through processes of self-knowledge and self-education.

In this regard, following the methodological paradigm of "educating oneself to educate," the SMC can provide knowledge and techniques for the biopsychosocial well-being of adults, primarily to trigger and increase their awareness of their understanding and reactions to the concepts of war and peace, in light of knowledge about brain functioning. Moreover, this approach could help adults support children's understanding of the concepts of war and peace through interaction and communication methods appropriate to their age and the different needs associated with their developmental stages. In continuity with the studies examined, which show the utility of providing adults with 'educational first aid kits' to help them guide children in making sense of events related to man-made disasters, kits designed based on the SMC would be a valuable tool to prevent and intervene in relation to risks, making them manageable and restoring a sense of security in children.

Regarding peace educators, the analyzed studies highlight the necessity of equipping them with knowledge and tools to create contexts that are easily accessible to all, where individual children and groups can express themselves freely, resolve interpersonal problems peacefully, respect diversity, and receive models of peace. This involves studying historical figures who have promoted peace and sharing practices and techniques for visualizing peace. In this direction, the Silence Practice Device (SPD) (Paoletti, 2018), which refers to the SMC, could be a valuable tool to guide visualizations where subjects can build a mental image of themselves experiencing peace, involving the body, emotions, and thoughts, offering them the opportunity to live in the present what they desire for the future, inspired by models of value. The SDP has proven to be a useful tool for supporting well-being, emotional self-regulation, and the ability to reframe experiences in proactive terms (Paoletti et al., 2023b). Through training designed from this theoretical framework, participants could be guided to focus on self-care (personal dimension, the "I") and simultaneously beyond themselves (social dimension, the "We," and the broader dimension of the human family, the "Other than us") (Morin, 2000; Paoletti, 2008; Paoletti et al., 2022a; Paoletti & Di Giuseppe, 2023), educating both adults and children on the value of peace, dialogue, reciprocity, and interconnection.

5. CONCLUSION

This review is the first to explore the existing literature on the dialogue between adults and children regarding war and peace, analyzing articles published in peer-reviewed scientific journals worldwide between 1985 and 2015. The review delves into three fundamental thematic categories: children's understanding of the concepts of war and peace, the dialogue between parents and children about war and peace, and educational practices aimed at peacebuilding. This work emphasizes the importance of considering, first and foremost, the cognitive and socio-emotional capacities of children relative to their age group, which allow for either a rudimentary or sophisticated understanding of war and peace. Furthermore, it highlights the functional characteristics of the dialogue between adults and children about war and peace, providing an overview of educational tools and strategies emerging from the literature to create peaceful generations and communities. Talking to children about war and peace can be challenging, but addressing this issue is essential for creating a peaceful and harmonious society in the future.

REFERENCES

Ahern, J., Galea, S., Resnick, H., & Vlahov, D. (2004). Television images and probable posttraumatic stress disorder after September 11: The role of background characteristics, event exposures, and perievent panic. *The Journal of Nervous and Mental Disease*, 192(3), 217–226. DOI: 10.1097/01.nmd.0000116465.99830.ca PMID: 15091303

Antonovsky, A. (1987). *Unravelling the mystery of health: How people manage stress and stay well.* Jossey-Bass.

Armstrong, R., Hall, B. J., Doyle, J., & Waters, E. (2011). 'Scoping the scope'of a cochrane review. *Journal of Public Health (Oxford, England)*, 33(1), 147–150. DOI: 10.1093/pubmed/fdr015 PMID: 21345890

Auger, C. P. (1998). *Information sources in grey literature (guides to information sources)* (4th ed.). Bowker Saur.

Bandura, A., & Walters, R. H. (1977). *Social learning theory.* Prentice Hall.

Becker-Blease, K. A., Finkelhor, D., & Turner, H. (2008). Media exposure predicts children's reactions to crime and terrorism. *Journal of Trauma & Dissociation*, 9(2), 225–248. DOI: 10.1080/15299730802048652 PMID: 19042776

Benzies, K. M., Premji, S., Hayden, K. A., & Serrett, K. (2006). State-of-theevidence reviews: Advantages and challenges of including grey literature. *Worldviews on Evidence-Based Nursing*, 3(2), 55–61. DOI: 10.1111/j.1741-6787.2006.00051.x PMID: 17040510

Berti, A. E., & Benesso, M. (1998). The concept of nation-state in Italian elementary school children: Spontaneous concepts and effects of teaching. *Genetic, Social, and General Psychology Monographs*, 120(2), 121–143. PMID: 9597745

Berti, A. E., & Bombi, A. S. (1988). *The child's construction of economics.* Cambridge University Press.

Berti, A. E., & Vanni, E. (2000). Italian Children's Understanding of War: A Domain-Specific Approach. *Social Development*, 9(4), 478–496. DOI: 10.1111/1467-9507.00139

Bolotin, J. P., & Duss, L. S. (2009). Teaching a pedagogy of peace: A study of peace educators in United States schools in the aftermath of September 11. *Journal of Peace Education*, 6(2), 189–207. DOI: 10.1080/17400200903086615

Bowlby, J. (1969). *Attachment.* Basic Books.

Bronfenbrenner, U. (1986). Ecology of the family as a context for human development: Research perspectives. *Developmental Psychology*, 22(6), 723–742. DOI: 10.1037/0012-1649.22.6.723

Brymer, M., Jacobs, A., Layne, C., Pynoos, R., Ruzek, J., & Steinberg, A.. (2006). *Psychological first aid*field operations guide* (2nd ed.). National Child Traumatic StressNetwork & National Center for PTSD.

Cantor, J., & Nathanson, A. I. (1996). Children's fright reactions to television news. *Journal of Communication*, 46(4), 139–152. DOI: 10.1111/j.1460-2466.1996.tb01510.x

Ceci, S. J., & Bruck, M. (1993). Suggestibility of the child witness: A historical review and synthesis. *Psychological Bulletin*, 113(3), 403–439. DOI: 10.1037/0033-2909.113.3.403 PMID: 8316609

Cooper, P. (1965). The development of the concept of war. *Journal of Peace Research*, 2(1), 1–17. DOI: 10.1177/002234336500200101

Covell, K., Rose-Krasnor, L., & Fletcher, K. (1994). Age differences in understanding peace, war, and conflict resolution. *International Journal of Behavioral Development*, 17(4), 717–737. DOI: 10.1177/016502549401700409

Covell, K. (1996). National and gender differences in adolescents' war attitudes. *International Journal of Behavioral Development*, 19(4), 871–883. DOI: 10.1177/016502549601900411

Danesh, H. B. (2006). Towards an integrative theory of peace education. *Journal of Peace Education*, 3(1), 55–78. DOI: 10.1080/17400200500532151

Deolmi, M., & Pisani, F. (2020). Psychological and psychiatric impact of COVID-19 pandemic among children and adolescents. *Acta Biomedica*, 91(4). Advance online publication. 10.23750%2Fabm.v91i4.10870 PMID: 33525229

DeMuth, D. H., & Melnick, J. (1998). What happens when they talk about it? Family reactions to nuclear war. *Peace and Conflict*, 4(1), 23–34. DOI: 10.1207/s15327949pac0401_3

Di Giuseppe, T., Perasso, G., Mazzeo, C., Maculan, A., Vianello, F., & Paoletti, P. (2022). *Envisioning the future: A neuropsycho-pedagogical intervention on resilience predictors among inmates during the pandemic*. Ricerche di Psicologia-Open., DOI: 10.3280/rip2022oa14724

Escalona, S. K. (1982). Growing up with the threat of nuclear war: Some indirect effects on personality development. *The American Journal of Orthopsychiatry*, 52(4), 600–607. DOI: 10.1111/j.1939-0025.1982.tb01449.x PMID: 7148981

Fargas-Malet, M., & Dillenburger, K. (2014). Children drawing their own conclusions: Children's perceptions of a "postconflict" society. *Peace and Conflict*, 20(2), 135–149. DOI: 10.1037/pac0000029

Gilligan, C. (1982). *In a different voice: Psychological theory and women's development*. Harvard University Press.

Hakvoort, I., & Hägglund, S. (2001). Concepts of peace and war as described by Dutch and Swedish girls and boys. *Peace and Conflict*, 7(1), 29–44. DOI: 10.1207/S15327949PAC0701_03

Hakvoort, I., & Oppenheimer, L. (1993). Children and adolescents' conceptions of peace, war, and strategies to attain peace: A Dutch case study. *Journal of Peace Research*, 30(1), 65–77. DOI: 10.1177/0022343393030001006

Hakvoort, I., & Oppenheimer, L. (1998). Understanding peace and war: A review of developmental psychology research. *Developmental Review*, 18(3), 353–389. DOI: 10.1006/drev.1998.0471

Hall, R. (1993). How children think and feel about war and peace: An Australian study. *Journal of Peace Research*, 30(2), 181–196. DOI: 10.1177/0022343393030002005

Joshi, P. T., Parr, A. F., & Efron, L. A. (2008). TV coverage of tragedies: What is the impact on children. *Indian Pediatrics*, 45(8), 629–634. PMID: 18723904

Jüni, P., Holenstein, F., Sterne, J., Bartlett, C., & Egger, M. (2002). Direction and impact of language bias in meta-analyses of controlled trials: Empirical study. *International Journal of Epidemiology*, 31(1), 115–123. DOI: 10.1093/ije/31.1.115 PMID: 11914306

Kohlberg, L. (1984). *The psychology of moral development: The nature and validity of moral stages*. Harper & Row.

Lahad, M., Shacham, M., & Ayalon, O. (2013). *The "BASIC-Ph" Model of Coping and Resiliency*. Jessica Kingsley Publishers.

Machin, D., & Van Leeuwen, T. (2009). Toys as discourse: Children's war toys and the war on terror. *Critical Discourse Studies*, 6(1), 51–63. DOI: 10.1080/17405900802560082

Maculan, A., Di Giuseppe, T., Vianello, F., & Vivaldi, S. (2022). Narrazioni e risorse. Gli operatori del sistema penale minorile al tempo del Covid-19. *Autonomie locali e servizi sociali. Quadrimestrale di studi e ricerche sul welfare*, 2(2022), 349-365. https://doi.org/DOI: 10.1447/105089

Mays, N., Roberts, E., & Popay, J. (2001). Synthesising research evidence. In Fulop, N., Allen, P., Clarke, A., & Black, N. (Eds.), *Studying the organisation and delivery of health services: Research methods*. Routledge.

McNeil, J. N. (1983). Young mothers' communication about death with their children. *Death Education*, 6(4), 323–339. DOI: 10.1080/07481188308252139 PMID: 10259896

Morin, E. (2001). *I sette saperi necessari all'educazione del futuro*. Raffaello Cortina Editore.

Myers-Bowman, K. S., Walker, K., & Myers-Walls, J. A. (2005). Differences Between War and Peace are Big": Children from Yugoslavia and the United States Describe Peace and War. *Peace and Conflict*, 11(2), 177–198. DOI: 10.1207/s15327949pac1102_4

Nishikawa-Pacher, A. (2022). Research questions with PICO: A universal mnemonic. *Publications / MDPI*, 10(3), 21. DOI: 10.3390/publications10030021

O'Malley, C. J., Blankemeyer, M., Walker, K. K., & Dellmann-Jenkins, M. (2007). Children's reported communication with their parents about war. *Journal of Family Issues*, 28(12), 1639–1662. DOI: 10.1177/0192513X07302726

Obidike, N. D., Bosah, I., & Olibie, E. (2015). Teaching peace concept to children. *International Journal of Multidisciplinary Research and Development*, 2(6), 24–26.

Paoletti, P. (2002). Flussi, Territori, Luogo [Flows, Territories, Place]. *Medica Publica (Oulu)*.

Paoletti, P. (2008). *Crescere nell'eccellenza*. Roma: Armando editore.

Paoletti, P., & Ben-Soussan, T. D. (2019). The sphere model of consciousness: From geometrical to neuro-psycho-educational perspectives. *Logica Univiversalis*, 13(3), 395–415. DOI: 10.1007/s11787-019-00226-0

Paoletti, P., & Diamond, A. (2020, 15 Aprile). *The Science of Education for Peace*. https://fondazionepatriziopaoletti.org/blog/the-science-of-education-for-peace-scarica-il-book-gratuito-e-semina-la-pace-dentro-e-intorno-a-te/

Paoletti, P., Di Giuseppe, T., Lillo, C., Ben-Soussan, T. D., Bozkurt, A., Tabibnia, G., Kelmendi, K., Warthe, G. W., Leshem, R., Bigo, V., Ireri, A., Mwangi, C., Bhattacharya, N., & Perasso, G. F. (2022a). What can we learn from the COVID-19 pandemic? Resilience for the future and neuropsychopedagogical insights. *Frontiers in Psychology*, 5403, 993991. Advance online publication. DOI: 10.3389/fpsyg.2022.993991 PMID: 36172227

Paoletti, P., Di Giuseppe, T., Lillo, C., Serantoni, G., Perasso, G., Maculan, A., & Vianello, F. (2022b). La resilienza nel circuito penale minorile in tempi di pandemia: un'esperienza di studio e formazione basata sul modello sferico della coscienza su un gruppo di educatori. *Narrare i Gruppi,* 1-10.

Paoletti, P., Perasso, G. F., Lillo, C., Serantoni, G., Maculan, A., Vianello, F., & Di Giuseppe, T. (2023). Envisioning the future for families running away from war: Challenges and resources of Ukrainian parents in Italy. *Frontiers in Psychology*, 14, 1122264. Advance online publication. DOI: 10.3389/fpsyg.2023.1122264 PMID: 37008874

Paoletti, P., & Di Giuseppe, T. (2023). Il Modello sferico della coscienza: Io, Noi, Altro da noi. Presented at the event "Promuovere le Risorse Positive della Comunità Penitenziaria", 15 Marzo 2023, Università degli Studi di Genova.

Patton, M. Q. (1990). *Qualitative evaluation and research methods*. Sage.

Petticrew, M., & Roberts, H. (2008). *Systematic reviews in the social sciences: A practical guide*. John Wiley & Sons.

Piaget, J., & Inhelder, B. (1956). *The child's conception of space*. Routledge & Kegan Paul.

Pine, D. S., Costello, J., & Masten, A. (2005). Trauma, proximity, and developmental psychopathology: The effects of war and terrorism on children. *Neuropsychopharmacology*, 30(10), 1781–1792. DOI: 10.1038/sj.npp.1300814 PMID: 16012537

Pintimalli, A., Di Giuseppe, T., Serantoni, G., Glicksohn, J., & Ben-Soussan, T. D. (2020). Dynamics of the sphere model of consciousness: Silence, space, and self. *Frontiers in Psychology*, 11, 548813. DOI: 10.3389/fpsyg.2020.548813 PMID: 33071865

Putnam, F. W. (2002). Televised trauma and viewer PTSD: Implications for prevention. *Psychiatry*, 65(4), 310–312. DOI: 10.1521/psyc.65.4.310.20241 PMID: 12530334

Raviv, A., Oppenheimer, L., & Bar-Tal, D. (1999). *How children understand war and peace*. Jossey-Bass.

Repko, A. F., & Szostak, R. (2020). *Interdisciplinary research: Process and theory.* Sage Publications.

Rodd, J. (1985). Pre-school children's understanding of war. *Early Child Development and Care*, 22(2-3), 109–121. https://psycnet.apa.org/doi/10.1080/0300443850220202. DOI: 10.1080/0300443850220202

Rodrigo-Ruiz, D. (2016). Effect of teachers' emotions on their students: Some evidence. *Journal of Education & Social Policy*, 3(4), 73–79.

Rumrill, P. D., Fitzgerald, S. M., & Merchant, W. R. (2010). Using scoping literature reviews as a means of understanding and interpreting existing literature. *Work (Reading, Mass.)*, 35(3), 399–404. DOI: 10.3233/WOR-2010-0998 PMID: 20364059

Schwebel, M. (1982). Effects of the nuclear war threat on children and teenagers: Implications for professionals. *The American Journal of Orthopsychiatry*, 52(4), 608–618. https://psycnet.apa.org/doi/10.1111/j.1939-0025.1982.tb01450.x. DOI: 10.1111/j.1939-0025.1982.tb01450.x PMID: 7148982

Schultz, J. H., Langballe, Å., & Raundalen, M. (2014). Explaining the unexplainable: Designing a national strategy on classroom communication concerning the 22 July terror attack in Norway. *European Journal of Psychotraumatology*, 5(1), 22758. DOI: 10.3402/ejpt.v5.22758 PMID: 25018859

Shacham, M. (2015). Suddenly–war. Intervention program for Enhancing teachers and children's resilience Following war. *Revista de Cercetare si Interventie Sociala*, (48), 60–68.

Shapiro, S. (2002). Toward a critical pedagogy of peace education. In Salomon, G., & Nevo, B. (Eds.), *Peace education: The concept principles, and practices around the world* (pp. 63–72). Lawrence Erlbaum.

Sippel, L. M., Pietrzak, R. H., Charney, D. S., Mayes, L. C., & Southwick, S. M. (2015). How does social support enhance resilience in the trauma-exposed individual? *Ecology and Society*, 20(4), art10. DOI: 10.5751/ES-07832-200410

Spielmann, M. (1986). If peace comes...future expectations of Israeli children and youth. *Journal of Peace Research*, 23(1), 51–67. DOI: 10.1177/002234338602300105

Tephly, J. (1985). Young children's understanding of war and peace. *Early Child Development and Care*, 20(4), 271–285. DOI: 10.1080/0300443850200405

Van Westrhenen, N., & Fritz, E. (2014). Creative arts therapy as treatment for child trauma: An overview. *The Arts in Psychotherapy*, 41(5), 527–534. DOI: 10.1016/j.aip.2014.10.004

Vygotsky, L. S. (1978). *Mind in society: The development of higher psychological processes*. Harvard University Press.

Walker, K., Myers-Bowman, K. S., & Myers-Walls, J. A. (2003). Understanding war, visualizing peace: Children draw what they know. *Art Therapy: Journal of the American Art Therapy Association*, 20(4), 191–200. DOI: 10.1080/07421656.2003.10129605

Weisgram, E. S., & Dinella, L. M. (Eds.). (2018). *Gender typing of children's toys: How early play experiences impact development*. American Psychological Association., DOI: 10.1037/0000077-000

KEY TERMS AND DEFINITIONS

Peacebuilding: involves educational efforts aimed at fostering understanding, cooperation, and peaceful coexistence among individuals and communities. It focuses on teaching conflict resolution, promoting tolerance, and building positive relationships to prevent violence and promote social harmony.

Emotion regulation: is the ability to manage and respond to emotional experiences in a healthy way. It includes skills to identify, understand, and control emotions, ensuring appropriate responses to various situations.

Coping: refers to the strategies and behaviors individuals use to manage stress and adversity. Effective coping mechanisms can include problem-solving, seeking support, and adapting to challenging circumstances.

Resilience: is the capacity to recover and thrive despite difficulties and setbacks. It involves mental, emotional, and behavioral flexibility and the ability to maintain or regain well-being in the face of adversity.

Scaffolding: is a teaching method that provides successive levels of temporary support to help students achieve higher levels of understanding and skill acquisition. It involves guiding learners through tasks they cannot complete independently.

Compilation of References

Abry, T., Bryce, C. I., Swanson, J., Bradley, R. H., Fabes, R. A., & Corwyn, R. F. (2017). Classroom-level adversity: Associations with children's internalizing and externalizing behaviors across elementary school. *Developmental Psychology*, 53(3), 497–510. DOI: 10.1037/dev0000268 PMID: 28045283

Acharya, L., Jin, L., & Collins, W. (2018). College life is stressful today - Emerging stressors and depressive symptoms in college students. Journal of American college health. *Journal of American College Health*, 66(7), 655–664. DOI: 10.1080/07448481.2018.1451869 PMID: 29565759

Achenbach, T., & Rescorla, L. (2019). *Handbook for the SAEBA school-age questionnaires and profiles*. EHRC. https://archive.org/details/manualforasebasc0000ache

Achenbach, T. M. (1966). The classification of children's psychiatric symptoms: A factor-analytic study. *Psychological Monographs*, 80(7), 1–37. DOI: 10.1037/h0093906 PMID: 5968338

Achenbach, T. M., & Rescorla, L. A. (2001). *Manual for the ASEBA School-Age Forms and Profiles*. University of Vermont Research Center for Children, Youth, & Families.

Adelman, H. S., & Taylor, L. (2006). *The school leader's guide to student learning supports: New directions for addressing barriers to learning*. Corwin Press.

Adriaanse, M., Veling, W., Doreleijers, T., & van Domburgh, L. (2014). The link between ethnicity, social disadvantage and mental health problems in a school-based multiethnic sample of children in The Netherlands. *European Child & Adolescent Psychiatry*, 23(11), 1103–1113. DOI: 10.1007/s00787-014-0564-5 PMID: 24927803

Aduen, P. A., Rich, B. A., Sanchez, L., O'Brien, K., & Alvord, M. K. (2014). Resilience Builder Program therapy addresses core social deficits and emotion dysregulation in youth with high-functioning autism spectrum disorder. *Journal of Psychological Abnormalities in Children*, 3(2), 118–128. DOI: 10.4172/2329-9525.1000118

Aggeli, K., & Vlachou, M. (2004). Problem-solving techniques and methods in the classroom. In Kalantzi-Azizi, A., & Zafiropoulou, M. (Eds.), *School adjustment: Prevention and intervention* (pp. 26–50). Ellinika Grammata. (in Greek)

Ahern, J., Galea, S., Resnick, H., & Vlahov, D. (2004). Television images and probable posttraumatic stress disorder after September 11: The role of background characteristics, event exposures, and perievent panic. *The Journal of Nervous and Mental Disease*, 192(3), 217–226. DOI: 10.1097/01.nmd.0000116465.99830.ca PMID: 15091303

Alberta Learning. (2000). *Teaching students with emotional disorders and/or mental illnesses*. Alberta Learning, Special Programs Branch.

Alberto, P. A., & Troutman, A. C. (2013). *Applied behavior analysis for teachers* (9th ed.). Pearson.

Aldridge, J. M., & Fraser, B. J. (2016). Teachers' views of their school climate and its relationship with teacher self-efficacy and job satisfaction. *Learning Environments Research*, 19(2), 291–307. DOI: 10.1007/s10984-015-9198-x

Aldridge, J. M., Fraser, B. J., Fozdar, F., Ala'i, K., Earnest, J., & Afari, E. (2016). Students' perceptions of school climate as determinants of wellbeing, resilience and identity. *Improving Schools*, 19(1), 5–26. DOI: 10.1177/1365480215612616

Aldridge, J. M., & McChesney, K. (2018). The relationships between school climate and adolescent mental health and wellbeing: A systematic literature review. *International Journal of Educational Research*, 88, 121–145. DOI: 10.1016/j.ijer.2018.01.012

Aldridge, J. M., McChesney, K., & Afari, E. (2018). Relationships between school climate, bullying and delinquent behaviours. *Learning Environments Research*, 21(2), 153–172. DOI: 10.1007/s10984-017-9249-6

Alegría, M., Green, J. G., McLaughlin, K. A., & Loder, S. (2010). *Disparities in child and adolescent mental health and mental health services in the US*. National Research Council.

Al-Fraihat, D., Joy, M., & Sinclair, J. (2020). Evaluating E-learning systems success: An empirical study. *Computers in Human Behavior*, 102, 67–86. DOI: 10.1016/j.chb.2019.08.004

Alinsunurin, J. (2020). School learning climate in the lens of parental involvement and school leadership: lessons for inclusiveness among public schools. *Smart Learning Environments, 7*(25). https://doi.org/.DOI: 10.1186/s40561-020-00139-2

Allen, K., Kern, M. L., Vella-Brodrick, D., Hattie, J., & Waters, L. (2018). What schools need to know about fostering school belonging: A meta-analysis. *Educational Psychology Review*, 30(1), 1–34. DOI: 10.1007/s10648-016-9389-8

Alvord, M. K., & Grados, J. J. (2005). Enhancing resilience in children: A proactive approach. *Professional Psychology, Research and Practice*, 36(3), 238–245. DOI: 10.1037/0735-7028.36.3.238

Alvord, M. K., Zucker, B., & Grados, J. J. (2011). *Resilience Builder Program for children and adolescents: Enhancing social competence and self-regulation–A cognitive-behavioral group approach*. Research Press.

American Psychiatric Association. (2013). *Diagnostic and statistical manual of mental disorders* (5th ed.)., DOI: 10.1176/appi.books.9780890425596

American Psychological Association. (2014). *Publication manual of the American Psychological Association* (6th ed.). Author.

Amstadter, A., Myers, J. M., & Kendler, K. S. (2014). The interaction of stress and genetics in the prediction of resilience. *Journal of Personality and Social Psychology*, 107(5), 844–858. PMID: 25243415

Andermo, S., Hallgren, M., Nguyen, T. T. D., Jonsson, S., Petersen, S., Friberg, M., Romqvist, A., Stubbs, B., & Elinder, L. S. (2020). School-related physical activity interventions and mental health among children: A systematic review and meta-analysis. *Sports Medicine - Open*, 6(1), 1–27. DOI: 10.1186/s40798-020-00254-x PMID: 32548792

Anderson, C. M., & Borgmeier, C. (2010). Tier II interventions within the framework of School-Wide Positive Behavior Support: Essential features for design, implementation, and maintenance. *Behavior Analysis in Practice*, 3(1), 33–45. DOI: 10.1007/BF03391756 PMID: 22479670

Angus, G., & Nelson, R. B. (2021). School-Wide Positive Behavior Interventions and Supports and student academic achievement. *Contemporary School Psychology*, 25(4), 443–465. DOI: 10.1007/s40688-019-00245-0

Antonovsky, A. (1987). *Unravelling the mystery of health: How people manage stress and stay well*. Jossey-Bass.

Araúz Ledezma, A. B., Massar, K., & Kok, G. (2021). Social emotional learning and the promotion of equal personal relationships among adolescents in Panama: A study protocol. *Health Promotion International*, 36(3), 741–752. DOI: 10.1093/heapro/daaa114 PMID: 33051640

Argyriadi, A., & Argyriadis, A. (2022). Recommended Interventions for the Promotion of Language Development for Children With Learning Difficulties. In *Rethinking Inclusion and Transformation in Special Education* (pp. 143–159). IGI Global. DOI: 10.4018/978-1-6684-4680-5.ch009

Argyriadis, A., Efthymiou, E., & Argyriadis, A. (2023). Cultural Competence at Schools: The Effectiveness of Educational Leaders' Intervention Strategies. In *Inclusive Phygital Learning Approaches and Strategies for Students With Special Needs* (pp. 33-51). IGI Global.

Argyriadis, A., Ioannidou, L., Dimitrakopoulos, I., Gourni, M., Ntimeri, G., Vlachou, C., & Argyriadi, A. (2023, March). Experimental mindfulness intervention in an emergency department for stress management and development of positive working environment. [). MDPI.]. *Health Care*, 11(6), 879. PMID: 36981535

Argyriadis, A., Paoullis, P., Samsari, E., & Argyriadi, A. (2023). Self-Assessment Inclusion Scale (SAIS): A tool for measuring inclusive competence and sensitivity. *Perspectives in Education*, 41(4), 34–49. DOI: 10.38140/pie.v41i4.7294

Armstrong, R., Hall, B. J., Doyle, J., & Waters, E. (2011). 'Scoping the scope'of a cochrane review. *Journal of Public Health (Oxford, England)*, 33(1), 147–150. DOI: 10.1093/pubmed/fdr015 PMID: 21345890

Arnold, E., Goldston, D., Walsh, A., Reboussin, B., Daniel, S., Hickman, E., & Wood, F. B. (2005). Severity of emotional and behavioral problems among poor and typical readers. *Journal of Abnormal Child Psychology*, 33(2), 205–217. DOI: 10.1007/s10802-005-1828-9 PMID: 15839498

Astor, R. A., Guerra, N., & Van Acker, R. (2010). How can we improve school safety research? *Educational Researcher*, 39(1), 69–78. DOI: 10.3102/0013189X09357619

Attwood, T. (2006). The pattern of abilities and development of girls with Asperger's syndrome. In: Attwood T, Bolick T, Faherty C, et al. (Eds.), *Asperger's and Girls*. Arlington, TX: Future Horizons, Inc. Bailey, B. (2008). *Daily Routine Cards*. UK: Conscious Discipline.

Auerbach, S. (2010). Beyond coffee with the principal: Toward leadership for authentic school-family partnerships. *Journal of School Leadership*, 20(6), 728–757. DOI: 10.1177/105268461002000603

Auger, C. P. (1998). *Information sources in grey literature (guides to information sources)* (4th ed.). Bowker Saur.

Austin, V., & Sciarra, D. (2016). *Difficult students and disruptive behavior in the classroom: Teacher responses that work*. W. W. Norton & Company.

Baffsky, R., Ivers, R., Cullen, P., Batterham, P. J., Toumbourou, J., Calear, A. L., Werner-Seidler, A., McGillivray, L., & Torok, M. (2022). A cluster randomised effectiveness-implementation trial of an intervention to increase the adoption of PAX Good Behaviour Game, a mental health prevention program, in Australian primary schools: Study protocol. *Contemporary Clinical Trials Communications*, 28, 100923. DOI: 10.1016/j.conctc.2022.100923 PMID: 35669488

Bandura, A. (1977). *Social learning theory*. Prentice Hall.

Bandura, A. (1978). The self-system in reciprocal determinism. *The American Psychologist*, 33(4), 344–358. DOI: 10.1037/0003-066X.33.4.344

Bandura, A. (1986). *Social foundations of thought and action: A social cognitive theory*. Prentice-Hall.

Banks, J. A. (2015). *Cultural diversity and education*. Routledge. DOI: 10.4324/9781315622255

Bapst, M. S., Genoud, P. A., & Hascoët, M. (2023). Taking a step towards understanding interactions between teacher efficacy in behavior management and the social learning environment: A two-level multilevel analysis. *European Journal of Psychology of Education*, 38(3), 1129–1144. DOI: 10.1007/s10212-022-00647-4

Barber, B. K. (1996). Parental psychological control: Revisiting a neglected construct. *Child Development*, 67(6), 3296–3319. DOI: 10.2307/1131780 PMID: 9071782

Barker, K., Poed, S., & Whitefield, P. (2023). *School-wide Positive Behaviour Support: The Australian handbook*. Routledge.

Barker, K., Poed, S., & Whitefield, P. (Eds.). (2022). *School-Wide Positive Behavior Support: The Australian handbook*. Routledge. DOI: 10.4324/9781003186236

Barkley, R., & Benton, C. (2013). *Your defiant child: 8 steps to better behavior* (2nd ed.). The Guilford Press.

Barlow, D. H., Farchione, T. J., Fairholme, C. P., Ellard, K. K., Boisseau, C. L., Allen, L. B., & Ehrenreich-May, J. (2018). *Unified protocol for transdiagnostic treatment of emotional disorders: Therapist guide*. Oxford University Press.

Baron-Cohen, S. (2003). *The essential difference: Men, women and the extreme male brain*. Penguin Books.

Barrett, P. M., Cooper, M., & Guajardo, J. (2019). FRIENDS program: Prevention and early intervention for anxiety and depression. *Journal of Clinical Psychology*, 75(12), 2333–2347.

Barrett, S., Eber, L., McIntosh, K., Perales, K., & Romer, N. (2018). *Teaching social-emotional competencies within a PBIS framework.* OSEP Technical Assistance Center on Positive Behavioral Interventions and Supports.

Bastable, E., Massar, M. M., & McIntosh, K. (2020). A survey of team members' perceptions of coaching activities related to tier 1 SWPBIS implementation. *Journal of Positive Behavior Interventions*, 22(1), 51–61. DOI: 10.1177/1098300719861566

Baum, W. M. (2011). What is radical behaviorism? A review of Jay Moore's conceptual foundations of radical behaviorism. *Journal of the Experimental Analysis of Behavior*, 95(1), 119–126. DOI: 10.1901/jeab.2011.95-119

Bear, G. G. (2020). *Improving school climate: Practical strategies to reduce behavior problems and promote social and emotional learning.* Routledge. DOI: 10.4324/9781351170482

Bear, G. G., Gaskins, C., Blank, J., & Chen, F. F. (2011). Delaware school climate survey–student: Its factor structure, concurrent validity, and reliability. *Journal of School Psychology*, 49(2), 157–174. DOI: 10.1016/j.jsp.2011.01.001 PMID: 21530762

Beaudoin, H., & Roberge, G. (2015). Student perceptions of school climate and lived bullying behaviours. *Procedia: Social and Behavioral Sciences*, 174, 213–330. DOI: 10.1016/j.sbspro.2015.01.667

Becerra, R., Preece, D. A., & Gross, J. J. (2020). Assessing beliefs about emotions: Development and validation of the Emotion Beliefs Questionnaire. *PLoS One*, 15(4), e0231395. Advance online publication. DOI: 10.1371/journal.pone.0231395 PMID: 32287328

Beck, A. T. (1976). *Cognitive therapy and emotional disorders.* International Universities Press.

Becker-Blease, K. A., Finkelhor, D., & Turner, H. (2008). Media exposure predicts children's reactions to crime and terrorism. *Journal of Trauma & Dissociation*, 9(2), 225–248. DOI: 10.1080/15299730802048652 PMID: 19042776

Beck, J. S. (2011). *Cognitive Behavior Therapy: Basics and Beyond* (2nd ed.). Guilford Press.

Behavioral Interventions and Supports and Social Emotional Learning Weist, M. D., Lever, N. A., Bradshaw, C. P., & Owens, J. S. (Eds.), *Handbook of school mental health: Research, training, practice, and policy* (pp. 101–118). Springer.

Beiser, M. (2009). Resettling refugees and safeguarding their mental health: Lessons learned from the Canadian refugee resettlement project. *Transcultural Psychiatry*, 46(4), 539–583. DOI: 10.1177/1363461509351373 PMID: 20028677

Bella-Awusah, T., Ani, C., Ajuwon, A., & Omigbodun, O. (2016). Effectiveness of brief school - based, group cognitive behavioral therapy for depressed adolescents in South West Nigeria. *Child and Adolescent Mental Health*, 21(1), 44–50. DOI: 10.1111/camh.12104 PMID: 32680363

Benbenishty, R., Astor, R. A., Roziner, I., & Wrabel, S. L. (2016). Testing the causal links between school climate, school violence, and school academic performance: A cross-lagged panel autoregressive model. *Educational Researcher*, 45(3), 197–206. DOI: 10.3102/0013189X16644603

Benigno, J., Brown, L., & Geist, K. (2018). Come together: Music therapy and speech language pathology students' perspectives on collaboration during an inclusive camp for children with ADS. *Music Therapy Perspectives*, 36(1), 12–25.

Benjet, C., Kazdin, A. E., & Spence, S. H. (2019). Prevention of mental health problems: Worldwide priorities. *International Journal of Mental Health Systems*, 13(1), 1–14.

Benner, A. D., Wang, Y., Shen, Y., Boyle, A. E., Polk, R., & Cheng, Y.-P. (2018). Racial/ethnic discrimination and well-being during adolescence: A meta-analytic review. *The American Psychologist*, 73(7), 855–883. DOI: 10.1037/amp0000204 PMID: 30024216

Benner, G. J., Nelson, J. R., Sanders, E. A., & Ralston, N. C. (2012). Behavior intervention for students with externalizing behavior problems: Primary-level standard protocol. *Exceptional Children*, 78(2), 181–198. DOI: 10.1177/001440291207800203

Benson, P. L., Scales, P. C., & Syvertsen, A. K. (2011). The contribution of the developmental assets framework to positive youth development theory and practice. *Advances in Child Development and Behavior*, 41, 197–230. DOI: 10.1016/B978-0-12-386492-5.00008-7 PMID: 23259193

Benzies, K. M., Premji, S., Hayden, K. A., & Serrett, K. (2006). State-of-theevidence reviews: Advantages and challenges of including grey literature. *Worldviews on Evidence-Based Nursing*, 3(2), 55–61. DOI: 10.1111/j.1741-6787.2006.00051.x PMID: 17040510

Berman, A. L. (2009). Depression and suicide. In Gotlib, I. H., & Hammen, C. L. (Eds.), *Handbook of depression* (2nd ed., pp. 510–530). The Guilford Press.

Bernal, G., & Domenech Rodríguez, M. M. (2012). *Cultural adaptations: Tools for evidence-based practice with diverse populations.* American Psychological Association. DOI: 10.1037/13752-000

Bernard, M. E. (2004). The relationship of young children's social-emotional competence to behavior and academic achievement in the later school years. *Journal of School Psychology*, 42(4), 261–282.

Berti, A. E., & Benesso, M. (1998). The concept of nation-state in Italian elementary school children: Spontaneous concepts and effects of teaching. *Genetic, Social, and General Psychology Monographs*, 120(2), 121–143. PMID: 9597745

Berti, A. E., & Bombi, A. S. (1988). *The child's construction of economics.* Cambridge University Press.

Berti, A. E., & Vanni, E. (2000). Italian Children's Understanding of War: A Domain-Specific Approach. *Social Development*, 9(4), 478–496. DOI: 10.1111/1467-9507.00139

Betancourt, T. S., McBain, R., Newnham, E. A., & Brennan, R. T. (2011). The intergenerational impact of war: longitudinal relationships between caregiver and child mental health in postconflict Sierra Leone. *Journal of Child Psychology and Psychiatry, 52*(9), 1086-1095.

Betancourt, J. R., Green, A. R., Carrillo, J. E., & Ananeh-Firempong, O.II. (2005). Defining cultural competence: A practical framework for addressing racial/ethnic disparities in health and health care. *Public Health Reports*, 118(4), 293–302. DOI: 10.1016/S0033-3549(04)50253-4 PMID: 12815076

Betancourt, T. S., McBain, R., Newnham, E. A., & Brennan, R. T. (2011). The intergenerational impact of war: Longitudinal relationships between caregiver and child mental health in postconflict Sierra Leone. *Journal of Child Psychology and Psychiatry, and Allied Disciplines*, 52(9), 1086–1095. PMID: 25665018

Bethune, K. S. (2017). Effects of coaching on teachers' implementation of Tier 1 School-Wide Positive Behavioral Interventions and Support strategies. *Journal of Positive Behavior Interventions*, 19(3), 131–142. DOI: 10.1177/1098300716680095

Biddle, S. J., & Asare, M. (2011). Physical activity and mental health in children and adolescents: A review of reviews. *British Journal of Sports Medicine*, 45(11), 886–895. DOI: 10.1136/bjsports-2011-090185 PMID: 21807669

Biederman, J., Ball, S. W., Monuteaux, M. C., Mick, E., Spencer, T. J., McCreary, M., Cote, M., & Faraone, S. V. (2008). New insights into the co-morbidity between ADHD and major depression in adolescent and young adult females. *Journal of the American Academy of Child and Adolescent Psychiatry*, 47(4), 426–434. DOI: 10.1097/CHI.0b013e31816429d3 PMID: 18388760

Biegel, G. M., Brown, K. W., Shapiro, S. L., & Schubert, C. M. (2009). Mindfulness-based stress reduction for the treatment of adolescent psychiatric outpatients: A randomized clinical trial. *Journal of Consulting and Clinical Psychology*, 77(5), 855–866. DOI: 10.1037/a0016241 PMID: 19803566

Bien, T. (2006). *Mindful therapy: A guide for therapists and helping professionals.* Wisdom Publications.

Blackman, G. L., Ostrander, R., & Herman, K. C. (2005). Children with ADHD and depression: A multisource, multimethod assessment of clinical, social, and academic functioning. *Journal of Attention Disorders*, 8(4), 195–207. DOI: 10.1177/1087054705278777 PMID: 16110050

Bluth, K., & Eisenlohr-Moul, T. A. (2017). Response to a mindfulness intervention in teens: Impact of interpersonal stress and distress. *Journal of Adolescence*, 60, 104–113.

Bluth, K., & Eisenlohr-Moul, T. A. (2017). Response to a mindfulness intervention in teens: The role of emotion regulation and callous-unemotional traits. *Mindfulness*, 8, 249–255.

Bolotin, J. P., & Duss, L. S. (2009). Teaching a pedagogy of peace: A study of peace educators in United States schools in the aftermath of September 11. *Journal of Peace Education*, 6(2), 189–207. DOI: 10.1080/17400200903086615

Boustani, M. M., Frazier, S. L., Becker, K. D., Bechor, M., Dinizulu, S. M., Hede-mann, E. R., Ogle, R. R., & Pasalich, D. S. (2015). Common elements of adolescent prevention programs: Minimizing burden while maximizing the reach. *Administration and Policy in Mental Health*, 42(2), 209–219. DOI: 10.1007/s10488-014-0541-9 PMID: 24504979

Bowlby, J. (1969). *Attachment.* Basic Books.

Brackett, M. A., & Rivers, S. E. (2014). Transforming students' lives with social and emotional learning. In Pekrun, R., & Linnenbrink-Garcia, L. (Eds.), *International Handbook of Emotions in Education* (pp. 368–388). Routledge.

Bradshaw, C.P., Bottiani, J. K., Osher, D., & Sugai, G. (2014). The integration of Positive

Bradshaw, C. P., Cohen, J., Espelage, D. L., & Nation, M. (2021). Addressing school safety through comprehensive school climate approaches. *School Psychology Review*, 50(2–3), 221–236. DOI: 10.1080/2372966X.2021.1926321

Bradshaw, C. P., Koth, C. W., Bevans, K. B., Ialongo, N., & Leaf, P. J. (2008). The impact of school-wide positive behavioral interventions and supports (PBIS) on the organizational health of elementary schools. *School Psychology Quarterly*, 23(4), 462–473. DOI: 10.1037/a0012883

Bradshaw, C. P., Koth, C. W., Thornton, L. A., & Leaf, P. J. (2009). Altering school climate through school-wide positive behavioral interventions and supports: Findings from a group-randomized effectiveness trial. *Prevention Science*, 10(2), 100–115. DOI: 10.1007/s11121-008-0114-9 PMID: 19011963

Bradshaw, C. P., Mitchell, M. M., & Leaf, P. J. (2010). Examining the effects of Schoolwide Positive Behavioral Interventions and Supports on student outcomes: Results from a randomized controlled effectiveness trial in elementary schools. *Journal of Positive Behavior Interventions*, 12(3), 133–148. DOI: 10.1177/1098300709334798

Bradshaw, C. P., Pas, E. T., Debnam, K. J., & Johnson, S. L. (2021). A randomized controlled trial of MTSS-B in high schools: Improving classroom management to prevent EBDs. *Remedial and Special Education*, 42(1), 44–59. DOI: 10.1177/0741932520966727

Bradshaw, C. P., Waasdorp, T. E., & Leaf, P. J. (2015). Examining variation in the impact of school-wide positive behavioral interventions and supports: Findings from a randomized controlled effectiveness trial. *Journal of Educational Psychology*, 107(2), 546–557. DOI: 10.1037/a0037630

Bradshaw, C., Waasdorp, T., & Leaf, P. (2012). Examining the variation in the impact of School-wide Positive Behavioral Interventions and Supports. *Pediatrics*, 10(5), 1136–1145. DOI: 10.1542/peds.2012-0243

Brand, S., Felner, R. D., Seitsinger, A., Burns, A., & Bolton, N. (2008). A large-scale study of the assessment of the social environment of middle and secondary schools: The validity and utility of teachers' ratings of school climate, cultural pluralism, and safety problems for understanding school effects and school improvement. *Journal of School Psychology*, 46(5), 507–535. DOI: 10.1016/j.jsp.2007.12.001 PMID: 19083370

Braswell, L., & Kendall, P. C. (1988). Cognitive-behavioral methods with children. In Dobson, K. S. (Ed.), *Handbook of cognitive-behavioral therapies* (pp. 167–213). The Guilford Press.

Braun, V., & Clarke, V. (2006). Using thematic analysis in psychology. *Qualitative Research in Psychology*, 3(2), 77–101. DOI: 10.1191/1478088706qp063oa

Briesch, A. M., & Briesch, J. M. (2016). Meta-analysis of behavioral self-management interventions in single-case research. *School Psychology Review*, 45(1), 3–18. DOI: 10.17105/SPR45-1.3-18

Brock, S. E., Nickerson, A. B., Reeves, M. A., Jimerson, S. R., Lieberman, R., & Feinberg, T. (2009). *School crisis prevention and intervention: The PREPaRE model*. National Association of School Psychologists.

Bromley, E., Johnson, J. G., & Cohen, P. (2006). Personality strengths in adolescence and decreased risk of developing mental health problems in early adulthood. *Comprehensive Psychiatry*, 47(4), 315–324. DOI: 10.1016/j.comppsych.2005.11.003 PMID: 16769307

Bronfenbrenner, U. (1979). *The ecology of human development experiments*. Harvard University Press. DOI: 10.4159/9780674028845

Bronfenbrenner, U. (1986). Ecology of the family as a context for human development: Research perspectives. *Developmental Psychology*, 22(6), 723–742. DOI: 10.1037/0012-1649.22.6.723

Brown Epstein, H. A. (2022). Adolescent mental health literacy: Definitions and program highlights. *Journal of Consumer Health on the Internet*, 26(1), 102–108. DOI: 10.1080/15398285.2022.2029244

Brown, B. (2013). The value of persona dolls in tacking sensitive issues. *Mag online library, 1*(12).

Brown, J. L., Jennings, P. A., Rasheed, D. S., Cham, H., Doyle, S. L., & Frank, J. L. (2023). Direct and moderating impacts of the CARE mindfulness-based professional learning program for teachers on children's academic and social-emotional outcomes. *Applied Developmental Science, 25*(1-20). DOI: 10.1080/10888691.2023.2268327

Brown, C., Anderson, J., & Garrison, D. (2017). School-based interventions for children with chronic asthma: A meta-analysis. *The Journal of School Health*, 87(3), 185–195.

Brown, G. I. (1971). *Human teaching for human learning. An introduction to confluent education*. Viking Press.

Brown, J., & Green, T. (2017). Implementing resilience interventions in schools: A case study approach. *Journal of School Psychology*, 62, 103–121.

Brown, L. H., Strauman, T., Barrantes-Vidal, N., Silvia, P. J., & Kwapil, T. R. (2011). An experience-sampling study of depressive symptoms and their social context. *The Journal of Nervous and Mental Disease*, 199(6), 403–409. DOI: 10.1097/NMD.0b013e31821cd24b PMID: 21629020

Brown, T. E. (2009). *ADHD comorbidities*. American Psychiatric Publishing.

Bruhn, A. L., & McDaniel, S. C. (2021). Tier 2: Critical issues in systems, practices, and data. *Journal of Emotional and Behavioral Disorders*, 29(1), 34–43. DOI: 10.1177/1063426620949859

Bruijns, B. A., Vanderloo, L. M., Johnson, A. M., Adamo, K. B., Burke, S. M., Carson, V., Heydon, R., Irwin, J. D., Naylor, P.-J., Timmons, B. W., & Tucker, P. (2022). Change in pre-and in-service early childhood educators' knowledge, self-efficacy, and intentions following an e-learning course in physical activity and sedentary behaviour: A pilot study. *BMC Public Health*, 22(1), 1–13. DOI: 10.1186/s12889-022-12591-5 PMID: 35125100

Brymer, M., Jacobs, A., Layne, C., Pynoos, R., Ruzek, J., & Steinberg, A.. (2006). *Psychological first aid*field operations guide* (2nd ed.). National Child Traumatic StressNetwork & National Center for PTSD.

Buli, B. G., Larm, P., Nilsson, K. W., Hellstrom-Olsson, C., & Giannotta, F. (2024). Trends in mental health problems among Swedish adolescents: Do school-related factors play a role? *PLoS One*, 19(3), e0300294. DOI: 10.1371/journal.pone.0300294 PMID: 38457463

Burgoon, J. K., Berger, C. R., & Waldron, V. R. (2000). Mindfulness and interpersonal communication. *The Journal of Social Issues*, 56(1), 105–127. Advance online publication. DOI: 10.1111/0022-4537.00154

Burke, C. A. (2010). Mindfulness-based approaches with children and adolescents: A preliminary review of current research in an emergent field. *Journal of Child and Family Studies*, 19(2), 133–144. DOI: 10.1007/s10826-009-9282-x

Burke, J. D., Loeber, R., Lahey, B. B., & Rathouz, P. J. (2005). Developmental transitions among affective and behavioral disorders in adolescent boys. *Journal of Child Psychology and Psychiatry, and Allied Disciplines*, 46(11), 1200–1210. DOI: 10.1111/j.1469-7610.2005.00422.x PMID: 16238667

Burnett-Zeigler, I., Walton, M. A., Ilgen, M., Barry, K. L., Chermack, S. T., Zucker, R. A., Zimmerman, M. A., Booth, B. M., & Blow, F. C. (2012). Prevalence and correlates of mental health problems and treatment among adolescents seen in primary care. *The Journal of Adolescent Health*, 50(6), 559–564. DOI: 10.1016/j.jadohealth.2011.10.005 PMID: 22626481

Burns, M. K., & Ysseldyke, J. E. (2009). Reported prevalence of evidence-based instructional practices in special education. *The Journal of Special Education*, 43(1), 3–11. DOI: 10.1177/0022466908315563

Burt, S. A., Clark, D. A., Gershoff, E. T., Klump, K. L., & Hyde, L. W. (2021). Twin differences in harsh parenting predict youth's antisocial behavior. *Psychological Science*, 32(3), 395–409. DOI: 10.1177/0956797620968532 PMID: 33577745

Butler, N., Quigg, Z., Bates, R., Jones, L., Ashworth, E., Gowland, S., & Jove, M. (2022). The contributing role of family, school, and peer supportive relationships in protecting the mental well-being of children and adolescents. *School Mental Health*, 14(3), 776–788. DOI: 10.1007/s12310-022-09502-9 PMID: 35154501

Caldarella, P., Larsen, R. A. A., Williams, L., Downs, K. R., Wills, H. P., & Wehby, J. H. (2020). Effects of teachers' praise-to-reprimand ratios on elementary students' on-task behaviour. *Educational Psychology*, 40(10), 1306–1322. DOI: 10.1080/01443410.2020.1711872

Caldarella, P., Shatzer, R. H., Gray, K. M., Young, R. K., & Young, E. L. (2011). The effects of School-wide Positive Behavior Support on middle school climate and student outcomes. *RMLE Online: Research in Middle Level Education*, 35(4), 1–14. DOI: 10.1080/19404476.2011.11462087

Calm Classroom. (2018). Calm Classroom: Mindfulness-based program for students and educators. Calm Classroom. Retrieved from https://www.calmclassroom.com

Calzada, E. J., Huang, K.-Y., Anicama, C., Fernandez, Y., & Brotman, L. M. (2013). Family and teacher characteristics as predictors of parent involvement in education during early childhood among Afro-Caribbean and Latino immigrant families. *Urban Education*, 50(7), 870–896. DOI: 10.1177/0042085914534862 PMID: 26417116

Cambridge University Press. (n.d.). Behavior. In *Cambridge Dictionaries Online*. https://dictionary.cambridge.org/dictionary/english/abortion

Campanarou, M. (2007). *Diagnostic issues of speech therapy*. Hellenic Publications.

Campbell, F., Blank, L., Cantrell, A., Baxter, S., Blackmore, C., Dixon, J., & Goyder, E. (2022). Factors that influence mental health of university and college students in the UK: A systematic review. *BMC Public Health*, 22(1), 1778. Advance online publication. DOI: 10.1186/s12889-022-13943-x PMID: 36123714

Campinha-Bacote, J. (2002). The process of cultural competence in the delivery of healthcare services: A model of care. *Journal of Transcultural Nursing*, 13(3), 181–184. DOI: 10.1177/10459602013003003 PMID: 12113146

Cantor, J., & Nathanson, A. I. (1996). Children's fright reactions to television news. *Journal of Communication*, 46(4), 139–152. DOI: 10.1111/j.1460-2466.1996.tb01510.x

Cappella, E., Kim, H. Y., Neal, J. W., & Jackson, D. R. (2012). Classroom peer relationships and behavioral engagement in elementary school: The role of social network equity. *American Journal of Community Psychology*, 50(1-2), 70–88. DOI: 10.1007/s10464-011-9485-2 PMID: 24081319

Carneiro, A., Dias, P., & Soares, I. (2016). Risk factors for internalizing and externalizing problems in the preschool years: Systematic literature review based on the child behavior checklist 11/2-5. *Journal of Child and Family Studies*, 25, 2941–2953. DOI: 10.1007/s10826-016-0456-z

Carr, A. (2016). *The handbook of child and adolescent clinical psychology: A contextual approach* (3rd ed.). Routledge.

Carr, E. G. (1999). *Positive behavior support for people with developmental disabilities: A research synthesis*. AAMR.

Carroll, J. M., & Iles, J. E. (2006). An assessment of anxiety levels in dyslexic students in higher education. *The British Journal of Educational Psychology*, 76(Pt3), 651–662. DOI: 10.1348/000709905X66233 PMID: 16953967

Carroll, J. M., Maughan, B., Goodman, R., & Meltzer, H. (2005). Literacy difficulties and psychiatric disorders: Evidence for comorbidity. *Journal of Child Psychology and Psychiatry, and Allied Disciplines*, 46(5), 524–532. DOI: 10.1111/j.1469-7610.2004.00366.x PMID: 15845132

CASEL. (2015). *Effective social and emotional learning programs: Middle and high school education*. Author.

Castro-Camacho, L., Díaz, M. M., & Barbosa, S. (2022). Effect of a group prevention program based on the unified protocol for college students in Colombia: A quasi-experimental study. *Journal of Behavioral and Cognitive Therapy*, 32(2), 111–123. DOI: 10.1016/j.jbct.2021.04.001

Castro, F. G., Barrera, M.Jr, & Martinez, C. R.Jr. (2010). The cultural adaptation of prevention interventions: Resolving tensions between fidelity and fit. *Prevention Science*, 5(1), 41–45. DOI: 10.1023/B:PREV.0000013980.12412.cd PMID: 15058911

Cavioni, V., Grazzani, I. and Ornaghi, V., 2020. Mental health promotion in schools: A comprehensive theoretical framework.

CDC. (2022). Promoting and protecting mental health in schools and learning environments. Retrieved from https://www.cdc.gov/healthyyouth/mental-health-action -guide/pdf/DASH_MH_Action_Guide_508.pdf

Ceci, S. J., & Bruck, M. (1993). Suggestibility of the child witness: A historical review and synthesis. *Psychological Bulletin*, 113(3), 403–439. DOI: 10.1037/0033-2909.113.3.403 PMID: 8316609

Cefai, C. (2020). *Social and emotional learning in the Mediterranean: Cross-cultural perspectives and approaches.* Brill Sense. https://books.google.ae/books ?id=y_T_DwAAQBAJ&printsec=frontcover&source=gbs_ViewAPI&redir_esc= y#v=onepage&q&f=false

Center on PBIS. (2023). *PBIS: An evidence-based framework for making schools safe, positive, predictable, and equitable.* Center on PBIS, University of Oregon. www.pbis.org

Center on PBIS. (2024). *PBIS improves student & adult mental health and wellbeing.* Center on PBIS, University of Oregon. www.pbis.org

Center on Positive Behavioral Interventions and Supports & Center for Parent Information & Resources. (2020). *Supporting families with PBIS at home.* University of Oregon. www.pbis.org

Center on Positive Behavioral Interventions and Supports. (2024). *PBIS: An evidence-based framework for making schools safe, positive, predictable, and equitable.* Center on PBIS, University of Oregon. www.pbis.org

Chaby, L., Chetouani, M., Plaza, M., & Cohen, D. (2012). *Exploring multimodal social-emotional behaviors in autism spectrum disorders: an interface between social signal processing and psychopathology.* IEEE., DOI: 10.1109/SocialCom-PASSAT.2012.111

Chaffee, R. K., Johnson, A. H., & Volpe, R. J. (2017). A meta-analysis of class-wide interventions for supporting student behavior. *School Psychology Review*, 46(2), 149–164. DOI: 10.17105/SPR-2017-0015.V46-2

Champ, M., & Xiong, Q. (2018). The effects of music therapy on cognition, psychiatric symptoms, and activities of daily living in patients with Alzheimer's disease. *Journal of Alzheimer's Disease*, 64(4), 1–12. PMID: 29991131

Charlton, C. T., Moulton, S., Sabey, C. V., & West, R. (2021). A systematic review of the effects of schoolwide intervention programs on student and teacher perceptions of school climate. *Journal of Positive Behavior Interventions*, 23(3), 185–200. DOI: 10.1177/1098300720940168

Charman, T., & Petrova, I. (2000). The internal structure of the Child Depression Inventory in Russian and UK schoolchildren. *Journal of Youth and Adolescence*, 30(1), 41–51. DOI: 10.1023/A:1005220820982

Chen, G., Gully, S. M., & Eden, D. (2001). Validation of a new general self-efficacy scale. *Organizational Research Methods*, 4(1), 62–83. DOI: 10.1177/109442810141004

Chen, S., & Li, X. (2021). Resilience in Chinese children with chronic health conditions: A mixed-methods study. *Journal of Pediatric Nursing*, 56, 45–52.

Childs, K. E., Kincaid, D., George, H. P., & Gage, N. A. (2016). The relationship between school-wide implementation of Positive Behavior Intervention and Supports and student discipline outcomes. *Journal of Positive Behavior Interventions*, 18(2), 89–99. DOI: 10.1177/1098300715590398

Chiumento, A., Hosny, W., Gaber, E., Emadeldin, M., El Barabry, W., Hamoda, H. M., & Alonge, O. (2022). Exploring the acceptability of a WHO school-based mental health program in Egypt: A qualitative study. *SSM. Mental Health*, 2, 100075. Advance online publication. DOI: 10.1016/j.ssmmh.2022.100075

Cho Blair, K. S., Park, E. Y., & Kim, W. H. (2021). A meta-analysis of Tier 2 interventions implemented within School-Wide Positive Behavioral Interventions and Supports. *Psychology in the Schools*, 58(1), 141–161. DOI: 10.1002/pits.22443

Cohen, J. (2006). Social, emotional, ethical, and academic education: Creating a climate for learning, participation in democracy, and well-being. *Harvard Educational Review*, 76(2), 201–237. DOI: 10.17763/haer.76.2.j44854x1524644vn

Cohen, J., McCabe, E. M., Michelli, N. M., & Pickeral, T. (2009). School climate: Research, policy, practice, and teacher education. *Teachers College Record*, 111(1), 180–213. DOI: 10.1177/016146810911100108

Coley, R. L., Sims, J., Dearing, E., & Spielvogel, B. (2018). Locating economic risks for adolescent mental and behavioral health: Poverty and affluence in families, neighborhoods, and schools. *Child Development*, 89(2), 360–369. DOI: 10.1111/cdev.12771 PMID: 28245340

Collaborative for Academic Social and Emotional Learning. (2003). *Safe and sound: An educational leader's guide to evidence-based social and emotional learning (SEL) programs*. Author.

Collaborative for Academic. Social and Emotional Learning (CASEL). (n.d.). *Program guide*. https://pg.casel.org/

Coll, C. G.. (2021). An integrative model for the study of developmental competencies in minority children. *Child Development*, 71(4), 1124–1140.

Collie, R. J., Shapka, J. D., & Perry, N. E. (2012). School climate and social–emotional learning: Predicting teacher stress, job satisfaction, and teaching efficacy. *Journal of Educational Psychology*, 104(4), 1189–1204. DOI: 10.1037/a0029356

Collins, F. S., & Fleming, R. (2017). Sound health: An NIH-Kennedy Center Initiative to explore Music and the Mind. *Journal of the American Medical Association*, 317(24), 2470–2471. DOI: 10.1001/jama.2017.7423 PMID: 28586832

Colomeischi, A. A., Duca, D. S., Bujor, L., Rusu, P. P., Grazzani, I., & Cavioni, V. (2022). Impact of a school mental health program on children's and adolescents' socio-emotional skills and psychosocial difficulties. *Children (Basel, Switzerland)*, 9(11), 1661. DOI: 10.3390/children9111661 PMID: 36360389

Colvin, G., & Fernandez, E. (2000). Sustaining effective behavior support systems in an elementary school. *Journal of Positive Behavior Interventions*, 2(4), 251–253. DOI: 10.1177/109830070000200414

Conklin, M., & Jairam, D. (2021). The effects of co-teaching zones of regulation on elementary students' social, emotional, and academic risk behaviors. *Advanced Journal of Social Science*, 8(1), 171–192. DOI: 10.21467/ajss.8.1.171-192

Conley, C. S., & Durlak, J. A. (2017). Universal mental health promotion and prevention programs for students. In S. Bährer-Kohler & F. J. Carod-Artal (Eds.), Global mental health: Prevention and promotion (pp. 127–139). Springer International Publishing/Springer Nature. DOI: 10.1007/978-3-319-59123-0_12

Conley, C. S., Durlak, J. A., & Dickson, D. A. (2013). An Evaluative Review of Outcome Research on Universal Mental Health Promotion and Prevention Programs for Higher Education Students. *Journal of American College Health*, 61(5), 286–301. DOI: 10.1080/07448481.2013.802237 PMID: 23768226

Conley, C. S., Durlak, J. A., & Kirsch, A. C. (2015). A meta-analysis of universal mental health prevention programs for higher education students. *Prevention Science*, 16(4), 487–507. DOI: 10.1007/s11121-015-0543-1 PMID: 25744536

Connor, K. M., & Davidson, J. R. T. (2003). Development of a new resilience scale: The Connor-Davidson Resilience Scale (CD-RISC). *Depression and Anxiety*, 18(2), 76–82. DOI: 10.1002/da.10113 PMID: 12964174

Constantin, F. A. (2018). Music therapy explained by the principles of neuroplasticity. Bulletin of the Transilvania University of Brasov, Series VIII. *Performing Arts*, 11(1), 19–24.

Cook, C. R., Fiat, A., Larson, M., Daikos, C., Slemrod, T., Holland, E. A., Thayer, A. J., & Renshaw, T. (2018). Positive greetings at the door: Evaluation of a low-cost, high-yield proactive classroom management strategy. *Journal of Positive Behavior Interventions*, 20(3), 149–159. DOI: 10.1177/1098300717753831

Cook, C. R., Frye, M., Slemrod, T., Lyon, A. R., Renshaw, T. L., & Zhang, Y. (2015). An integrated approach to universal prevention: Independent and combined effects of PBIS and SEL on youths' mental health. *School Psychology Quarterly*, 30(2), 166–183. DOI: 10.1037/spq0000102 PMID: 25602629

Cook-Cottone, C. P. (2015). *Mindfulness and yoga for self-regulation*. Springer. DOI: 10.1891/9780826198631

Cooper, J., Heron, T., & Heward, W. (2020). *Applied behavior analysis* (3rd ed.). Pearson Education.

Cooper, P. (1965). The development of the concept of war. *Journal of Peace Research*, 2(1), 1–17. DOI: 10.1177/002234336500200101

Corcoran, T., & Edward Thomas, M. K. (2021). School-wide positive behaviour support as evidence-making interventions. *Research in Education*, 111(1), 108–125. DOI: 10.1177/00345237211034884

Cornell, D., & Huang, F. (2019). Collecting and analyzing local school safety and climate data. In Mayer, M. J., & Jimerson, S. R. (Eds.), *School safety and violence prevention: Science, practice, policy* (pp. 151–175). American Psychological Association. DOI: 10.1037/0000106-007

Côté-Lussier, C., & Fitzpatrick, C. (2016). Feelings of safety at school, socioemotional functioning, and classroom engagement. *The Journal of adolescent health: official publication of the Society for Adolescent Medicine, 58*(5), 543–550.

Council of the European Union. (2022). *Council recommendation of 28 November 2022 on pathways to school success and replacing the council Recommendation of 28 June 2011 on policies to reduce early school leaving.*https://eur-lex.europa.eu/legal-content/EN/TXT/PDF/?uri=CELEX:32022H1209(01)

Covell, K. (1996). National and gender differences in adolescents' war attitudes. *International Journal of Behavioral Development*, 19(4), 871–883. DOI: 10.1177/016502549601900411

Covell, K., Rose-Krasnor, L., & Fletcher, K. (1994). Age differences in understanding peace, war, and conflict resolution. *International Journal of Behavioral Development*, 17(4), 717–737. DOI: 10.1177/016502549401700409

Creswell, J. W., & Plano Clark, V. L. (2017). *Designing and conducting mixed methods research*. Sage Publications.

Crone, D., Hawken, L., & Horner, R. (2015). *Building positive behavior support systems in schools: Functional behavioral assessment* (2nd ed.). The Guilford Press.

Cross, T. L., Bazron, B. J., Dennis, K. W., & Isaacs, M. R. (1989). *Toward a culturally competent system of care: A monograph on effective services for minority children who are severely emotionally disturbed* (Vol. 1). Georgetown University Child Development Center.

Crowley, B. Z., Cornell, D., & Konold, T. (2021). School climate moderates the association between sexual harassment and student well-being. *School Mental Health*, 13(4), 695–706. DOI: 10.1007/s12310-021-09449-3

Csikszentmihalyi, M. (1990). *Flow: The Psychology of Optimal Experience*. Harper & Row.

Cumming, T. M., & O'Neill, S. C. (2019). Using data-based individualization to intensify behavioral interventions. *Intervention in School and Clinic*, 54(5), 280–285. DOI: 10.1177/1053451218819203

Cunningham, L. K., Hartwell, B., & Kreppner, J. (2019). Exploring the impact of nurture groups on children's social skills: A mixed-methods approach. *Educational Psychology in Practice*, 35(4), 368–383. DOI: 10.1080/02667363.2019.1615868

D'Alessandro, A. M., Butterfield, K. M., Hanceroglu, L., & Roberts, K. P. (2022). Listen to the children: Elementary school students' perspectives on a mindfulness intervention. *Journal of Child and Family Studies*, 31(8), 2108–2120. DOI: 10.1007/s10826-022-02292-3 PMID: 35505672

D'Zurilla, T. J., & Goldfried, M. R. (1971). Problem solving and behavior modification. *Journal of Abnormal Psychology*, 78(1), 107–126. DOI: 10.1037/h0031360 PMID: 4938262

Daily, S. M., Mann, M. J., Kristjansson, A. L., Smith, M. L., & Zullig, K. J. (2019). School climate and academic achievement in middle and high school students. *The Journal of School Health*, 89(3), 173–180. DOI: 10.1111/josh.12726 PMID: 30680750

Dambrun, M., & Ricard, M. (2011). Self-centeredness and selflessness: A theory of self-based psychological functioning and its consequences for happiness. *Review of General Psychology*, 15(2), 138–157. DOI: 10.1037/a0023059

Damsgaard, M. T., Holstein, B. E., Koushede, V., Madsen, K. R., Meilstrup, C., Nelausen, M. K., Nielsen, L., & Rayce, S. B. (2014). Close relations to parents and emotional symptoms among adolescents: Beyond socio-economic impact? *International Journal of Public Health*, 59(5), 721–726. DOI: 10.1007/s00038-014-0600-8 PMID: 25178736

Danesh, H. B. (2006). Towards an integrative theory of peace education. *Journal of Peace Education*, 3(1), 55–78. DOI: 10.1080/17400200500532151

Daniele, K., Gambacorti Passerini, M. B., Palmieri, C., & Zannini, L. (2022). Educational interventions to promote adolescents' mental health: A scoping review. *Health Education Journal*, 81(5), 597–613. DOI: 10.1177/00178969221105359

Darling-Hammond, L., & Cook-Harvey, C. M. (2018). *Educating the Whole Child: Improving School Climate to Support Student Success*. Learning Policy Institute. DOI: 10.54300/145.655

Davidson, R. J., & McEwen, B. S. (2012). Social influences on neuroplasticity: Stress and interventions to promote well-being. *Nature Neuroscience*, 15(5), 689–695. DOI: 10.1038/nn.3093 PMID: 22534579

Daviss, W. B., Weinman, D. R., Diler, R. S., & Birmaher, B. (2006b). *Risk Factors for Co-morbid Depression in Adolescents with ADHD*. Poster presented at 53rd Annual Meeting of the American Academy of Child and Adolescent Psychiatry; (abstract), San Diego, CA.

de Leeuw, R. R., de Boer, A. A., & Minnaert, A. E. M. G. (2020). The proof of the intervention is in the implementation: A systematic review about implementation fidelity of classroom-based interventions facilitating social participation of students with social-emotional problems or behavioural difficulties. *International Journal of Educational Research Open*, 1, 100002. Advance online publication. DOI: 10.1016/j.ijedro.2020.100002 de Witte, M., Spruit, A., van Hooren, S., Moonen, X., & Stams, G. J. (2020). Effects of music interventions on stress-related outcomes: A systematic review and two meta-analyses. *Health Psychology Review*, 14(2), 294–324. DOI: 10.1080/17437199.2019.1627897 PMID: 31167611

Dearing, E., Kreider, H., Simpkins, S., & Weiss, H. B. (2006). Family involvement in school and low-income children's literacy performance: Longitudinal associations between and within families. *Journal of Educational Psychology*, 98(4), 653–664. DOI: 10.1037/0022-0663.98.4.653

Deater-Deckard, K., & Dodge, K. A. (1997). Externalizing behavior problems and discipline revisited: Nonlinear effects and variation by culture, context, and gender. *Psychological Inquiry*, 8(3), 161–175. DOI: 10.1207/s15327965pli0803_1

Deci, E. L., & Ryan, R. M. (2012). Self-determination theory. Handbook of theories of social psychology, 1(20), 416-436.

Deltour, C., Dachet, D., Monseur, C., & Baye, A. (2021). Does SWPBIS increase teachers' collective efficacy? Evidence from a quasi-experiment. *Frontiers in Education*, 6, 720065. DOI: 10.3389/feduc.2021.720065

Dember, W. N. (1974). Motivation and the cognitive revolution. *American Psychologist, 29*(3), 161–168. [REMOVED HYPERLINK FIELD]DOI: 10.1037/h0035907

DeMuth, D. H., & Melnick, J. (1998). What happens when they talk about it? Family reactions to nuclear war. *Peace and Conflict*, 4(1), 23–34. DOI: 10.1207/s15327949pac0401_3

Deolmi, M., & Pisani, F. (2020). Psychological and psychiatric impact of COVID-19 pandemic among children and adolescents. *Acta Biomedica*, 91(4). Advance online publication. 10.23750%2Fabm.v91i4.10870 PMID: 33525229

Department for Education, 2019. ITT Core Content Framework. Crown copyright.

Di Giuseppe, T., Perasso, G., Mazzeo, C., Maculan, A., Vianello, F., & Paoletti, P. (2022). *Envisioning the future: A neuropsycho-pedagogical intervention on resilience predictors among inmates during the pandemic*. Ricerche di Psicologia-Open., DOI: 10.3280/rip2022oa14724

Didaskalou, E., & Millward, A. (2002). Breaking the policy log-jam: Comparative perspectives on policy formulation and development for pupils with emotional and behavioral difficulties. *Oxford Review of Education*, 28(1), 109–121. DOI: 10.1080/03054980120113661

Dincer, B. (2021). Investigating the school climate perceptions and school motivations of middle school students. *International Journal of Educational Methodology*, 7(2), 361–372. DOI: 10.12973/ijem.7.2.361

Dingle, G. A., & Fay, C. (2017). Tuned In: The effectiveness for young adults of a group emotion regulation program using music listening. *Psychology of Music*, 45(4), 513–529. DOI: 10.1177/0305735616668586

Doe, S., & Lee, P. (2019). Technological advancements in measuring and enhancing resilience. *The Journal of Applied Psychology*, 104(3), 432–447.

Doll, B. (2013). Enhancing resilience in classrooms. In Goldstein, S., & Brooks, R. B. (Eds.), *Handbook of Resilience in Children* (pp. 399–410). Springer. DOI: 10.1007/978-1-4614-3661-4_23

Doll, B., Zucker, St., & Brehm, K. (2014). *Resilient classrooms: Creating healthy environments for learning*. The Guilford Press.

Dolton, A., Adams, S., & O'Reilly, M. (2020). In the child's voice: The experiences of primary school children with social, emotional and mental health difficulties. *Clinical Child Psychology and Psychiatry*, 25(2), 419–434. DOI: 10.1177/1359104519859923 PMID: 31257914

Dougherty, L. R., Klein, D. N., Durbin, C. E., Hayden, E. P., & Olino, T. M. (2010). Temperamental positive and negative emotionality and children's depressive symptoms: A longitudinal prospective study from age three to age ten. *Journal of Social and Clinical Psychology*, 29(4), 462–488. DOI: 10.1521/jscp.2010.29.4.462

Dray, J., Bowman, J., Campbell, E., Freund, M., Hodder, R. K., Wolfenden, L., & Wiggers, J. (2014). Systematic review of universal resilience interventions targeting child and adolescent mental health in the school setting: Review protocol. *BMJ Open*, 4(7), e004718. PMID: 24861548

Drevon, D. D., Hixson, M. D., Wyse, R. D., & Rigney, A. M. (2019). A meta-analytic review of the evidence for check-in check-out. *Psychology in the Schools*, 56(3), 393–412. DOI: 10.1002/pits.22195

Duncan, M. J., Patte, K. A., & Leatherdale, S. T. (2021). Mental health associations with academic performance and education behaviors in Canadian secondary school students. *Canadian Journal of School Psychology*, 36(4), 335–357. DOI: 10.1177/0829573521997311

Dunning, D. L., Griffiths, K., Kuyken, W., Crane, C., Foulkes, L., Parker, J., & Dalgleish, T. (2019). Research Review: The effects of mindfulness-based interventions on cognition and mental health in children and adolescents – a meta-analysis of randomized controlled trials. *Journal of Child Psychology and Psychiatry, and Allied Disciplines*, 60(3), 244–258. DOI: 10.1111/jcpp.12980 PMID: 30345511

Durlak, J. A., Weissberg, R. P., Dymnicki, A. B., Taylor, R. D., & Schellinger, K. B. (2011). The impact of enhancing students' social and emotional learning: A meta-analysis of school-based universal interventions. Child development, 82(1), 405-432.Elias, M. J., Zins, J. E., Weissberg, R. P., Frey, K. S., Greenberg, M. T., Haynes, N. M., ... & Shriver, T. P. (1997). Promoting social and emotional learning: Guidelines for educators. ASCD.

Durlak, J. A., Mahoney, J. L., & Boyle, A. E. (2022). What we know, and what we need to find out about universal, school-based social and emotional learning programs for children and adolescents: A review of meta-analyses and directions for future research. *Psychological Bulletin*, 148(11-12), 765–782. DOI: 10.1037/bul0000383

Durlak, J. A., Weissberg, R. P., Dymnicki, A. B., Taylor, R. D., & Schellinger, K. B. (2011). The impact of enhancing students' social and emotional learning: A meta-analysis of school-based universal interventions. *Child Development*, 82(1), 405–432. DOI: 10.1111/j.1467-8624.2010.01564.x PMID: 21291449

Eber, L., Barrett, S., Perales, K., Jeffrey-Pearsall, J., Pohlman, K., Putnam, R., Splett, J., & Weist, M. D. (2019). Advancing Education Effectiveness: Interconnecting School Mental Health and School-Wide PBIS, Volume 2: An Implementation Guide. Center for Positive Behavior Interventions and Supports. University of Oregon Press.

Elias, M. J., Zins, J. E., Weissberg, R. P., Frey, K. S., Greenberg, M. T., Haynes, N. M., & Shriver, T. P. (1997). *Promoting social and emotional learning: Guidelines for educators*. ASCD.

El-Khodary, B., & Samara, M. (2019). Effectiveness of a school-based intervention on the students' mental health after exposure to war-related trauma. *Frontiers in Psychiatry*, 10, 1031. DOI: 10.3389/fpsyt.2019.01031 PMID: 32273852

Ellis, A. (1962). *Reason and emotion in psychotherapy*. Lyle Stuart.

Ellis, K., Gage, N. A., Kramer, D., Baton, E., & Angelosante, C. (2022). School climate in rural and urban schools and the impact of SWPBIS. *Rural Special Education Quarterly*, 41(2), 73–83. DOI: 10.1177/87568705221098031

Elrod, B. G., Rice, K. G., & Meyers, J. (2022). PBIS fidelity, school climate, and student discipline: A longitudinal study of secondary schools. *Psychology in the Schools*, 59(2), 376–397. DOI: 10.1002/pits.22614

Ennis, R. P., Jolivette, K., Swoszowski, N. C., & Johnson, M. L. (2012). Secondary prevention efforts at a residential facility for students with emotional and behavioral disorders: Function-based check-in, check-out. *Residential Treatment for Children & Youth*, 29(2), 79–102. DOI: 10.1080/0886571X.2012.669250

Ennis, R. P., Royer, D. J., Lane, K. L., & Dunlap, K. D. (2020). Behavior-specific praise in pre-K–12 settings: Mapping the 50-year knowledge base. *Behavioral Disorders*, 45(3), 131–147. DOI: 10.1177/0198742919843075

Epstein, J. L., & Sheldon, S. B. (2002). Present and accounted for: Improving student attendance through family and community involvement. *The Journal of Educational Research*, 95(5), 308–318. DOI: 10.1080/00220670209596604

Epstein, R. A., Fonnesbeck, C., Potter, S., Rizzone, K. H., & McPheeters, M. (2015). Psychosocial interventions for child disruptive behaviors: A meta-analysis. *Pediatrics*, 136(5), 947–960. DOI: 10.1542/peds.2015-2577 PMID: 26482672

Ergas, O. (2019). Mindfulness in, as and of education: Three roles of mindfulness in education. *Journal of Philosophy of Education*, 53(2), 2. DOI: 10.1111/1467-9752.12349

Erskine, H. E., Baxter, A., Patton, G. C., Moffitt, T. E., Patel, V., Whiteford, H., & Scott, J. F. (2017). The global coverage of prevalence data for mental disorders in children and adolescents. *Epidemiology and Psychiatric Sciences*, 26(4), 395–402. DOI: 10.1017/S2045796015001158 PMID: 26786507

Erskine, H. E., Moffitt, T. E., Copeland, W. E., Costello, E. J., Ferrari, A. J., Patton, G., Degenhardt, L., Vos, T., Whiteford, H. A., & Scott, J. G. (2015). A heavy burden on young minds: The global burden of mental health and substance use disorders in children and youth. *Psychological Medicine*, 45(7), 1551–1563. DOI: 10.1017/S0033291714002888 PMID: 25534496

Escalona, S. K. (1982). Growing up with the threat of nuclear war: Some indirect effects on personality development. *The American Journal of Orthopsychiatry*, 52(4), 600–607. DOI: 10.1111/j.1939-0025.1982.tb01449.x PMID: 7148981

Eschenbeck, H., Kaess, M., Lehner, L., Hofmann, H., Bauer, S., Becker, K., Diestelkamp, S., Moessner, M., Rummel-Kluge, C., Salize, H.-J., Thomasius, R., Bertsch, K., Bilic, S., Brunner, R., Feldhege, J., Gallinat, C., Herpertz, S. C., Koenig, J., & Lustig, S.. (2019). School-based mental health promotion in children and adolescents with StresSOS using online or face-to-face interventions: Study protocol for a randomized controlled trial within the ProHEAD Consortium. *Trials*, 20(1), 64. DOI: 10.1186/s13063-018-3159-5 PMID: 30658675

Estrapala, S., Rila, A., & Bruhn, A. L. (2021). A systematic review of tier 1 PBIS implementation in high schools. *Journal of Positive Behavior Interventions*, 23(4), 288–302. DOI: 10.1177/1098300720929684

European Council. (2022). Pathways to school success. *Official Journal of the European Union, C*, 496, 1–15. https://eur-lex.europa.eu/legal content/EN/TXT/ PDF/?uri=CELEX:32022H1209(01)

Falcon, S., Izzard, S., & Bastable, E. (2021). Effects of an equity-focused PBIS approach to school improvement on exclusionary discipline and school climate. *Preventing School Failure*, 65(4), 354–361. DOI: 10.1080/1045988X.2021.1937027

Fargas-Malet, M., & Dillenburger, K. (2014). Children drawing their own conclusions: Children's perceptions of a "postconflict" society. *Peace and Conflict*, 20(2), 135–149. DOI: 10.1037/pac0000029

Fazel, M., Hoagwood, K., Stephan, S., & Ford, T. (2014). Mental health interventions in schools in high-income countries. *The Lancet. Psychiatry*, 1(5), 377–387. DOI: 10.1016/S2215-0366(14)70312-8 PMID: 26114092

Fazel, M., Reed, R. V., Panter-Brick, C., & Stein, A. (2012). Mental health of displaced and refugee children resettled in low-income and middle-income countries: Risk and protective factors. *Lancet*, 379(9812), 250–265. DOI: 10.1016/S0140-6736(11)60051-2 PMID: 21835460

Felver, J. C., Celis-de Hoyos, C. E., Tezanos, K., & Singh, N. N. (2016). A systematic review of mindfulness-based interventions for youth in school settings. *Mindfulness*, 7(1), 34–45. DOI: 10.1007/s12671-015-0389-4

Fenwick-Smith, A., Dahlberg, E. E., & Thompson, S. C. (2018). Systematic review of resilience-enhancing, universal, primary school-based mental health promotion programs. *BMC Psychology*, 6(1), 1–17. DOI: 10.1186/s40359-018-0242-3 PMID: 29976252

Fergus, S., & Zimmerman, M. A. (2005). Adolescent resilience: A framework for understanding healthy development in the face of risk. *Annual Review of Public Health*, 26(1), 399–419. DOI: 10.1146/annurev.publhealth.26.021304.144357 PMID: 15760295

Fernandez-Castillo, A., & Rojas, M. E. G. (2009). Atencion selectiva, ansiedad, sintomatologia depressive y rendimiento academico en adolescentes. *Electronic Journal of Research in Educational Psychology*, 7(1), 49–76.

Ferro, M. A., & Boyle, M. H. (2015). The impact of chronic physical illness, maternal depressive symptoms, family functioning, and self-esteem on symptoms of anxiety and depression in children. *Journal of Abnormal Child Psychology*, 43(1), 177–187. DOI: 10.1007/s10802-014-9893-6 PMID: 24938212

Filcheck, H. A., McNeil, C. B., Greco, L. A., & Bernard, R. S. (2004). Using a whole-class token economy and coaching of teacher skills in a preschool classroom to manage disruptive behavior. *Psychology in the Schools*, 41(3), 351–361. DOI: 10.1002/pits.10168

Firose, M., Musthafa, M.M., Marikar, & F.M.M.T. (2023). Mental health and self-esteem correlated with the academic achievements of youths from Sri Lankan schools. *Psihiatru.ro, 73(2)*, 27-32.

Fisher, B. C. (2007). *Attention Deficit Disorder: Practical Coping Mechanisms* (2nd ed.). Healthcare.

Fixsen, D. L., Naoom, S. F., Blase, K. A., Friedman, R. M., & Wallace, F. (2005). *Implementation research: A synthesis of the literature* (FMHI Publication No. 231). University of South Florida, Louis de la Parte Florida Mental Health Institute, National Implementation Research Network.

Flannery, K. B., Fenning, P., Kato, M. M., & McIntosh, K. (2014). Effects of school-wide positive behavioral interventions and supports and fidelity of implementation on problem behavior in high schools. *School Psychology Quarterly*, 29(2), 111–124. DOI: 10.1037/spq0000039 PMID: 24188290

Flook, L., Goldberg, S. B., Pinger, L., Bonus, K., & Davidson, R. J. (2013). Mindfulness for teachers: A pilot study to assess effects on stress, burnout, and teaching efficacy. *Mind, Brain and Education : the Official Journal of the International Mind, Brain, and Education Society*, 7(3), 182–195. DOI: 10.1111/mbe.12026 PMID: 24324528

Flores, G. (2000). Culture and the patient-physician relationship: Achieving cultural competency in health care. *The Journal of Pediatrics*, 136(1), 14–23. DOI: 10.1016/S0022-3476(00)90043-X PMID: 10636968

Ford, B. Q., & Gross, J. J. (2019). Why beliefs about emotion matter: An emotion-regulation perspective. *Current Directions in Psychological Science*, 28(1), 74–81. DOI: 10.1177/0963721418806697

Fox, R. A., Leif, E. S., Moore, D. W., Furlonger, B., Anderson, A., & Sharma, U. (2022). A systematic review of the facilitators and barriers to the sustained implementation of school-wide positive behavioral interventions and supports. *Education & Treatment of Children*, 45(1), 105–126. DOI: 10.1007/s43494-021-00056-0

Francis, K. (2007). *Pervasive Developmental Disorders or autism spectrum disorders. Disability Specialization Guide (EPEAEK)*. Panteion University of Social and Political Sciences. In Greek

Frank, J. L., Jennings, P. A., & Greenberg, M. T. (2016). Validation of the Mindfulness in Teaching Scale. *Mindfulness*, 7(1), 155–163. DOI: 10.1007/s12671-015-0461-0

Freeman, J., Simonsen, B., McCoach, D. B., Sugai, G., Lombardi, A., & Horner, R. (2016). Relationship between school-wide positive behavior interventions and supports and academic, attendance, and behavior outcomes in high schools. *Journal of Positive Behavior Interventions*, 18(1), 41–51. DOI: 10.1177/1098300715580992

Freeman, J., Sugai, G., Simonsen, B., & Everett, S. (2017). MTSS coaching: Bridging knowing to doing. *Theory into Practice*, 56(1), 29–37. DOI: 10.1080/00405841.2016.1241946

Freeman, R., Simacek, J., Jeffrey-Pearsall, J., Lee, S., Khalif, M., & Oteman, Q. (2024). Development of the tiered onsite evaluation tool for organization-wide person-centered Positive Behavior Support. *Journal of Positive Behavior Interventions*, 26(3), 131–141. DOI: 10.1177/10983007231200540

Freiberg, H. J., & Stein, T. A. (1999). Measuring, improving and sustaining healthy learning environments. In Freiberg, H. J. (Ed.), *School climate: Measuring, improving and sustaining healthy learning environments* (pp. 11–29). Falmer Press.

Gable, R. A., Hester, P. H., Rock, M. L., & Hughes, K. G. (2009). Rules, praise, ignoring, and reprimands revisited. *Intervention in School and Clinic*, 44(4), 195–254. DOI: 10.1177/1053451208328831

Galanaki, E. (1997). Applications of systems theory in school: The reframing technique. [in Greek]. *Tetradia Psychiatrikis*, 59, 67–79.

Galanaki, E. (2000a). Systemic approach of the school. In Kalantzi-Azizi, A., & Besevegis, E. G. (Eds.), *Training/awareness-raising issues for child and adolescent mental health professionals* (pp. 215–220). Ellinika Grammata. (in Greek)

Galanaki, E. (2000b). Systems theory as a framework for dealing with the child's behavior problems at school. [in Greek]. *Educational Review*, 30, 7–25.

Gándara, P., & Hopkins, M. (Eds.). (2010). *Forbidden language: English learners and restrictive language policies*. Teachers College Press.

Garcia, M. E., Williams, S., & Haddad, F. (2019). Familismo: Implications for assessment and treatment of Latino families. *Journal of Family Therapy*, 41(3), 352–371.

Gardner, F., & Shaw, D. S. (2008). Behavioral problems of infancy and preschool children. In M. Rutter, D. Bishop, D. Pine, S. Scott, J. Stevenson, E. Taylor, & A. Thapar (Eds.), *Rutter's child and adolescent psychiatry* (5th ed., pp. 882–894). Wiley-Blackwell. DOI: 10.1002/9781444300895.ch53

Garmezy, N. (1991). Resiliency and vulnerability to adverse developmental outcomes associated with poverty. *The American Behavioral Scientist*, 34(4), 416–430. DOI: 10.1177/0002764291034004003

Gay, G. (2018). *Culturally responsive teaching: Theory, research, and practice*. Teachers College Press.

Gearing, R. E., MacKenzie, M. J., Ibrahim, R. W., Brewer, K. B., Batayneh, J. S., & Schwalbe, C. S. (2018). Adaptation and translation of mental health interventions in middle eastern arab countries: A systematic review of barriers to and strategies for effective treatment implementation. *The International Journal of Social Psychiatry*, 59(7), 671–681. DOI: 10.1177/0020764012452349 PMID: 22820177

Gena, A. (2002). *Autism and Pervasive Developmental Disorders. Evaluation-Diagnosis-Treatment*. Leader Books. In Greek

Geretsegger, M., Quoc, E., Riedl, H., Smetana, M., & Stegemann, T. (2019). Music therapy and other music-based interventions in pediatric health care: An overview. *Medicines (Basel, Switzerland)*, 6(25), 1–12. PMID: 30769834

Gerzberg, R. (2018). The quality of research in the field of mindfulness in education is growing exponentially. *Mindful Magazine*. Retrieved from https://www.mindful.org

Giannakopoulos, G., Kazantzi, M., Dimitrakaki, C., Tsiantis, J., Kolaitis, G., Trzesniewski, K. H., Donnellan, M. B., Moffitt, T. E., Robins, R. W., Poulton, R., & Caspi, A. (2006). Low self-esteem during adolescence predicts poor health, criminal behavior, and limited economic prospects during adulthood. *Developmental Psychology*, 42(2), 381–390. DOI: 10.1037/0012-1649.42.2.381 PMID: 16569175

Gillham, J. E., Reivich, K. J., Freres, D. R., Chaplin, T. M., Shatté, A. J., Samuels, B., Elkon, A. G. L., Litzinger, S., Lascher, M., Gallop, R., & Seligman, M. E. P. (2007). School-based prevention of depressive symptoms: A randomized controlled study of the effectiveness and specificity of the Penn Resiliency Program. *Journal of Consulting and Clinical Psychology*, 75(1), 9–19. DOI: 10.1037/0022-006X.75.1.9 PMID: 17295559

Gilligan, C. (1982). *In a different voice: Psychological theory and women's development*. Harvard University Press.

Gimbert, B. G., Miller, D., Herman, E., Breedlove, M., & Molina, C. E. (2021). Social emotional learning in schools: the importance of educator competence. *Journal of Research in Leadership Education, 18*(3-39). https://doi.org/DOI: 10.1177/19427751211014920

Gion, C., Peshak George, H., Nese, R., McGrath Kato, M., Massar, M., & McIntosh, K. (2020). School-wide Positive Behavioral Interventions and Supports. In Reschly, A. L., Pohl, A. J., & Christenson, S. L. (Eds.), *Student engagement: Effective academic, behavioral, cognitive, and affective interventions at school* (pp. 171–184). Springer. DOI: 10.1007/978-3-030-37285-9_10

Gladney, D., Lo, Y.-y., Kourea, L., & Johnson, H. N. (2021). Using multilevel coaching to improve general education teachers' implementation fidelity of culturally responsive social skill instruction. *Preventing School Failure*, 65(2), 175–184. Advance online publication. DOI: 10.1080/1045988X.2020.1864715

Glymitsa, E. (2019). Andreas doesn't want to wear his shoes. In Zafiropoulou, M. (Ed.), *The "difficult" child at home and at school* (pp. 108–123). Pedio. (in Greek)

Goei, S. L., & Kourea, L. (2017). Positive Behaviour Support Europe Network. *Remediaal*, 17(4-5), 5–8.

Goh, A. E., & Bambara, L. M. (2012). Individualized positive behavior support in school settings: A meta-analysis. *Remedial and Special Education*, 33(5), 271–286. DOI: 10.1177/0741932510383990

Goldberg, J. M., Sklad, M., Elfrink, T. R., Schreurs, K. M., Bohlmeijer, E. T., & Clarke, A. M. (2019). Effectiveness of interventions adopting a whole school approach to enhancing social and emotional development: A meta-analysis. *European Journal of Psychology of Education*, 34(4), 755–782. DOI: 10.1007/s10212-018-0406-9

Goldrich, C. (2015). *8 keys to parenting children with ADHD*. W. W. Norton & Company.

Gonzalez, R., & Padilla, A. M. (1997). The academic resilience of Mexican American high school students. *Hispanic Journal of Behavioral Sciences*, 19(3), 301–317. DOI: 10.1177/07399863970193004

Goodman, R. (1997). The Strengths and Difficulties Questionnaire: A research note. *Journal of Child Psychology and Psychiatry, and Allied Disciplines*, 38(5), 581–586. DOI: 10.1111/j.1469-7610.1997.tb01545.x PMID: 9255702

Gorski, P. C. (2016). *Reaching and teaching students in poverty: Strategies for erasing the opportunity gap*. Teachers College Press.

Grantham, R., & Primrose, F. (2017). Investigating the fidelity and effectiveness of nurture groups in the secondary school context. *Emotional & Behavioural Difficulties*, 22(3), 219–236. DOI: 10.1080/13632752.2017.1331986

Grant, N., Meyer, J. L., & Strambler, M. J. (2023). Measuring social and emotional learning implementation in a research-practice partnership. *Frontiers in Psychology*, 14, 1052877. DOI: 10.3389/fpsyg.2023.1052877 PMID: 37564314

Grasley-Boy, N. M., Reichow, B., van Dijk, W., & Gage, N. (2021). A systematic review of tier 1 PBIS implementation in alternative education settings. *Behavioral Disorders*, 46(4), 199–213. DOI: 10.1177/0198742920915648

Gray, C. (1994). *Comic Strip conversations*. Future Horizons.

Grazia, V., & Molinari, L. (2020). School climate multidimensionality and measurement: A systematic literature review. *Research Papers in Education*, 36(5), 561–587. DOI: 10.1080/02671522.2019.1697735

Green, A. L., Ferrande, S., Boaz, T. L., Kutash, K., & Wheeldon-Reese, B. (2021). Social and emotional learning during early adolescence: Effectiveness of a classroom-based SEL program for middle school students. *Psychology in the Schools*, 58(6), 1056–1069. DOI: 10.1002/pits.22487

Greenberg, J., Putman, H., & Walsh, K. (2014). Training our future teachers: Classroom management. https://files.eric.ed.gov/fulltext/ED556312.pdf

Greenberg, M. T., Kusché, C. A., Cook, E. T., & Quamma, J. P. (1995). Promoting emotional competence in school-aged children: The effects of the PATHS curriculum. *Development and Psychopathology*, 7(1), 117–136. DOI: 10.1017/S0954579400006374

Greenberg, M., Domitrovich, C., Weissberg, R., & Durlak, J. (2017). Social and emotional learning as a public health approach to education. *The Future of Children*, 27(1), 13–32. DOI: 10.1353/foc.2017.0001

Grigorenko, P. (2001). Developmental dyslexia: An update on genes, brains and environments. *Journal of Child Psychology and Psychiatry, and Allied Disciplines*, 42(1), 91–125. DOI: 10.1111/1469-7610.00704 PMID: 11205626

Guhn, A., Sterzer, F., Haack, F. H., & Köhler, S. (2018). Affective and cognitive reactivity to mood induction in chronic depression. *Journal of Affective Disorders*, 229, 275–281. DOI: 10.1016/j.jad.2017.12.090 PMID: 29329060

Habayeb, S., Rich, B., & Alvord, M. K. (2017). Targeting heterogeneity and comorbidity in children with autism spectrum disorder through the resilience builder group therapy program. *Child and Youth Care Forum*, 46(4), 539–557. DOI: 10.1007/s10566-017-9394-1

Hakvoort, I., & Hägglund, S. (2001). Concepts of peace and war as described by Dutch and Swedish girls and boys. *Peace and Conflict*, 7(1), 29–44. DOI: 10.1207/S15327949PAC0701_03

Hakvoort, I., & Oppenheimer, L. (1993). Children and adolescents' conceptions of peace, war, and strategies to attain peace: A Dutch case study. *Journal of Peace Research*, 30(1), 65–77. DOI: 10.1177/0022343393030001006

Hakvoort, I., & Oppenheimer, L. (1998). Understanding peace and war: A review of developmental psychology research. *Developmental Review*, 18(3), 353–389. DOI: 10.1006/drev.1998.0471

Hall, G. C. N. (2001). Psychotherapy research with ethnic minorities: Empirical, ethical, and conceptual issues. *Journal of Consulting and Clinical Psychology*, 69(3), 502–510. DOI: 10.1037/0022-006X.69.3.502 PMID: 11495179

Hallis, L., Cameli, L., Bekkouche, N. S., & Knäuper, B. (2017). Combining cognitive therapy with acceptance and commitment therapy for depression: A group therapy feasibility study. *Journal of Cognitive Psychotherapy*, 31(3), 171–190. DOI: 10.1891/0889-8391.31.3.171 PMID: 32755936

Hall, R. (1993). How children think and feel about war and peace: An Australian study. *Journal of Peace Research*, 30(2), 181–196. DOI: 10.1177/0022343393030002005

Hanicke, T., & Broadbent, J. (2016). The influence of academic self-efficacy on academic performance. A systematic review. *Educational Research Review*, 17, 63–84. DOI: 10.1016/j.edurev.2015.11.002

Han, Z. R., Wang, J., Luo, J., & Zhang, J. (2023). The role of resilience and hope in enhancing mental health among adolescents: A cross-cultural study. *Journal of Adolescence*, 92, 52–63.

Harpin, V., Mazzone, L., Raynaud, J. P., Kahle, J. R., & Hodgkins, P. (2013). Long-term outcomes of ADHD: A systematic review of self-esteem and social function. *Journal of Attention Disorders*, 20(4), 295–305. DOI: 10.1177/1087054713486516 PMID: 23698916

Harris, A., Jennings, P. A., Katz, D. A., Abenavoli, R. M., & Greenberg, M. T. (2016). Promoting stress management and wellbeing in educators: Feasibility and efficacy of a school-based yoga and mindfulness intervention. *Mindfulness*, 7(1), 143–154. DOI: 10.1007/s12671-015-0451-2

Hartmann, W. E., Wendt, D. C., Saftner, M. D., Marcus, J. D., & Momper, S. L. (2019). Advancing community-based participatory research with culturally grounded technology: Development of the healing pathways app. *Journal of Psychotherapy Integration*, 29(1), 14.

Hattie, J. (2009). The black box of tertiary assessment: An impending revolution. Tertiary assessment & higher education student outcomes: Policy, practice & research, 259, 275.

Hatzichristou, X. (2009). *Introduction to school psychology* (8th ed.). Greek Letters. In Greek

Hawken, L. S., Crone, D. A., Bundock, K., & Horner, R. H. (2020). *Responding to problem behavior in schools*. Guilford Publications.

Hawken, L. S., & Horner, R. H. (2003). Evaluation of a targeted intervention within a schoolwide system of behavior support. *Journal of Behavioral Education*, 12(3), 225–240. DOI: 10.1023/A:1025512411930

Hayes, S. C., Strosahl, K. D., & Wilson, K. G. (2012). *Acceptance and Commitment Therapy: The Process and Practice of Mindful Change*. Guilford Press. DOI: 10.1037/17335-000

Haynes, N. M., Emmons, C., & Ben-Avie, M. (1997). School climate as a factor in student adjustment and achievement. *Journal of Educational & Psychological Consultation*, 8(3), 321–329. DOI: 10.1207/s1532768xjepc0803_4

Henderson, N., & Milstein, M. M. (2003). *Resiliency in schools: Making it happen for students and educators* (updated ed.). Corwin Press.

Henry, J. D., & Crawford, J. R. (2005). The short-form version of the Depression Anxiety Stress Scales (DASS-21): Construct validity and normative data in a large non-clinical sample. *British Journal of Clinical Psychology*, 44(Pt 2), 227–239. DOI: 10.1348/014466505X29657 PMID: 16004657

Hepburn, L. (2022). Installation of school-wide positive behaviour support in government schools: Queensland experiences. *International Journal of Positive Behavioural Support*, 12(1), 13–20.

Hernandez-Ruiz, E. (2017). Collaboration and assistance in music therapy practice: Roles, relationships, challenges. *Music Therapy Perspectives*, 38(1), e9–e10. DOI: 10.1093/mtp/mix008

Hershfeldt, P. A., Pell, K., Sechrest, R., Pas, E. T., & Bradshaw, C. P. (2012). Lessons learned coaching teachers in behavior management: The PBIS*plus* Coaching Model. *Journal of Educational & Psychological Consultation*, 22(4), 280–299. DOI: 10.1080/10474412.2012.731293 PMID: 23599661

Hess, R. S., & Copeland, E. P. (2001). Students' stress, coping strategies, and school completion: A longitudinal perspective. *School Psychology Quarterly*, 16(4), 389–405. DOI: 10.1521/scpq.16.4.389.19899

Heward, W. L., Alber-Morgan, S. R., & Konrad, M. (2016). *Exceptional children: An introduction to special education* (11th ed.). Pearson.

Holmes, S. (2019). Play-based interview techniques with young children. In *Using innovative methods in early years research* (pp. 92–108). Routledge. DOI: 10.4324/9780429423871-8

Holmes, S. E., & Sinclair, V. (2024). pending. What is working? A Qualitative Comparative Analysis of approaches to pupil well-being in a MAT in NorthWest England. *British Educational Research Journal*.

Homme, L. E. (1965). Perspectives in psychology: XXIV Control of coverants, the operants of the mind. *The Psychological Record*, 15(4), 501–511. DOI: 10.1007/BF03393622

Horn, I. S., & Little, J. W. (2010). Attending to problems of practice: routines and resources for professional learning in teachers' workplace interactions. *American Educational Research Journal, 47*(181-217). https://doi.org/DOI: 10.3102/0002831209345158

Horner, R. H., & Kittelman, A. (2021). Advancing the large-scale implementation of Applied Behavior Analysis. *Behavior and Social Issues*, 30(1), 94–105. DOI: 10.1007/s42822-021-00049-z

Horner, R. H., & Monzalve, M. M. (2018). A framework for building safe and effective school environments: Positive behavioral interventions and supports. *Pedagogická Orientace*, 28(4), 663–685. DOI: 10.5817/PedOr2018-4-663

Horner, R. H., & Sugai, G. (2015). School-wide PBIS: An example of Applied Behavior Analysis implemented at a scale of social importance. *Behavior Analysis in Practice*, 8(1), 80–85. DOI: 10.1007/s40617-015-0045-4 PMID: 27703887

Horner, R. H., Sugai, G., & Anderson, C. M. (2010). Examining the evidence base for school-wide positive behavior support. *Focus on Exceptional Children*, 42(8). Advance online publication. DOI: 10.17161/foec.v42i8.6906

Horner, R. H., Sugai, G., & Lewis, T. (2015). *Is school-wide positive behavior support an evidence-based practice?* Center on PBIS.

Horner, R., Sugai, G., Smolkowski, K., Todd, A., Nakasato, J., & Esperanza, J. (2009). A randomized control trial of School-wide Positive Behavior Support in elementary schools. *Journal of Positive Behavior Interventions*, 11(3), 113–144. DOI: 10.1177/1098300709332067

Hoza, B., Waschbusch, D. A., Pelham, W. E., Molina, B. S., & Milich, R. (2005). Attention deficit/hyperactivity disordered and control boys' responses to social success and failure. *Child Development*, 71(2), 432–446. DOI: 10.1111/1467-8624.00155 PMID: 10834475

Huang, Y., Edwards, J., & Laurel-Wilson, M. (2020). The shadow of context: Neighborhood and school socioeconomic disadvantage, perceived social integration, and the mental and behavioral health of adolescents. *Health & Place*, 66, 102425. DOI: 10.1016/j.healthplace.2020.102425 PMID: 32911129

Hulac, D. M., & Briesch, A. M. (2017). *Evidence-based strategies for effective classroom management*. The Guilford Press.

Huppert, F. A., & Johnson, D. M. (2010). A controlled trial of mindfulness training in schools: The importance of practice for an impact on well-being. *The Journal of Positive Psychology*, 5(4), 264–274. DOI: 10.1080/17439761003794148

Huth, T., Munson, J., Adams, R., Gunderson, A., & Gonzalez, V. (2021). South Korean Popular Music Industry: Globalization of Identity and Exploitation.

Ihbour, S., Essaidi, O., Laaroussi, M., Najimi, M., & Chigr, F. (2023). Links between reading acquisition level, emotional difficulties, and academic performance in school-aged children. *The Journal of Mental Health Training, Education and Practice*, 18(2), 135–145. DOI: 10.1108/JMHTEP-05-2021-0040

Ioannidou, L., & Michael, K. (2022). Mental resilience in schools. The necessity of developing prevention and intervention programs. *Mental Health and Human Resilience International Journal*, 6(2), 000199. DOI: 10.23880/mhrij-16000199

Jagers, R. J., Rivas-Drake, D., & Williams, B. (2019). Transformative social and emotional learning (SEL): Toward SEL in service of educational equity and excellence. *Educational Psychologist*, 54(3), 162–184. DOI: 10.1080/00461520.2019.1623032

Janowsky, D. S., & Davis, J. M. (2005). Diagnosis and treatment of depression in patients with mental retardation. *Current Psychiatry Reports*, 7(6), 421–428. DOI: 10.1007/s11920-005-0062-z PMID: 16318819

Janssen, I., & LeBlanc, A. G. (2010). Systematic review of the health benefits of physical activity and fitness in school-aged children and youth. *The International Journal of Behavioral Nutrition and Physical Activity*, 7(1), 1–16. DOI: 10.1186/1479-5868-7-40 PMID: 20459784

Jennings, P. A., Brown, J. L., Frank, J. L., Doyle, S., Oh, Y., & Davis, R. (2017). Impacts of the CARE for Teachers program on teachers' social and emotional competence and classroom interactions. *Journal of Educational Psychology, 109*(1010-1028). DOI: 10.1037/edu0000187

Jennings, P. A., Brown, J. L., Frank, J. L., Doyle, S., Oh, Y., Davis, R., & Greenberg, M. T. (2017). Impacts of the CARE for Teachers program on teachers' social and emotional competence and classroom interactions. *Journal of Educational Change*, 18(4), 489–507.

Jennings, P. A., & DeMauro, A. A. (2017). *The Mindful School: Transforming School Culture through Mindfulness and Compassion*. The Guilford Press.

Jennings, P. A., Frank, J. L., Snowberg, K. E., Coccia, M. A., & Greenberg, M. T. (2013). Improving classroom learning environments by cultivating awareness and resilience in education (CARE): Results of a randomized controlled trial. *School Psychology Quarterly*, 28(4), 374–390. DOI: 10.1037/spq0000035 PMID: 24015983

Jeynes, W. H. (2012). A meta-analysis of the efficacy of different types of parental involvement programs for urban students. *Urban Education*, 47(4), 706–742. DOI: 10.1177/0042085912445643

Johns Hopkins Bloomberg School of Public Health & United Nations Children's Fund. (2022). *On My Mind: How adolescents experience and perceive mental health around the world*. JHU and UNICEF.

Johnson, D., & Thompson, A. (2008). Methodological approaches in resilience research. *Journal of Clinical Psychology*, 64(9), 1054–1068.

Jones, A., & Shindler, J. (2016). Exploring the school climate-student achievement connection: Making sense of why the first precedes the second. *Educational Leadership and Administration*, 27, 35–51.

Jones, A., Smith, P., & Brown, L. (2022). Culturally tailored interventions for building resilience in children with chronic illnesses. *International Journal of Child Health and Human Development*, 15(2), 120–136.

Jones, S. M., & Bouffard, S. M. (2012). Social and emotional learning in schools: From programs to strategies. *Social Policy Report*, 26(4), 3–22. DOI: 10.1002/j.2379-3988.2012.tb00073.x

Jones, S. M., Greenberg, M., & Crowley, M. (2015). Early social-emotional functioning and public health: The relationship between kindergarten social competence and future wellness. *American Journal of Public Health*, 105(11), 2283–2290. DOI: 10.2105/AJPH.2015.302630 PMID: 26180975

Joshi, P. T., Parr, A. F., & Efron, L. A. (2008). TV coverage of tragedies: What is the impact on children. *Indian Pediatrics*, 45(8), 629–634. PMID: 18723904

Jossou, T., Medenou, D., Et-tahir, A., Ahouandjinou, H., Edoh, T., Houessouvo, R., & Pecchia, L. (2022). A review about technology in mental health sensing and assessment. *ITM Web of Conferences, 46*. https://doi.org/DOI: 10.1051/itm-conf/20224601005

Jüni, P., Holenstein, F., Sterne, J., Bartlett, C., & Egger, M. (2002). Direction and impact of language bias in meta-analyses of controlled trials: Empirical study. *International Journal of Epidemiology*, 31(1), 115–123. DOI: 10.1093/ije/31.1.115 PMID: 11914306

Kabat-Zinn, J. (2013). Full catastrophe living, *revised edition: How to cope with stress, pain and illness using mindfulness meditation*. New York, NY: Bantam Books.

Kabat-Zinn, J. (2016). *Mindfulness for Beginners: Reclaiming the Present Moment—and Your Life*. Sounds True.

Kakouros, E., & Maniadaki, K. (2006). *Child and Adolescent Psychopathology: A Developmental Approach*. Dadranos. In Greek

Kalantzi-Azizi A., & Galanaki, E. (2001). Psychotherapy as a system and the need for "openings": Examples of the systemic perspective of the cognitive behavioral psychotherapy. *Psychology: The Journal of the Hellenic Psychological Society, 8*(2), 153–172. (in Greek). https://doi.org/DOI: 10.12681/psy_hps.24111

Kalantzi-Azizi, A., & Zafeiropoulou, M. (Eds.). (2011). *Adjustment to school-Prevention and coping with difficulties.* Pedio.

Kallapiran, K., Koo, S., Kirubakaran, R., & Hancock, K. (2015). Review: Effectiveness of mindfulness in improving mental health symptoms of children and adolescents: A meta-analysis. *Child and Adolescent Mental Health*, 20(4), 182–194. DOI: 10.1111/camh.12113 PMID: 32680348

Karmba, C., & Zafiropoulou, M. (2002). Cognitive behavior modification and learning disabilities. In Scrimali, T., & Grimaldi, L. (Eds.), *Cognitive psychotherapy toward a new millennium: Scientific foundations and clinical practice* (pp. 219–222). Kluwer Academic/Plenum Publishers.

Kazak, A. E., Simms, S., & Rourke, M. T. (2003). Family systems practice in pediatric psychology. *Journal of Pediatric Psychology*, 27(2), 133–143. DOI: 10.1093/jpepsy/27.2.133 PMID: 11821497

Kearney, C. A., & Graczyk, P. A. (2014). A response to intervention model to promote school attendance and decrease school absenteeism. *Child and Youth Care Forum*, 43(1), 1–25. DOI: 10.1007/s10566-013-9222-1

Kearney, C. A., & Graczyk, P. A. (2020). A multidimensional, multitiered system of supports model to promote school attendance and address school absenteeism. *Clinical Child and Family Psychology Review*, 23(3), 316–337. DOI: 10.1007/s10567-020-00317-1 PMID: 32274598

Kelm, J. L., McIntosh, K., & Cooley, S. (2014). Effects of implementing school-wide positive behavioural interventions and supports on problem behaviour and academic achievement in a Canadian elementary school. *Canadian Journal of School Psychology*, 29(3), 195–212. DOI: 10.1177/0829573514540266

Kempe, C., Gustafson, S., & Samuelsson, S. (2011). A longitudinal study of early reading difficulties and subsequent problem behaviors. *Scandinavian Journal of Psychology*, 52(3), 242–250. DOI: 10.1111/j.1467-9450.2011.00870.x PMID: 21332486

Kern, L., Gaier, K., Kelly, S., Nielsen, C. M., Commisso, C. E., & Wehby, J. H. (2020). An evaluation of adaptations made to Tier 2 social skill training programs. *Journal of Applied School Psychology*, 36(2), 155–172. DOI: 10.1080/15377903.2020.1714858

Kincade, L., Cook, C., & Goerdt, A. (2020). Meta-analysis and common practice elements of universal approaches to improving student-teacher relationships. *Review of Educational Research*, 90(5), 710–748. DOI: 10.3102/0034654320946836

Klik, K. A., Cárdenas, D., & Reynolds, K. J. (2023). School climate, school identification and student outcomes: A longitudinal investigation of student well-being. *The British Journal of Educational Psychology*, 93(3), 806–824. DOI: 10.1111/bjep.12597 PMID: 37068920

Klingbeil, D. A., Renshaw, T. L., Willenbrink, J. B., Copek, R. A., Chan, K. T., Haddock, A., Yassine, J., & Clifton, J. (2017). Mindfulness-based interventions with youth: A comprehensive meta-analysis of group-design studies. *Journal of School Psychology*, 63, 77–103. DOI: 10.1016/j.jsp.2017.03.006 PMID: 28633940

Koelsch, S. (2020). A coordinate-based meta-analysis of music-evoked emotions. *NeuroImage*, 223, 117350. DOI: 10.1016/j.neuroimage.2020.117350 PMID: 32898679

Kohlberg, L. (1984). *The psychology of moral development: The nature and validity of moral stages*. Harper & Row.

Koliadis, E. A. (2010). Cognitive-behavioral/cognitive techniques. In Koliadis, E. A. (Ed.), *Behavior at school: We explore possibilities - We cope with problems* (pp. 184–208). Grigoris. (in Greek)

Konold, T., Cornell, D., Shukla, K., & Huang, F. (2017). Racial/ethnic differences in perceptions of school climate and its association with student engagement and peer aggression. *Journal of Youth and Adolescence*, 46(6), 1289–1303. DOI: 10.1007/s10964-016-0576-1 PMID: 27663576

Kourea, L., & Goei, S. (2018). *Developing network efforts in PBS across Europe*. Poster presentation at the 15th International Conference of the Association for Positive Behavior Support (APBS), Denver, CO.

Kourea, L., Lo, Y.-y., Scardina, T., & Phtiaka, H. (2016). Implementing schoolwide positive behavior support across diverse elementary schools in the United States and in Cyprus. [University of Nevada-Las Vegas & University of Nicosia.]. *Proceedings of the Building Bridges Among Researchers and Practitioners: Special Education Conference*, II, 16–24.

Kourea, L., & Phtiaka, H. (2023). Initial exploration and implementation efforts of SWPBIS Tier 1 in Cyprus: Results from two model demonstration sites. *Exceptionality*, 31(5), 395–415. DOI: 10.1080/09362835.2023.2266534

Kourkoutas, E., Stavrou, P. D., & Plexousakis, S. (2018). Teachers' emotional and educational reactions toward children with behavioral problems: Implication for school-based counseling work with teachers. *Journal of Psychology and Behavioural Science*, 6(2), 17–34. DOI: 10.15640/jpbs.v6n2a3

Kourkoutas, H. (2011). *Behavioral problems in children: Interventions in the context of the family and the school*. Topos. (in Greek)

Kovacs, M. (1992). *Children's Depression Inventory*. Multi-Health Systems.

Kraft, M. A., Blazar, D., & Hogan, D. (2018). The effect of teacher coaching on instruction and achievement: A meta-analysis of the causal evidence. *Review of Educational Research*, 88(4), 547–588. DOI: 10.3102/0034654318759268

Kubiszewski, V., & Carrizales, A. (2024). Effects of school-wide positive behavioral interventions and supports on students' perceptions of teachers' practices. *European Journal of Psychology of Education*. Advance online publication. DOI: 10.1007/s10212-024-00848-z

Kumm, S., Mathur, S. R., Cassavaugh, M., & Butts, E. (2020). Using the PBIS Framework to meet the mental health needs of youth in juvenile justice facilities. *Remedial and Special Education*, 41(2), 80–87. DOI: 10.1177/0741932519880336

Kumpfer, K. L., Magalhães, C., & Xie, J. (2012). Cultural adaptations of evidence-based family interventions to strengthen families and improve children's developmental outcomes. *European Journal of Developmental Psychology*, 9(1), 104–116. DOI: 10.1080/17405629.2011.639225

Kurth, J. A., & Enyart, M. (2016). Schoolwide positive behavior supports and students with significant disabilities: Where are we? *Research and Practice for Persons with Severe Disabilities : the Journal of TASH*, 41(3), 216–222. DOI: 10.1177/1540796916633083

Kutsyuruba, B., Klinger, D., & Hussain, A. (2015). Relationships among school climate, school safety, and student achievement and well-being: A review of the literature. *Review of Education*, 3(2), 103–135. DOI: 10.1002/rev3.3043

Kuyken, W., Weare, K., Ukoumunne, O. C., Vicary, R., Motton, N., Burnett, R., Cullen, C., Hennelly, S., & Huppert, F. (2013). Effectiveness of the mindfulness in schools programme: Non-randomised controlled feasibility study. *The British Journal of Psychiatry*, 203(2), 126–131. DOI: 10.1192/bjp.bp.113.126649 PMID: 23787061

Kuypers, L. M. (2013). The zones of regulation: A framework to foster self-regulation. *Sensory Integration Special Interest Section Quarterly, 36*(4), 1y I. https://www.scribd.com/document/379956599/The-Zones-of-Regulation-A-Framework-to-Foster-Self-regulation-2013

La Salle-Finley, T. (2024). *School climate and PBIS fidelity.* Center on PBIS, University of Oregon.

Lacoe, J. (2020). Too scared to learn? The academic consequences of feeling unsafe in the classroom. *Urban Education,* 55(10), 1385–1418. DOI: 10.1177/0042085916674059

Ladson-Billings, G. (1995). Toward a theory of culturally relevant pedagogy. *American Educational Research Journal,* 32(3), 465–491. DOI: 10.3102/00028312032003465

Lahad, M., Shacham, M., & Ayalon, O. (2013). *The "BASIC-Ph" Model of Coping and Resiliency.* Jessica Kingsley Publishers.

Landrum, T. J., & Kauffman, J. M. (2006). Behavioral approaches to classroom management. In Evertson, C. M., & Weinstein, C. S. (Eds.), *Handbook of classroom management: Research, practice, and contemporary issues* (pp. 47–71). Erlbaum.

Lane, K. L., Capizzi, A. M., Fisher, M. H., & Ennis, R. P. (2012). Secondary prevention efforts at the middle school level: An application of the behavior education program. *Education & Treatment of Children,* 35(1), 51–90. DOI: 10.1353/etc.2012.0002

Lee, A., & Gage, N. A. (2020). Updating and expanding systematic reviews and meta-analyses on the effects of school-wide positive behavior interventions and supports. *Psychology in the Schools,* 57(5), 783–804. DOI: 10.1002/pits.22336

Lee, E., Reynolds, K. J., Subasic, E., Bromhead, D., Lin, H., Marinov, V., & Smithson, M. (2017). Development of a dual school climate and school identification measure–student (SCASIM-St). *Contemporary Educational Psychology,* 49, 91–106. DOI: 10.1016/j.cedpsych.2017.01.003

Lee, Y., & Kim, S. (2020). The effects of social-emotional learning on resilience and school adjustment in elementary school students. *International Journal of Educational Research,* 100, 101543.

Lei, H., Cui, Y., & Chiu, M. M. (2016). Affective teacher-student relationships and students' externalizing behavior problems: A meta-analysis. *Frontiers in Psychology,* 1311, 7. DOI: 10.3389/fpsyg.2016.01311 PMID: 27625624

Leirbakk, M.J., Clench-Aas, J., & Ruth, K., Raanaas. (. (2015). ADHD with Co- Occurring Depression/Anxiety in Children: The Relationship with Somatic Complaints and Parental Socio-Economic Position. *Journal of Psychological Abnormalities*, 4, 137. DOI: 10.4172/2329-9525.1000125

Leubner, D., & Hinterberger, T. (2017). Reviewing the effectiveness of music interventions in treating depression. *Frontiers in Psychology*, 8, 1109. Advance online publication. DOI: 10.3389/fpsyg.2017.01109 PMID: 28736539

Levy, I. P. (2019). Hip-hop and spoken word therapy in urban school counseling. *Professional School Counseling*, 22(1b), 2156759X1983443. Advance online publication. DOI: 10.1177/2156759X19834436

Leyfer, O. T., Folstein, S. E., Bacalman, S., Davis, N. O., Dinh, E., Morgan, J., Tager-Flusberg, H., & Lainhart, J. E. (2006). Comorbid psychiatric disorders in children with autism: Interview development and rates of disorders. *Journal of Autism and Developmental Disorders*, 36(7), 849–861. DOI: 10.1007/s10803-006-0123-0 PMID: 16845581

Li, J., Li, J., Zhang, W., Wang, G., & Qu, Z. (2023). Effectiveness of a school-based, lay counselor-delivered cognitive behavioral therapy for Chinese children with posttraumatic stress symptoms: A randomized controlled trial. *The Lancet Regional Health. Western Pacific*, 33, 100699. Advance online publication. DOI: 10.1016/j.lanwpc.2023.100699 PMID: 36785644

Lindner, P., Miloff, A., Hamilton, W., Reuterskiöld, L., Andersson, G., & Carlbring, P. (2017). Creating state-of-the-art, next-generation virtual reality exposure therapies for anxiety disorders using consumer hardware platforms: Design considerations and future directions. *Cognitive Behaviour Therapy*, 46(5), 404–420. DOI: 10.1080/16506073.2017.1280843 PMID: 28270059

Lindsay, J., & Dockrell, J. (2002). The behaviour and selfesteem of children with specific speech and language difficulties. *The British Journal of Educational Psychology*, 70(Pt4), 583–601. PMID: 11191188

Lindsey, B., & White, M. (2009). Tier 2 behavioral interventions for at-risk students. *School social work: Practice, policy, and research*, 665-673.

Lindstrom Johnson, S., Burke, J. G., & Gielen, A. C. (2012). Urban students' perceptions of the school environment's influence on school violence. *Children & Schools*, 34(2), 92–102. DOI: 10.1093/cs/cds016 PMID: 26726297

Little, B. (2018). Reciprocal determinism. In Zeigler-Hill, V., & Shackelford, T. (Eds.), *Encyclopedia of personality and individual differences*. Springer., DOI: 10.1007/978-3-319-28099-8_1807-1

Li, Z., Yu, C., & Nie, Y. (2021). The association between school climate and aggression: A moderated mediation model. *International Journal of Environmental Research and Public Health*, 18(16), 8709. DOI: 10.3390/ijerph18168709 PMID: 34444470

Lombardi, E., Traficante, D., Bettoni, R., Offredi, I., Giorgetti, M., & Vernice, M. (2019). The impact of school climate on well-being experience and school engagement: A study with high-school students. *Frontiers in Psychology*, 10, 2482. DOI: 10.3389/fpsyg.2019.02482 PMID: 31749747

Lombardo, M. V., & Baron-Cohen, S. (2011). The role of the self in mindblindness in autism. *Consciousness and Cognition*, 20(1), 130–140. DOI: 10.1016/j.concog.2010.09.006 PMID: 20932779

Lopata, C., Toomey, J. A., Fox, J. D., Volker, M. A., Chow, S. Y., Thomeer, M. L., Lee, G. K., Rodgers, J. D., McDonald, C. A., & Smerbeck, A. M. (2010). Anxiety and depression in children with HFASDs: Symptom levels and source differences. *Journal of Abnormal Child Psychology*, 38(6), 765–776. DOI: 10.1007/s10802-010-9406-1 PMID: 20354899

Lopez, A., Williams, J. K., & Newsom, K. (2015). PBIS in Texas juvenile justice Department's division of education and state programs: Integrating programs and developing systems for sustained implementation. *Residential Treatment for Children & Youth*, 32(4), 344–353. DOI: 10.1080/0886571X.2015.1113460

Lougy, R. A., Deruvo, S. L., & Rosenthal, D. (2007). *Teaching young children with ADHD: Succesful strategies and Practical Interventions for Prek - 3*. Corwin Press.

Low, Y. T. A., Wong, D. F. K., Kwok, S., Man, K. W., & Ip, S. Y. (2023). Effectiveness of a culturally specific school-based cognitive-behavioural group therapy for primary school children with anxiety problems in Hong Kong. *Asia Pacific Journal of Social Work and Development*, ●●●, 1–14. DOI: 10.1080/29949769.2023.2296894

Lubans, D., Richards, J., Hillman, C., Faulkner, G., Beauchamp, M., Nilsson, M., Kelly, P., Smith, J., Raine, L., & Biddle, S. (2016). Physical activity for cognitive and mental health in youth: A systematic review of mechanisms. *Pediatrics*, 138(3), 1. DOI: 10.1542/peds.2016-1642 PMID: 27542849

Luby, J. L., Heffelfinger, A. K., Mrakotsky, C., Brown, K. M., Hessler, M. J., Wallis, J. M., & Spitznagel, E. L. (2003). The clinical picture of depression in preschool children. *Journal of the American Academy of Child and Adolescent Psychiatry*, 42(3), 340–348. DOI: 10.1097/00004583-200303000-00015 PMID: 12595788

Luthar, S. S., Cicchetti, D., & Becker, B. (2000). The construct of resilience: A critical evaluation and guidelines for future work. *Child Development*, 71(3), 543–562. DOI: 10.1111/1467-8624.00164 PMID: 10953923

Lyon, A. R., & Bruns, E. J. (2019). From evidence to impact: Joining our best school mental health practices with our best implementation strategies. *School Mental Health*, 11(1), 106–114. DOI: 10.1007/s12310-018-09306-w PMID: 31709018

Maag, J., & Reid, R. (2006). Depression among students with Learning Disabilities: Assesing the Risk. *Journal of Learning Disabilities*, 39(1), 3–10. DOI: 10.1177/00222194060390010201 PMID: 16512079

Maccoby, E. E. (2000). Parenting and its effects on children: On reading and misreading behavior genetics. *Annual Review of Psychology*, 51(1), 1–27. DOI: 10.1146/annurev.psych.51.1.1 PMID: 10751963

Machin, D., & Van Leeuwen, T. (2009). Toys as discourse: Children's war toys and the war on terror. *Critical Discourse Studies*, 6(1), 51–63. DOI: 10.1080/17405900802560082

Maculan, A., Di Giuseppe, T., Vianello, F., & Vivaldi, S. (2022). Narrazioni e risorse. Gli operatori del sistema penale minorile al tempo del Covid-19. *Autonomie locali e servizi sociali. Quadrimestrale di studi e ricerche sul welfare*, 2(2022), 349-365. https://doi.org/DOI: 10.1447/105089

Madianos, M. (2003). *Clinical psychiatry. Learning Difficulties – Dyslexia*. Kastaniotis Publications. In Greek

Madigan, K., Cross, R. W., Smolkowski, K., & Strycker, L. A. (2016). Association between schoolwide positive behavioural interventions and supports and academic achievement: A 9-year evaluation. *Educational Research and Evaluation*, 22(7–8), 402–421. DOI: 10.1080/13803611.2016.1256783

Madireddy, S., & Madireddy, S. (2020). Strategies for schools to prevent psychosocial stress, stigma, and suicidality risks among LGBTQ+ students. *American Journal of Educational Research*, 8(9), 659–667. DOI: 10.12691/education-8-9-7

Mahoney, J. L., Weissberg, R. P., Greenberg, M. T., Dusenbury, L., Jagers, R. J., Niemi, K., Schlinger, M., Schlund, J., Shriver, T. P., VanAusdal, K., & Yoder, N. (2021). Systemic social and emotional learning: Promoting educational success for all preschool to high school students. *The American Psychologist*, 76(7), 1128–1142. DOI: 10.1037/amp0000701 PMID: 33030926

Malchiodi, C. A. (2003). *Handbook of art therapy*. U.K Guilford publications.

Malikiosi-Loizou, M. (2017). *Counselling Psychology*. Pedio. In Greek

Malinen, O.-P., & Savolainen, H. (2016). The effect of perceived school climate and teacher efficacy in behavior management on job satisfaction and burnout: A longitudinal study. *Teaching and Teacher Education*, 60, 144–152. DOI: 10.1016/j.tate.2016.08.012

Maloney, J. E., Lawlor, M. S., Schonert-Reichl, K. A., & Whitehead, J. (2016). A Mindfulness-Based Social and Emotional Learning Curriculum for School-Aged Children: The MindUP Program. In Schonert-Reichl, K., & Roeser, R. (Eds.), *Handbook of Mindfulness in Education. Mindfulness in Behavioral Health*. Springer., DOI: 10.1007/978-1-4939-3506-2_20

Manzano-Sánchez, D., Gómez-Mármol, A., Valero-Valenzuela, A., & Jiménez-Parra, J. F. (2021). School climate and responsibility as predictors of antisocial and prosocial behaviors and violence: A study towards self-determination theory. *Behavioral Sciences (Basel, Switzerland)*, 11(3), 36. DOI: 10.3390/bs11030036 PMID: 33802667

Marc, R., Crundwell, A., & Killu, K. (2010). Responding to a student's depression. *Interventions That Work*, 68(2), 46–51.

Maria, O., Kleifgen, J. A., & Falchi, L. (2008). *From English language learners to emergent bilinguals. Equity Matters: Research Review No. 1*. Teachers College, Columbia University.

Martínez-García, A. (2022). Contributions of universal school-based mental health promotion to the wellbeing of adolescents and preadolescents: A systematic review of educational interventions. *Health Education*, 122(5), 564–583. DOI: 10.1108/HE-07-2021-0106

Martinez, J., Vasquez, L., & Pena, E. (2020). Culturally relevant diabetes management for Hispanic children: Outcomes of a tailored intervention. *Journal of Pediatric Nursing*, 53, 45–52.

Maslow, A. H. (1968). Toward a psychology of being (2nd ed.). D. Van Nostrand.

Maslow, A. H. (1987). *Motivation and personality* (3rd ed.). Addison-Wesley.

Mason, A., & Mason, M. (2005). Understanding College Students with Learning Disabilities. *Pediatric Clinics of North America*, 52(1), 61–70. DOI: 10.1016/j. pcl.2004.11.001 PMID: 15748924

Masten, A. S., & Gewirtz, A. H. (2006). Resilience in development: The importance of early childhood. In R. E. Tremblay, R. G. Barr, & R. DeV. Peters (Eds.), *Encyclopedia on Early Childhood Development* (pp. 1-6). Montreal, Quebec: Centre of Excellence for Early Childhood Development.

Masten, A. S. (2014). Global perspectives on resilience in children and youth. *Child Development*, 85(1), 6–20. DOI: 10.1111/cdev.12205 PMID: 24341286

Masten, A. S. (2014). *Ordinary magic: Resilience in development*. Guilford Press.

Masten, A. S., & Coatsworth, J. D. (1998). The development of competence in favorable and unfavorable environments: Lessons from research on successful children. *The American Psychologist*, 53(2), 205–220. DOI: 10.1037/0003-066X.53.2.205 PMID: 9491748

Maxwell, L. E. (2016). School building condition, social climate, student attendance and academic achievement: A mediation model. *Journal of Environmental Psychology*, 46, 206–216. DOI: 10.1016/j.jenvp.2016.04.009

Maxwell, S., Reynolds, K. J., Lee, E., Subasic, E., & Bromhead, D. (2017). The impact of school climate and school identification on academic achievement: Multilevel modeling with student and teacher data. *Frontiers in Psychology*, 8, 2069. DOI: 10.3389/fpsyg.2017.02069 PMID: 29259564

Mayes, S. D., Calhoun, S. L., Bixler, E. O., Vgontzas, A. N., Mahr, F., Hillwig-Garcia, J., Elamir, B., Edhere-Ekezie, L., & Parvin, M. (2009). ADHD subtypes and co morbid anxiety, depression, and oppositional-defiant disorder: Differences in sleep problems. *Journal of Pediatric Psychology*, 34(3), 328–337. DOI: 10.1093/jpepsy/jsn083 PMID: 18676503

Maynard, B. R., Kjellstrand, E. K., & Thompson, A. M. (2014). Effects of check and connect on attendance, behavior, and academics: A randomized effectiveness trial. *Research on Social Work Practice*, 24(3), 296–309. DOI: 10.1177/1049731513497804

Mays, N., Roberts, E., & Popay, J. (2001). Synthesising research evidence. In Fulop, N., Allen, P., Clarke, A., & Black, N. (Eds.), *Studying the organisation and delivery of health services: Research methods*. Routledge.

McDaniel, S. C., Bruhn, A. L., & Mitchell, B. (2015). A Tier 2 framework for identification and intervention. *Beyond Behavior*, 24(1), 10–17. DOI: 10.1177/107429561502400103

McDaniel, S. C., Bruhn, A. L., & Troughton, L. (2017). A brief social skills intervention to reduce challenging classroom behavior. *Journal of Behavioral Education*, 26(1), 53–74. DOI: 10.1007/s10864-016-9259-y

McFerran, K. (2010). *Adolescents, music and music therapy: Methods and techniques for clinicians, educators and students*. Jessica Kingsley., DOI: 10.1080/01609513.2011.561044

McIntosh, K., Bennett, J. L., & Price, K. (2011). Evaluation of social and academic effects of School-wide Positive Behaviour Support in a Canadian school district. *Exceptionality Education International*, 21(1), 46–60. DOI: 10.5206/eei.v21i1.7669

McIntosh, K., Girvan, E. J., McDaniel, S. C., Santiago-Rosario, M. R., St. Joseph, S., Fairbanks Falcon, S., & Bastable, E. (2021). Effects of an equity-focused PBIS approach to school improvement on exclusionary discipline and school climate. *Preventing School Failure*, 65(4), 354–361.

McIntosh, K., Mercer, S., Hume, A., Frank, F., Turri, M., & Mathews, S. (2013). Factors relate to sustained implementation of schoolwide positive behavior support. *Exceptional Children*, 79(3), 293–311.

McLeod, J. D., Uemura, R., & Rohrman, S. (2012). Adolescent mental health, behavio problems, and academic achievement. *Journal of Health and Social Behavior*, 53(4), 482–497. DOI: 10.1177/0022146512462888 PMID: 23197485

McMullen, J. M., George, M., Ingman, B. C., Pulling Kuhn, A., Graham, D. J., & Carson, R. L. (2020). A systematic review of community engagement outcomes research in school-based health interventions. *The Journal of School Health*, 90(12), 985–994. DOI: 10.1111/josh.12962 PMID: 33184891

McNeil, J. N. (1983). Young mothers' communication about death with their children. *Death Education*, 6(4), 323–339. DOI: 10.1080/07481188308252139 PMID: 10259896

McNulty, M. A. (2003). Dyslexia and the life course. *Journal of Learning Disabilities*, 36(4), 363–381. DOI: 10.1177/00222194030360040701 PMID: 15490908

Meichenbaum, D. (1977). Cognitive behavior modification. *Scandinavian Journal of Behaviour Therapy*, 6(4), 185–192. DOI: 10.1080/16506073.1977.9626708

Meiklejohn, J., Phillips, C., Freedman, M. L., Griffin, M. L., Biegel, G., Roach, A., Frank, J., Burke, C., Pinger, L., Soloway, G., Isberg, R., Sibinga, E., Grossman, L., & Saltzman, A. (2012). Integrating mindfulness training into K-12 education: Fostering the resilience of teachers and students. *Mindfulness*, 3(4), 291–307. DOI: 10.1007/s12671-012-0094-5

Melegari, M. G., Sette, S., Vittori, E., Mallia, L., Devoto, A., Lucidi, F., Ferri, R., & Bruni, O. (2018). Relations Between Sleep and Temperament in Preschool Children With ADHD. *Journal of Attention Disorders*. Advance online publication. DOI: 10.1177/1087054718757645 PMID: 29468918

Mendes de Oliveira, C., Santos Almeida, C. R., & Hofheinz Giacomoni, C. (2022). School-based positive psychology interventions that promote well-being in children: A systematic review. *Child Indicators Research*, 15(5), 1583–1600. DOI: 10.1007/s12187-022-09935-3

Miller, J. K. (2018). *Thriving with ADHD Workbook for Kids: 60 Fun Activities to Help Children Self-Regulate, Focus, and Succeed (Health and Wellness Workbooks for Kids)*. United Kingdom: Callisto Kids. Mitsiu- Daktila, G. (2008). *Neuropsychologies of learning disorders: diagnosis and treatm*ent. Athens: Dardanos. In Greek.

Miller, A. E., & Racine, S. E. (2022). Emotion regulation difficulties as common and unique predictors of impulsive behaviors in university students. *Journal of American College Health*, 70(5), 1387–1395. DOI: 10.1080/07448481.2020.1799804 PMID: 32790500

Miller, F. G., Swenson Wagner, N., & Robers, A. C. (2023). Examining behavior specific praise as an individual behavior management strategy in a high-need educational setting. *Preventing School Failure*, 1–11. DOI: 10.1080/1045988X.2023.2269891

Miller, G. A. (2003). The cognitive revolution: A historical perspective. *Trends in Cognitive Sciences*, 7(3), 141–144. DOI: 10.1016/S1364-6613(03)00029-9 PMID: 12639696

Miller, G. E., Chen, E., & Zhou, E. S. (2007). If it goes up must it come down? Chronic stress and the hypothalamic-pituitary-adrenocortical axis in humans. *Psychological Bulletin*, 133(1), 25–45. DOI: 10.1037/0033-2909.133.1.25 PMID: 17201569

Miller, G. E., Chen, E., & Zhou, E. S. (2022). Effects of chronic stress on mental health: Implications for resilience interventions. *Annual Review of Clinical Psychology*, 18, 27–50.

Mindful Schools. (2018). https://help.mindfulschools.org/hc/en-us

Mingebach, T., Kamp-Becker, I., Christiansen, H., & Weber, L. (2018). Meta-meta-analysis on the effectiveness of parent-based interventions for the treatment of child externalizing behavior problems. *PLoS One*, 13(9), e0202855. DOI: 10.1371/journal.pone.0202855 PMID: 30256794

Missouri Department of Elementary and Secondary Education. (2018). *Missouri Schoolwide Positive Behavior Support, Tier 1 Team Workbook 2018-2019*.https://pbismissouri.org/wpcontent/uploads/2018/05/MO-SW-PBS-Tier-1-2018.pdf

Missouri School-wide Positive Behavior Support. (2019). *Missouri Schoolwide Positive Behavior handbook*. MO SWPBS.

Mitchell, B. S., Bruhn, A. L., & Lewis, T. J. (2015). Essential features of Tier 2 & 3 school-wide positive behavioral supports. In Jimerson, S. R., Burns, M. K., & VanDerHeyden, A. M. (Eds.), *Handbook of response to intervention: The science and practice of assessment and intervention* (2nd ed., pp. 539–562). Springer.

Mitchell, B. S., Stormont, M., & Gage, N. A. (2011). Tier two interventions implemented within the context of a tiered prevention framework. *Behavioral Disorders*, 36(4), 241–261. DOI: 10.1177/019874291103600404

Molinari, L., & Grazia, V. (2023). Students' school climate perceptions: Do engagement and burnout matter? *Learning Environments Research*, 26(1), 1–18. DOI: 10.1007/s10984-021-09384-9

Molnar, A., & Lindquist, B. (2009). *Changing problem behavior in schools*. Information Age Publishing.

Moos, R. H. (1979). *Evaluating educational environments: Procedures, measures, findings and policy implications*. Jossey-Bass.

Morgan, D. P., & Jenson, W. R. (1988). *Teaching behaviorally disordered students: Preferred practices*. Prentice Hall.

Morin, E. (2001). *I sette saperi necessari all'educazione del futuro*. Raffaello Cortina Editore.

Moroz, K. B., & Jones, K. M. (2002). The effects of positive peer reporting on children's social involvement. *School Psychology Review*, 31(2), 235–245. DOI: 10.1080/02796015.2002.12086153

Mugnaini, D., Lassi, S., Lamalrfa, G., & Albertini, G. (2009). Internalizing correlates of dyslexia. *World Journal of Pediatrics*, 5(4), 255–264. DOI: 10.1007/s12519-009-0049-7 PMID: 19911139

Muhajirah, M. (2020). Basic of learning theory: Behaviorism, cognitivism, constructivism, and humanism. *International Journal of Asian Education*, 1(1), 37–42. DOI: 10.46966/ijae.v1i1.23

Mundy, P., Gwaltney, M., & Henderson, H. (2010). Self-referenced processing, neurodevelopment and joint attention in autism. *Autism*, 14(5), 408–429. DOI: 10.1177/1362361310366315 PMID: 20926457

Murano, D., Sawyer, J. E., & Lipnevich, A. A. (2020). A meta-analytic review of preschool social and emotional learning interventions. *Review of Educational Research*, 90(2), 227–263. DOI: 10.3102/0034654320914743

Myers-Bowman, K. S., Walker, K., & Myers-Walls, J. A. (2005). Differences Between War and Peace are Big": Children from Yugoslavia and the United States Describe Peace and War. *Peace and Conflict*, 11(2), 177–198. DOI: 10.1207/s15327949pac1102_4

Nakamura, J., & Csikszentmihalyi, M. (2014). *Flow and the Foundations of Positive Psychology: The Collected Works of Mihaly Csikszentmihalyi*. Springer.

Napoli, M., Krech, P. R., & Holley, L. C. (2005). Mindfulness training for elementary school students: The attention academy. *Journal of Applied School Psychology*, 21(1), 99–125. DOI: 10.1300/J370v21n01_05

Närhi, V., Kiiski, T., Peitso, S., & Savolainen, H. (2014). Reducing disruptive behaviours and improving learning climates with class-wide positive behaviour support in middle schools. *European Journal of Special Needs Education*, 30(2), 274–285. DOI: 10.1080/08856257.2014.986913

National Center on Safe Supportive Learning Environments. (n.d.). *School climate improvement.* https://safesupportivelearning.ed.gov/school-climate-improvement

National Institutes of Health. (2018). Sound Health: An NIH-Kennedy Center Partnership [Research Plan]. National Institutes of Health. https://www.nih.gov/sound-health/research-plan

National School Climate Council. (2007). *The school climate challenge: narrowing the gap between school climate research and school climate policy, practice guidelines and teacher education policy.* http://www.ecs. org/school-climate

Neitzel, J., & Bogin, J. (2008). *Steps for implementation: Functional behavior assessment.* The National Professional Development Center on Autism Spectrum Disorders, Frank Porter Graham Child Development Institute, The University of North Carolina.

Nelen, M. J., Willemse, T. M., van Oudheusden, M. A., & Goei, S. L. (2020). Cultural challenges in adapting SWPBIS to a Dutch context. *Journal of Positive Behavior Interventions*, 22(2), 105–115. DOI: 10.1177/1098300719876096

Nelson, J. M., & Harwood, H. (2011). Learning disabilities and anxiety: A meta-analysis. *Journal of Learning Disabilities*, 44(1), 3–17. DOI: 10.1177/0022219409359939 PMID: 20375288

Nese, R. N. T., Kittelman, A., Strickland-Cohen, M. K., & McIntosh, K. (2023). Examining teaming and Tier 2 and 3 practices within a PBIS Framework. *Journal of Positive Behavior Interventions*, 25(1), 16–27. DOI: 10.1177/10983007211051090

Nguyen, L., Helen, R. M., & Tsai, J. L. (2020). The effects of cultural adaptation on intervention efficacy: A meta-analytic review. *Journal of Consulting and Clinical Psychology*, 88(8), 694–705.

Nie, Y. G., Liu, Y., & Wu, D. (2022). The impact of school climate on student well-being: The mediating role of resilience. *Journal of School Psychology*, 90, 25–38.

Nisar, H., Elgin, D., Bradshaw, C., Dolan, V., Frey, A., Horner, R., Owens, J., Perales, K., & Sutherland, K. (2022). *Promoting social and behavioral success for learning in elementary schools: Practice recommendations for elementary school educators, school and district administrators, and parents*. 2M Research Services. Contract No. 92990019F0319.

Nishikawa-Pacher, A. (2022). Research questions with PICO: A universal mnemonic. *Publications / MDPI*, 10(3), 21. DOI: 10.3390/publications10030021

Noltemeyer, A., Palmer, K., James, A., & Petrasek, M. (2019). Disciplinary and achievement outcomes associated with school-wide positive behavioral interventions and supports implementation level. *School Psychology Review*, 48(1), 81–87. DOI: 10.17105/SPR-2017-0131.V48-1

Noltemeyer, A., Ward, R., & Mcloughlin, C. (2015). Relationship between school suspension and student outcomes: A meta-analysis. *School Psychology Review*, 44(2), 224–240. DOI: 10.17105/spr-14-0008.1

O'Malley, C. J., Blankemeyer, M., Walker, K. K., & Dellmann-Jenkins, M. (2007). Children's reported communication with their parents about war. *Journal of Family Issues*, 28(12), 1639–1662. DOI: 10.1177/0192513X07302726

O'Neill, R. E., Allbin, R. W., Storey, K., Horner, R. H., & Sprague, J. R. (2015). *Functional assessment and program development for problem behavior*. Cengage Learning.

Oberle, E., Guhn, M., Gadermann, A. M., Thomson, K., & Schonert-Reichl, K. A. (2018). Positive mental health and supportive school environments: A population-level longitudinal study of dispositional optimism and school relationships in early adolescence. *Social Science & Medicine*, 214, 154–161. DOI: 10.1016/j.socscimed.2018.06.041 PMID: 30072159

Obidike, N. D., Bosah, I., & Olibie, E. (2015). Teaching peace concept to children. *International Journal of Multidisciplinary Research and Development*, 2(6), 24–26.

Oder, T., & Eisenschmidt, E. (2018). Teachers' perceptions of school climate as an indicator of their beliefs of effective teaching. *Cambridge Journal of Education*, 48(1), 3–20. DOI: 10.1080/0305764X.2016.1223837

Office of Safe and Healthy Students (OSHS). (2016). *Quick guide on making school climate improvements*. U.S. Department of Education. https://safesupportivelearning .ed.gov/SCIRP/Quick-Guide

Office of Special Education Programs (OSEP) Technical Assistance Center on Positive Behavioral Interventions and Supports. (2019). *Positive Behavioral Interventions & Supports*. U.S. Department of Education, Office of Special Education www.pbis.org

Ogbu, J. U. (1992). Understanding cultural diversity and learning. *Educational Researcher*, 21(8), 5–14. DOI: 10.3102/0013189X021008005

Ogden, T., Sørlie, M.-A., Arnesen, A., & Meek-Hansen, W. (2012). The PALS School-Wide Positive Behaviour Support model in Norwegian primary schools – Implementation and evaluation. In J. Visser, H. Daniels, and T. Cole, (Ed.) *Transforming troubled lives: Strategies and interventions for children with social, emotional and behavioural difficulties (International Perspectives on Inclusive Education, Vol. 2)* (pp. 39-55). Emerald Group Publishing Limited. DOI: 10.1108/S1479-3636(2012)0000002006

Ohkubo, K., Tsukimoto, H., Otsui, K., Tanaka, Y., Noda, W., & Niwayama, K. (2022). Effectiveness and social validity of Tier 1 intervention with school-wide positive behavioural support in a public elementary school in Japan. *International Journal of Positive Behavioural Support*, 12(2), 4–18.

Olweus, D. (2005). A useful evaluation design, and effects of the Olweus Bullying Prevention Program. *Psychology, Crime & Law*, 11(4), 389–402. DOI: 10.1080/10683160500255471

Olweus, D., Limber, S. P., Flerx, V. C., Mullin, N., Riese, J., & Snyder, M. (2007). *Olweus Bullying Prevention Program: Schoolwide guide*. Hazelden.

Olweus, D., Solberg, M. E., & Breivik, K. (2020). Long-term school-level effects of the Olweus Bullying Prevention Program (OBPP). *Scandinavian Journal of Psychology*, 61(1), 108–116. DOI: 10.1111/sjop.12486 PMID: 30277582

Onnela, A., Hurtig, T., & Ebeling, H. (2021). A psychoeducational mental health promotion intervention in comprehensive school: Recognising problems and reducing stigma. *Health Education Journal*, 80(5), 554–566. DOI: 10.1177/0017896921994134

Otsui, K., Niwayama, K., Ohkubo, K., Tanaka, Y., & Noda, W. (2022). Introduction and development of school-wide positive behavioural support in Japan. *International Journal of Positive Behavioural Support*, 12(2), 19–28.

Ow, N., Marchand, K., Glowacki, K., Alqutub, D., Mathias, S., & Barbic, S. P. (2022). YESS: A feasibility study of a supported employment program for youths with mental health disorders. *Frontiers in Psychiatry*, 13, 856905. Advance online publication. DOI: 10.3389/fpsyt.2022.856905 PMID: 36213923

Pachter, L. M., & Coll, C. G. (2009). Racism and child health: A review of the literature and future directions. *Journal of Developmental and Behavioral Pediatrics*, 30(3), 255–263. DOI: 10.1097/DBP.0b013e3181a7ed5a PMID: 19525720

Pachter, L. M., Coll, C. G., & Weller, S. C. (2010). Integration of culture in parent interventions for young children with behavioral problems: A meta-analysis. *Journal of Clinical Child and Adolescent Psychology*, 35(4), 762–772.

Palmer, K., & Noltemeyer, A. (2019). Professional development in schools: Predictors of effectiveness and implications for statewide PBIS trainings. *Teacher Development*, 23(5), 511–528. DOI: 10.1080/13664530.2019.1660211

Pandey, A., Hale, D., Das, S., Goddings, A. L., Blakemore, S. J., & Viner, R. M. (2018). Effectiveness of universal self-regulation-based interventions in children and adolescents a systematic review and meta-analysis. *Journal American Medical Association Pediatrics, 172*(6), 566cs, 17https://doi.org/DOI: 10.1001/jamapediatrics.2018.0232

Paoletti, P. (2008). *Crescere nell'eccellenza.* Roma: Armando editore.

Paoletti, P., & Di Giuseppe, T. (2023). Il Modello sferico della coscienza: Io, Noi, Altro da noi. Presented at the event "Promuovere le Risorse Positive della Comunità Penitenziaria", 15 Marzo 2023, Università degli Studi di Genova.

Paoletti, P., & Diamond, A. (2020, 15 Aprile). *The Science of Education for Peace.* https://fondazionepatriziopaoletti.org/blog/the-science-of-education-for-peace -scarica-il-book-gratuito-e-semina-la-pace-dentro-e-intorno-a-te/

Paoletti, P., Di Giuseppe, T., Lillo, C., Serantoni, G., Perasso, G., Maculan, A., & Vianello, F. (2022b). La resilienza nel circuito penale minorile in tempi di pandemia: un'esperienza di studio e formazione basata sul modello sferico della coscienza su un gruppo di educatori. *Narrare i Gruppi,* 1-10.

Paoletti, P. (2002). Flussi, Territori, Luogo [Flows, Territories, Place]. *Medica Publica (Oulu).*

Paoletti, P., & Ben-Soussan, T. D. (2019). The sphere model of consciousness: From geometrical to neuro-psycho-educational perspectives. *Logica Univiversalis*, 13(3), 395–415. DOI: 10.1007/s11787-019-00226-0

Paoletti, P., Di Giuseppe, T., Lillo, C., Ben-Soussan, T. D., Bozkurt, A., Tabibnia, G., Kelmendi, K., Warthe, G. W., Leshem, R., Bigo, V., Ireri, A., Mwangi, C., Bhattacharya, N., & Perasso, G. F. (2022a). What can we learn from the COVID-19 pandemic? Resilience for the future and neuropsychopedagogical insights. *Frontiers in Psychology*, 5403, 993991. Advance online publication. DOI: 10.3389/fpsyg.2022.993991 PMID: 36172227

Paoletti, P., Perasso, G. F., Lillo, C., Serantoni, G., Maculan, A., Vianello, F., & Di Giuseppe, T. (2023). Envisioning the future for families running away from war: Challenges and resources of Ukrainian parents in Italy. *Frontiers in Psychology*, 14, 1122264. Advance online publication. DOI: 10.3389/fpsyg.2023.1122264 PMID: 37008874

Papadatos, I. (2010). *Mental disorders and learning disabilities of children and adolescents*. Gutenberg Editions.

Papageorgiou, B. (2005). *Child and adolescent psychiatry*. University Studio Press. In Greek

Pargament, K. I. (2011). *Spiritually integrated psychotherapy: Understanding and addressing the sacred*. Guilford press.

Parhiala, P., Ranta, K., Gergov, V., Kontunen, J., Law, R., La Greca, A. M., Torppa, M., & Marttunen, M. (2020). Interpersonal counseling in the treatment of adolescent depression: A randomized controlled effectiveness and feasibility study in school health and welfare services. *School Mental Health*, 12(2), 265–283. DOI: 10.1007/s12310-019-09346-w

Parker, J. D., Summerfeldt, L. J., Hogan, M. J., & Majeski, S. A. (2004). Emotional intelligence and academic success: Examining the transition from high school to university. *Personality and Individual Differences*, 36(1), 163–172. DOI: 10.1016/S0191-8869(03)00076-X

Park, J., Lee, H. J., & Kim, Y. (2019). School-wide positive behavior support in six special schools of South Korea: Processes and outcomes across years. *International Journal of Developmental Disabilities*, 65(5), 337–346. DOI: 10.1080/20473869.2019.1647729 PMID: 34141357

Parsonson, B. S. (2012). Evidence-based classroom behaviour management strategies. *Kairanga, 13*(1), 16–23. https://api.semanticscholar.org/CorpusID:17274857

Pascoe, M., Bailey, A. P., Craike, M., Carter, T., Patten, R., Stepto, N., & Parker, A. (2020). Physical activity and exercise in youth mental health promotion: A scoping review. *BMJ Open Sport & Exercise Medicine*, 6(1), e000677. DOI: 10.1136/bmjsem-2019-000677 PMID: 32095272

Patton, K., & Parker, M. (2017). Teacher education communities of practice: more than a culture of collaboration. *Teaching and Teacher Education, 67*(351-360). https://doi.org/DOI: 10.1016/j.tate.2017.06.013

Patton, M. Q. (1990). *Qualitative evaluation and research methods*. Sage.

Pavlov, I. P. (1927). *Conditioned reflexes: An investigation of the physiological activity of the cerebral cortex*. Oxford University Press.

Perry, A. C. (1919). *The management of a city school*. The Macmillan Company.

Perry, D. W., Marston, G. M., Hinder, S. A., Munden, A., & Roy, A. (2001). The phenomenology of depressive illness in people with a learning disability and autism. *Autism*, 5(3), 265–275. DOI: 10.1177/1362361301005003004 PMID: 11708586

Petticrew, M., & Roberts, H. (2008). *Systematic reviews in the social sciences: A practical guide*. John Wiley & Sons.

Pezirkianidis, C., Karakasidou, E., Lakioti, A., Stalikas, A., & Galanakis, M. (2018). Psychometric Properties of the Depression, Anxiety, Stress Scales-21 (DASS-21) in a Greek Sample. *Psychology (Irvine, Calif.)*, 9(15), 2933–2950. DOI: 10.4236/psych.2018.915170

Phinney, J. S., Horenczyk, G., Liebkind, K., & Vedder, P. (2001). Ethnic identity, immigration, and well-being: An interactional perspective. *The Journal of Social Issues*, 57(3), 493–510. DOI: 10.1111/0022-4537.00225

Piaget, J., & Inhelder, B. (1956). *The child's conception of space*. Routledge & Kegan Paul.

Pianta, R. C. (1992). *The Child-Parent Relationship Scale*. University of Virginia.

Pianta, R. C. (1999). How the parts affect the whole: Systems theory in classroom relationships. In Pianta, R. C. (Ed.), *Enhancing relationships between children and teachers* (pp. 23–43). American Psychological Association., DOI: 10.1037/10314-002

Pianta, R. C., Hamre, B. K., & Allen, J. P. (2012). Teacher-student relationships and engagement: Conceptualizing, measuring, and improving the capacity of classroom interactions. In *Handbook of research on student engagement* (pp. 365–386). Springer US. DOI: 10.1007/978-1-4614-2018-7_17

Pine, D. S., Costello, J., & Masten, A. (2005). Trauma, proximity, and developmental psychopathology: The effects of war and terrorism on children. *Neuropsychopharmacology*, 30(10), 1781–1792. DOI: 10.1038/sj.npp.1300814 PMID: 16012537

Pinquart, M., & Shen, Y. (2011). Behavior problems in children and adolescents with chronic physical illness: A meta-analysis. *Journal of Pediatric Psychology*, 36(9), 1003–1016. DOI: 10.1093/jpepsy/jsr042 PMID: 21810623

Pintimalli, A., Di Giuseppe, T., Serantoni, G., Glicksohn, J., & Ben-Soussan, T. D. (2020). Dynamics of the sphere model of consciousness: Silence, space, and self. *Frontiers in Psychology*, 11, 548813. DOI: 10.3389/fpsyg.2020.548813 PMID: 33071865

Plank, S. B., Bradshaw, C. P., & Young, H. (2009). An application of "broken-windows" and related theories to the study of disorder, fear, and collective efficacy in schools. *American Journal of Education*, 115(2), 227–247. DOI: 10.1086/595669

Pliszka, S. (2007). Practice parameter for the assessment and treatment of children and adolescents with attention-deficit/hyperactivity disorder. *Journal of the American Academy of Child and Adolescent Psychiatry*, 46(7), 894–921. DOI: 10.1097/chi.0b013e318054e724 PMID: 17581453

Pliszka, S. R. (2011). *Treating ADHD and Comorbid Disorders: Psychosocial and Psychopharmacological Interventions*. Guilford Press.

Pollard, A. J., & Prendergast, M. (2004). Depressive pseudodementia in a child with autism. *Developmental Medicine and Child Neurology*, 46(7), 485–489. DOI: 10.1111/j.1469-8749.2004.tb00510.x PMID: 15230463

Powers, K., Hagans, K., & Linn, M. (2017). A mixed-method efficacy and fidelity study of Check and Connect. *Psychology in the Schools*, 54(9), 1019–1033. DOI: 10.1002/pits.22038

Priest, N., Paradies, Y., Trenerry, B., Truong, M., Karlsen, S., & Kelly, Y. (2013). A systematic review of studies examining the relationship between reported racism and health and wellbeing for children and young people. *Social Science & Medicine*, 95, 115–127. DOI: 10.1016/j.socscimed.2012.11.031 PMID: 23312306

Proulx, K. (2008). Experiences of women with integrative approaches to stress management: A qualitative study. *Stress and Health*, 24(4), 311–322. DOI: 10.1002/smi.1184

Public Health England, 2021

Purkey, W. W. (1991). *Invitational teaching, learning, and living. Analysis and action series* (ED340689). https://files.eric.ed.gov/fulltext/ED340689.pdf

Purkey, W. W. (1970). *Self-concept and school achievement*. Prentice-Hall.

Purkey, W. W. (1978). *Inviting school success: A self-concept approach to teaching and learning*. Wadsworth Publishing Company.

Putnam, F. W. (2002). Televised trauma and viewer PTSD: Implications for prevention. *Psychiatry*, 65(4), 310–312. DOI: 10.1521/psyc.65.4.310.20241 PMID: 12530334

Pyne, J. (2019). Suspended attitudes: Exclusion and emotional disengagement from school. *Sociology of Education*, 92(1), 59–82. DOI: 10.1177/0038040718816684

Randall, W. M., Rickard, N. S., & Vella-Brodrick, D. A. (2014). Emotional outcomes of regulation strategies used during personal music listening: A mobile experience sampling study. *Musicae Scientiae*, 18(3), 275–291. DOI: 10.1177/1029864914536430

Raviv, A., Oppenheimer, L., & Bar-Tal, D. (1999). *How children understand war and peace*. Jossey-Bass.

Reaves, J. S., & Cozzens, J. A. (2018). Teacher perceptions of climate, motivation, and self-efficacy: Is there really a connection? *Journal of Education and Training Studies*, 6(12), 48–67. DOI: 10.11114/jets.v6i12.3566

Reback, R. (2010). Schools' mental health services and young children's emotions, behavior, and learning. *Journal of Policy Analysis and Management*, 29(4), 698–725. DOI: 10.1002/pam.20528 PMID: 20964104

Rechtschaffen, D. (2016). *The mindful education workbook. Lessons for teaching mindfulness to students*. W. W. Norton.

Repko, A. F., & Szostak, R. (2020). *Interdisciplinary research: Process and theory*. Sage Publications.

Reppa G.P., (2021). *"Mindfulness Method: Learn how to enjoy your life. Theory and practical applications"*. Athens: Papazisis publication.

Reppa, G.P. (2017). The Effects of a Yoga and Mindfulness Techniques Program on the Prosocial Behavior and the Emotional Regulation of Preschool Children: A Pilot Study. *Educational Research Applications*, (Educ Res Appl): ERCA-138. DOI: (pp:1-7)DOI: 10.29011/2575-7032/100038

Rice, F. (2010). Genetics of childhood and adolescent depression: Insights into etiological heterogeneity and challenges for future genomic research. *Genome Medicine*, 2(9), 68. DOI: 10.1186/gm189 PMID: 20860851

Richaud de Minzi, M. C. (2006). Family structure and children's perceptions of parental support. *Perceptual and Motor Skills*, 103(3), 843–853.

Rich, B. A., Shiffrin, N. D., Cummings, C. M., Zarger, M. M., Berghorst, L., & Alvord, M. K. (2018). Resilience-based intervention with underserved children: Impact on self-regulation in a randomized clinical trial in schools. *International Journal of Group Psychotherapy*, 69(1), 30–53. DOI: 10.1080/00207284.2018.1479187 PMID: 38449213

Richter, A., Sjunnestrand, M., Romare Strandh, M., & Hasson, H. (2022). Implementing school-based mental health services: A scoping review of the literature summarizing the factors that affect implementation. *International Journal of Environmental Research and Public Health*, 19(6), 3489. DOI: 10.3390/ijerph19063489 PMID: 35329175

Riesberg, A. (2022). *Reflection Journal: For Children*. Lulu.

Rimm-Kaufman, S. E., & Hulleman, C. S. (2015). Social and emotional learning in elementary school settings: Identifying mechanisms that matter. Handbook of social and emotional learning: Research and practice, 151-166.

Rodd, J. (1985). Pre-school children's understanding of war. *Early Child Development and Care*, 22(2-3), 109–121. https://psycnet.apa.org/doi/10.1080/0300443850220202. DOI: 10.1080/0300443850220202

Rodrigo-Ruiz, D. (2016). Effect of teachers' emotions on their students: Some evidence. *Journal of Education & Social Policy*, 3(4), 73–79.

Rodwin, A. H., Shimizu, R., Travis, R.Jr, James, K. J., Banya, M., & Munson, M. R. (2023). A systematic review of music-based interventions to improve treatment engagement and mental health outcomes for adolescents and young adults. *Child & Adolescent Social Work Journal*, 40(4), 537–566. DOI: 10.1007/s10560-022-00893-x PMID: 36407676

Roeser, R. W., Schonert-Reichl, K. A., Jha, A., Cullen, M., Wallace, L., Wilensky, R., Oberle, E., Thomson, K., Taylor, C., & Harrison, J. (2013). Mindfulness training and reductions in teacher stress and burnout: Results from two randomized, waitlist-control field trials. *Journal of Educational Psychology*, 105(3), 787–804. DOI: 10.1037/a0032093

Roeser, R. W., Skinner, E., Beers, J., & Jennings, P. A. (2013). Mindfulness training and teachers' professional development: An emerging area of research and practice. *Child Development Perspectives*, 6(2), 167–173. DOI: 10.1111/j.1750-8606.2012.00238.x

Ronen, T. (2003). *Cognitive constructivist psychotherapy with children and adolescents*. Kluwer Academic/Plenum Publishers. DOI: 10.1007/978-1-4419-9284-0

Rosenberg, M. (1965). *Society and the adolescent self-image*. Princeton University Press. DOI: 10.1515/9781400876136

Ross, S. W., Horner, R. H., & Higbee, T. (2009). Bully prevention in positive behavior support. *Journal of Applied Behavior Analysis*, 42(4), 747–759. DOI: 10.1901/jaba.2009.42-747 PMID: 20514181

Ross, S. W., Romer, N., & Horner, R. H. (2012). Teacher well-being and the implementation of school-wide positive behavior interventions and support. *Journal of Positive Behavior Interventions*, 14(2), 118–128. DOI: 10.1177/1098300711413820

Rothstein, H. R., Sutton, A. J., & Borenstein, M. (Eds.). (2005). *Publication bias in meta-analysis: Prevention, assessment and adjustments*. John Wiley & Sons. DOI: 10.1002/0470870168

Royer, D. J., Lane, K. L., Dunlap, K. D., & Ennis, R. P. (2019). A systematic review of teacher-delivered behavior-specific praise on K–12 student performance. *Remedial and Special Education*, 40(2), 112–128. DOI: 10.1177/0741932517751054

Rubie-Davies, C. M. (2007). Classroom interactions: Exploring the practices of high and low expectation teachers. *The British Journal of Educational Psychology*, 77(2), 289–306. DOI: 10.1348/000709906X101601 PMID: 17504548

Rubin, D. H. (2012). Joy returns last: Anhedonia and treatment resistance in depressed adolescents. *Journal of the American Academy of Child and Adolescent Psychiatry*, 51(4), 353–355. DOI: 10.1016/j.jaac.2012.01.012 PMID: 22449641

Ruch, D. A., Horowitz, L. M., Hughes, J. L., Sarkisian, K., Luby, J. L., Fontanella, C. A., & Bridge, J. A. (2024). Suicide in US preteens aged 8 to 12 years, 2001-2022. *JAMA Network Open*, 7(7), e2424664. DOI: 10.1001/jamanetworkopen.2024.24664 PMID: 39078634

Rudasill, K. M., Snyder, K. E., Levinson, H., & Adelson, L., J. (. (2018). Systems view of school climate: A theoretical framework for research. *Educational Psychology Review*, 30(1), 35–60. DOI: 10.1007/s10648-017-9401-y

Rumrill, P. D., Fitzgerald, S. M., & Merchant, W. R. (2010). Using scoping literature reviews as a means of understanding and interpreting existing literature. *Work (Reading, Mass.)*, 35(3), 399–404. DOI: 10.3233/WOR-2010-0998 PMID: 20364059

Rutherford, L. E., Hier, B. O., McCurdy, B. L., Mautone, J. A., & Eiraldi, R. (2023). Aspects of School-wide Positive Behavioral Interventions and Supports that predict school climate in urban settings. *Contemporary School Psychology*, 27(3), 534–544. DOI: 10.1007/s40688-022-00417-5

Rutter, M. (2012). Resilience as a dynamic concept. *Development and Psychopathology*, 24(2), 335–344. DOI: 10.1017/S0954579412000028 PMID: 22559117

Saarikallio, S., Gold, C., & McFerran, K. (2015). Development and validation of the Healthy-Unhealthy Music Scale. *Child and Adolescent Mental Health*, 20(4), 210–217. DOI: 10.1111/camh.12109 PMID: 26726295

Sadler, C. (2000). Effective behavior support implementation at the district level: Tigard-Tualatin school district. *Journal of Positive Behavior Interventions*, 2(4), 241–243. DOI: 10.1177/109830070000200411

Sahdra, B. K., Shaver, P. R., & Brown, K. W. (2010). A scale to measure non-attachment: A Buddhist complement to Western research on attachment and adaptive functioning. *Journal of Personality Assessment*, 92(2), 116–127. DOI: 10.1080/00223890903425960 PMID: 20155561

Sameroff, A. J. (2000). Dialectical processes in developmental psychopathology. In A. J. Sameroff, M. Lewis, & S. M. Miller (Eds.), *Handbook of developmental psychopathology*. Springer. https://doi.org/DOI: 10.1007/978-1-4615-4163-9_2

Samm, A., Värnik, A., Tooding, L.-M., Sisask, M., Kõlves, K., & von Knorring, A.-L. (2007). Children's Depression Inventory in Estonia. Single items and factor structure by age and gender. *European Child & Adolescent Psychiatry*, 17(3), 162–170. DOI: 10.1007/s00787-007-0650-z PMID: 17876502

Santiago-Rosario, M. R., McIntosh, K., Izzard, S., Cohen-Lissman, D., & Calhoun, T. E. (2023). *Is Positive Behavioral Interventions and Supports (PBIS) an evidence-based practice?* Center on PBIS. https://www.pbis.org/resource/is-school-wide-positive-behavior-support-an-evidence-based-practice

Saputra, W. N. E., Supriyanto, A., Astuti, B., Ayriza, Y., & Adiputra, S. (2020). The effect of student perception of negative school climate on poor academic performance of students in Indonesia. *International Journal of Learning. Teaching and Educational Research*, 19(2), 279–291.

Sauer-Zavala, S., Tirpak, J. W., Eustis, E. H., Woods, B. K., & Russell, K. (2021). Unified protocol for the transdiagnostic prevention of emotional disorders: Evaluation of a brief, online course for college freshmen. *Behavior Therapy*, 52(1), 64–76. DOI: 10.1016/j.beth.2020.01.010 PMID: 33483125

Schola Europaea/Office of the Secretary-General. (2022). *Pupils' Well-Being Policy Framework of the European Schools.* https://www.eursc.eu/BasicTexts/2022-01-D -6-en-2.pdf

Schonert-Reichl, K. A., & Lawlor, M. S. (2010). The effects of a mindfulness-based education program on pre- and early adolescents' well-being and social and emotional competence. *Mindfulness*, 1(3), 137–151. DOI: 10.1007/s12671-010-0011-8

Schriber, R. A., Robins, R. W., & Solomon, M. (2014). Personality and Self-Insight in Individuals with Autism Spectrum Disorder. *Journal of Personality and Social Psychology*, 106(1), 112–130. https://psycnet.apa.org/doi/10.1037/a0034950. DOI: 10.1037/a0034950 PMID: 24377361

Schuenemann, L., Scherenberg, V., von Salisch, M., & Eckert, M. (2022). "I'll worry about it tomorrow"–Fostering emotion regulation skills to overcome procrastination. *Frontiers in Psychology*, 13, 780675. DOI: 10.3389/fpsyg.2022.780675 PMID: 35391959

Schultz, J. H., Langballe, Å., & Raundalen, M. (2014). Explaining the unexplainable: Designing a national strategy on classroom communication concerning the 22 July terror attack in Norway. *European Journal of Psychotraumatology*, 5(1), 22758. DOI: 10.3402/ejpt.v5.22758 PMID: 25018859

Schussler, D. L., Jennings, P. A., Sharp, J. E., & Frank, J. L. (2016). Improving teacher awareness and well-being through CARE: A qualitative analysis of the underlying mechanisms. *Mindfulness*, 7(1), 130–142. DOI: 10.1007/s12671-015-0422-7

Schwarz, S. (2018). Factors of mental resilience in youth: A review of current research and future directions. *Journal of Child Psychology and Psychiatry, and Allied Disciplines*, 20(3), 123–138.

Schwebel, M. (1982). Effects of the nuclear war threat on children and teenagers: Implications for professionals. *The American Journal of Orthopsychiatry*, 52(4), 608–618. https://psycnet.apa.org/doi/10.1111/j.1939-0025.1982.tb01450.x. DOI: 10.1111/j.1939-0025.1982.tb01450.x PMID: 7148982

Sciarra, D. S., Austin, V. L., & Bienia, E. J. (2022). *Working with students with emotional and behavioral disorders: A guide for K-12 teachers and service providers*. Vernon Press.

Scott, T. (2017). *Teaching behavior*. Corwin., DOI: 10.4135/9781506337883

Seligman, M. E. P., & Csikszentmihalyi, M. (2000). Positive psychology: An introduction. *The American Psychologist*, 55(1), 5–14. DOI: 10.1037/0003-066X.55.1.5 PMID: 11392865

Shacham, M. (2015). Suddenly–war. Intervention program for Enhancing teachers and children's resilience Following war. *Revista de Cercetare si Interventie Sociala*, (48), 60–68.

Shapiro, S. (2002). Toward a critical pedagogy of peace education. In Salomon, G., & Nevo, B. (Eds.), *Peace education: The concept principles, and practices around the world* (pp. 63–72). Lawrence Erlbaum.

Shapiro, S. L., & Carlson, L. E. (2009). *The art and science of mindfulness: Integrating mindfulness into psychology and the helping professions*. American Psychological Association. DOI: 10.1037/11885-000

Sharpe, J., Bunting, B., & Heary, C. (2023). A latent class analysis of mental health symptoms in primary school children: Exploring associations with school attendance problems. *School Mental Health*, 15(4), 1128–1144. DOI: 10.1007/s12310-023-09610-0

Shaul, J. (2017). *The ASD and me picture book: Visual guide to understanding challenges and strengths for children on the Autism Spectrum*. Jessica Kinglsley Publishers.

Shelley, K., Hudson, J., & Schenk, K. (2011). Family-centered care in pediatric chronic illness: A review of the literature. *Journal of Pediatric Nursing*, 26(4), 339–345.

Shelton, L. (2018). *The Bronfenbrenner primer: A guide to develecology*. Routledge. DOI: 10.4324/9781315136066

Sheridan, S. M., Kunz, G. M., & Holmes, S. R. (2019). Family-school partnerships in context: Relations between parent-teacher partnership perceptions and student outcomes in a diverse, low-income population. *The Elementary School Journal*, 120(1), 47–73.

Sheridan, S. M., Smith, T. E., Kim, E. M., Beretvas, S. N., & Park, S. (2019). A meta-analysis of family-school interventions and children's social-emotional functioning: Moderators and components of efficacy. *Review of Educational Research*, 89(2), 296–332. DOI: 10.3102/0034654318825437

Shernoff, D. J., Kelly, S., Tonks, S. M., Anderson, B., Cavanagh, R. F., Sinha, S., & Abdi, B. (2016). Student engagement as a function of environmental complexity in high school classrooms. *Learning and Instruction*, 43, 52–60. DOI: 10.1016/j. learninstruc.2015.12.003

Shields-Lysiak, L., Boyd, M. P., Iorio Jr, J., & Vasquez, C. R. (2020). Classroom greetings: More than a simple hello. *Iranian Journal of Language Teaching Research*, 8(3 (Special Issue), 41–56. DOI: 10.30466/ijltr.2020.120933

Shi, J., Cheung, A. C. K., & Ni, A. (2022). The effectiveness of Promoting Alternative Thinking Strategies program: A meta-analysis. *Frontiers in Psychology*, 13, 1030572. Advance online publication. DOI: 10.3389/fpsyg.2022.1030572 PMID: 36571043

Sibinga, E. M., Webb, L., Ghazarian, S. R., & Ellen, J. M. (2016). School-based mindfulness instruction: An RCT. *Pediatrics*, 137(1), e20152532. DOI: 10.1542/ peds.2015-2532 PMID: 26684478

Simeonsson, R. J. (Ed.). (1994). *Risk, resilience & prevention: Promoting the well-being of all children*. Paul H. Brookes Publishing Co.

Simkiss, N. J., Gray, N. S., Dunne, C., & Snowden, R. J. (2021). Development and psychometric properties of the Knowledge and Attitudes to Mental Health Scales (KAMHS): A psychometric measure of mental health literacy in children and adolescents. *BMC Pediatrics*, 21(1), 508. Advance online publication. DOI: 10.1186/ s12887-021-02964-x PMID: 34774022

Simonoff, E., Pickles, A., Charman, T., Chandler, S., Loucas, T., & Baird, G. (2008). Psychiatric disorders in children with autism spectrum disorders: Prevalence, co-morbidity, and associated factors in a population-derived sample. *Journal of the American Academy of Child and Adolescent Psychiatry*, 47(8), 921–992. DOI: 10.1097/CHI.0b013e318179964f PMID: 18645422

Simonsen, B., Britton, L., & Young, D. (2010). Schoolwide positive behavior support in an alternative school setting. *Journal of Positive Behavior Interventions*, 12(3), 180–191. DOI: 10.1177/1098300708330495

Simonsen, B., & Sugai, G. (2019). School-wide positive behavioral interventions and supports: A systems-level application of behavioral principles. In Little, S. G., & Akin-Little, A. (Eds.), *Behavioral interventions in schools: Evidence-based positive strategies* (2nd ed., pp. 35–60). American Psychological Association., DOI: 10.1037/0000126-003

Simonsen, B., Sugai, G., & Negron, M. (2008). Schoolwide Positive Behavior Supports: Primary systems and practices. *Teaching Exceptional Children*, 40(6), 32–40. DOI: 10.1177/004005990804000604

Şimşir, Z. (2023). The effects of resilience and hope on mental health among adolescents: A longitudinal study. *Journal of Youth and Adolescence*, 52(4), 567–580.

Sippel, L. M., Pietrzak, R. H., Charney, D. S., Mayes, L. C., & Southwick, S. M. (2015). How does social support enhance resilience in the trauma-exposed individual? *Ecology and Society*, 20(4), art10. DOI: 10.5751/ES-07832-200410

Skinner, B. F. (1966). Contingencies of reinforcement in the design of a culture. *Behavioral Science*, 11(3), 159–166. DOI: 10.1002/bs.3830110302 PMID: 5935977

Skinner, S. R., McDonald, A., & Walters, T. (2005). A patient with autism and severe depression: Medical and ethical challenges for an adolescent medicine unit. *The Medical Journal of Australia*, 183(8), 422–424. DOI: 10.5694/j.1326-5377.2005. tb07108.x PMID: 16225449

Sklad, M., Diekstra, R., Ritter, M., Ben, J., & Gravesteijn, C. (2012). Effectiveness of school-based universal social, emotional and behavioral programs: Do they enhance students' development in the area of skill, behavior and adjustment? *Psychology in the Schools*, 49(9), 892–909. DOI: 10.1002/pits.21641

Skoric, D., Rakic, J. G., Jovanovic, V., Backovic, D., Soldatovic, I., & Zivojinovic, J. I. (2023). Psychosocial school factors and mental health of first-grade secondary school students—Results of the health behavior in school-aged children survey in Serbia. *PLoS One*, 18(11), e0293179. DOI: 10.1371/journal.pone.0293179 PMID: 37943735

Sloan, S., Winter, K., Connolly, P., & Gildea, A. (2020). The effectiveness of Nurture Groups in improving outcomes for young children with social, emotional, and behavioural difficulties in primary schools: An evaluation of Nurture Group provision in Northern Ireland. *Children and Youth Services Review*, 108, 104619. DOI: 10.1016/j.childyouth.2019.104619

Smith, A., Johnson, R., & Thompson, L. (2018). The impact of social-emotional learning on resilience in children with chronic health conditions. *Journal of School Psychology*, 66, 24–32.

Smith, P., & Jones, D. (2015). Enhancing resilience among students: A review of school-based interventions. *Educational Psychology*, 35(1), 1–20.

Smith, S. M., & Malaney, V. M. (2016). Mindfulness practices in education: Student responses from an ethnically diverse urban university. *Journal of Transformative Education*, 14(2), 171–188. DOI: 10.1177/1541344616655889

Smith, T. E., Sheridan, S. M., Kim, E. M., Park, S., & Beretvas, S. N. (2019). The effects of family-school partnership interventions on academic and social-emotional functioning: A meta-analysis exploring what works for whom. *Educational Psychology Review*, 32(2), 511–544. DOI: 10.1007/s10648-019-09509-w

Social and Emotional Aspects of Learning (SEAL). https://sealcommunity.org/

Sørlie, M.-A., & Ogden, T. (2007). Immediate impacts of PALS: A school-wide multi-level programme targeting behaviour problems in elementary school. *Scandinavian Journal of Educational Research*, 51(5), 471–492. DOI: 10.1080/00313830701576581

Southwick, S. M., Bonanno, G. A., Masten, A. S., Panter-Brick, C., & Yehuda, R. (2014). Resilience definitions, theory, and challenges: Interdisciplinary perspectives. *European Journal of Psychotraumatology*, 5(1), 25338. DOI: 10.3402/ejpt.v5.25338 PMID: 25317257

Southwick, S. M., & Charney, D. S. (2012). The science of resilience: Implications for the prevention and treatment of depression. *Science*, 338(6103), 79–82. DOI: 10.1126/science.1222942 PMID: 23042887

Sperlich, M., & Kabilamany, P. (2022). The survivor moms' companion trauma-specific perinatal psychoeducation intervention in a community outreach program: An open pilot. *Journal of Midwifery & Women's Health*, 67(5), 569–579. DOI: 10.1111/jmwh.13380 PMID: 35689499

Spielmann, M. (1986). If peace comes…future expectations of Israeli children and youth. *Journal of Peace Research*, 23(1), 51–67. DOI: 10.1177/002234338602300105

Sprague, J. R., Biglan, A., Rusby, J. C., Gau, J. M., & Vincent, C. G. (2017). Implementing school wide PBIS in middle schools: Results of a randomized trial. *Journal of Health Science & Education*, 1(2), 1–10.

Stalikas, A., & Mitskidou, C. (2011). Psychological resilience: Theory, research, and interventions. *Hellenic Journal of Psychology*, 8(1), 89–113.

Steele, H., & Steele, M. (2014). Attachment disorders: Theory, research, and treatment considerations. In M. Lewis & K. D. Rudolph (Eds.), *Handbook of developmental psychopathology* (3rd ed., pp. 357–370). Springer.

Stenseng, F., Belsky, J., Skalicka, V., & Wichstrøm, L. (2015). Peer Rejection and Attention Deficit Hyperactivity Disorder Symptoms: Reciprocal Relations Through Ages 4, 6, and 8. *Child Development*, 87(2), 365–373. DOI: 10.1111/cdev.12471 PMID: 26671073

Stevenson, H. C., Davis, G. Y., & Abdul-Kabir, S. (2019). Stickin' to, watchin' over, and gettin' with: An African American parent's guide to discipline. *Family Relations*, 49(4), 328–336.

Stewart, M. E., Barnard, L., Pearson, J., Hasan, R., & O'Brien, G. (2006). Presentation of depression in autism and Asperger syndrome: A review. *Autism*, 10(1), 103–116. DOI: 10.1177/1362361306062013 PMID: 16522713

Strickland-Cohen, M. K., Pinkelman, S. E., Jimerson, J. B., Berg, T. A., Pinkney, C. J., & McIntosh, K. (2018). Sustaining effective individualized behavior support: Barriers and enablers. *Preventing School Failure*, 63(1), 1–11. DOI: 10.1080/1045988X.2018.1456399

Sue, S. (2001). *Cultural competency: From philosophy to research and practice.* Springer.

Sugai, G., & Simonsen, B. (2012). *Positive behavioral interventions and supports: History, defining features, and misconceptions.* Center for PBIS & Center for Positive Behavioral Interventions and Supports, University of Connecticut. www.PBIS.org

Sugai, G., & Horner, R. (2020). Sustaining and scaling positive behavioral interventions and supports: Implementation drivers, outcomes, and considerations. *Psychology in the Schools*, 57(5), 882–903.

Sugai, G., & Horner, R. H. (2002). Introduction to the special series on positive behavior support in schools. *Journal of Emotional and Behavioral Disorders*, 10(3), 130–135. DOI: 10.1177/10634266020100030101

Sugai, G., & Horner, R. H. (2020). Sustaining and scaling Positive Behavioral Interventions and Supports: Implementation drivers, outcomes, and considerations. *Exceptional Children*, 86(2), 120–136. DOI: 10.1177/0014402919855331

Sugai, G., Horner, R. H., Dunlap, G., Hieneman, M., Lewis, T. J., Nelson, C. M., Scott, T., Liaupsin, C., Sailor, W., Turnbull, A. P., Turnbull, H. R.III, Wickham, D., Wilcox, B., & Ruef, M. (2000). Applying positive behavior support and functional behavioral assessment in schools. *Journal of Positive Behavior Interventions*, 2(3), 131–143. DOI: 10.1177/109830070000200302

Sugai, G., & Lewis, T. J. (1999). Developing positive behavioral support systems. In Sugai, G., & Lewis, T. J. (Eds.), *Developing positive behavioral support for students with challenging behavior* (pp. 15–23). Council for Children with Behavioral Disorders.

Sulkowski, M. L., & Joyce, D. J. (2012). School psychology goes to college: The emerging role of school psychology in college communities. *Psychology in the Schools*, 49(8), 809–815. DOI: 10.1002/pits.21634

Sun, J., & Stewart, D. (2010). How effective is the health-promoting school approach in building social capital in primary schools? *Health Education*, 110(4), 226–246.

Sun, Y., & Lee, J. (2023). School-based interventions to enhance resilience in children and adolescents: A systematic review. *The Journal of School Health*, 93(2), 45–63.

Sutherland, K. S., Conroy, M. A., McLeod, B. D., Kunemund, R., & McKnight, K. (2018). Common practice elements for improving social, emotional, and behavioral outcomes of young elementary school students. *Journal of Emotional and Behavioral Disorders*, 27(2), 76–85. DOI: 10.1177/1063426618784009

Tang, Y. Y., Yang, L., Leve, L. D., & Harold, G. T. (2012). Improving executive function and its neurobiological mechanisms through a mindfulness-based intervention: Advances within the field of developmental neuroscience. *Child Development Perspectives*, 6(4), 361–366. DOI: 10.1111/j.1750-8606.2012.00250.x PMID: 25419230

Tani, N., Fujihara, H., Ishii, K., Kamakura, Y., Tsunemi, M., Yamaguchi, C., Eguchi, H., Imamura, K., Kanamori, S., Kojimahara, N., & Ebara, T. (2024). What digital health technology types are used in mental health prevention and intervention? Review of systematic reviews for systematization of technologies. *Journal of Occupational Health*, 66(1), uiad003. Advance online publication. DOI: 10.1093/joccuh/uiad003 PMID: 38258936

Tanner-Smith, E. E., Fisher, B. W., Addington, L. A., & Gardella, J. H. (2018). Adding security, but subtracting safety? Exploring schools' use of multiple visible security measures. *American Journal of Criminal Justice*, 43(1), 102–119. DOI: 10.1007/s12103-017-9409-3

Taylor, J. C., Hanley, W., Deger, G., & Hunter, C., W. (. (2023). Promoting anti-racism practices and the cycle of critical consciousness within positive behavior interventions and supports frameworks. *Teaching Exceptional Children*, 55(5), 314–322. DOI: 10.1177/00400599221120242

Taylor, R. D., Oberle, E., Durlak, J. A., & Weissberg, R. P. (2017). Promoting positive youth development through school-based social and emotional learning interventions: A meta-analysis of follow-up effects. *Child Development*, 88(4), 1156–1171. DOI: 10.1111/cdev.12864 PMID: 28685826

Tephly, J. (1985). Young children's understanding of war and peace. *Early Child Development and Care*, 20(4), 271–285. DOI: 10.1080/0300443850200405

Thapa, A., Cohen, J., Guffey, S., & Higgins-D'Alessandro, A. (2013). A review of school climate research. *Review of Educational Research*, 83(3), 357–385. DOI: 10.3102/0034654313483907

The Hawn Foundation. (2018). *MindUp curriculum: Brain-focused strategies for learning—and living*. Scholastic Inc.

Thies, C., & Tscharntke, T. (1999). Landscape structure and biological control in agroecosystems. *Science*, 285(5429), 893–895. DOI: 10.1126/science.285.5429.893 PMID: 10436158

Thomas, C., & Zolkoski, S. (2020, June). Preventing stress among undergraduate learners: The importance of emotional intelligence, resilience, and emotion regulation. [). Frontiers Media SA]. *Frontiers in Education*, 5, 94. DOI: 10.3389/feduc.2020.00094

Thomson, C. J., Reece, J. E., & Di Benedetto, M. (2014). The relationship between music-related mood regulation and psychopathology in young people. *Musicae Scientiae*, 18(2), 150–165. DOI: 10.1177/1029864914521422

Thorndike, E. L. (1898). Animal Intelligence: An experimental study of associative processes in animals. *Psychological Monographs*, 2(4), i–109. DOI: 10.1037/h0092987

Todd, A. W., Campbell, A. L., Meyer, G. G., & Horner, R. H. (2008). The effects of a targeted intervention to reduce problem behaviors: Elementary school implementation of check in—check out. *Journal of Positive Behavior Interventions*, 10(1), 46–55. DOI: 10.1177/1098300707311369

Tomé, G., Almeida, A., Ramiro, L., & Gaspar, T. (2021). Intervention in schools promoting mental health and well-being: A systematic. *Global J Comm Psychol Pract*, 34, 3–23.

Tountas, Y. (2009). Screening for children's depression symptoms in Greece: The use of the Children's Depression Inventory in a nation - wide school - based sample. *European Child & Adolescent Psychiatry*, 18(8), 485–492. DOI: 10.1007/s00787-009-0005-z PMID: 19255802

Trikkas, G. (2005). *Clinical forms of depression*. In G. N. Christodoulou (Ed.), Depression (2nd Ed.) (pp. 13–22). Athens: BETA, medical arts. In Greek.

Tucker, P., Bruijns, B. A., Adamo, K. B., Burke, S. M., Carson, V., Heydon, R., Irwin, J. D., Johnson, A. M., Naylor, P. J., Timmons, B. W., & Vanderloo, L. M. (2022). Training Pre-Service Early Childhood Educators in Physical Activity (TEACH): Protocol for a Quasi-Experimental Study. *International Journal of Environmental Research and Public Health*, 19(7), 3890. DOI: 10.3390/ijerph19073890 PMID: 35409573

Tyre, A., Begay, K. K., Beaudoin, K., & Feuerborn, L. (2023). Understanding middle and high school student preferences for acknowledgements in the context of schoolwide PBIS. *Preventing School Failure*, 68(2), 139–148. DOI: 10.1080/1045988X.2023.2186339

Ungar, M. (2012). *The social ecology of resilience: A handbook of theory and practice*. Springer Science & Business Media. DOI: 10.1007/978-1-4614-0586-3

Ungar, M. (2013). Resilience, trauma, context, and culture. *Trauma, Violence & Abuse*, 14(3), 255–266. DOI: 10.1177/1524838013487805 PMID: 23645297

UNICEF. (2022). Promoting and protecting mental health in schools and learning environments. Retrieved from https://www.unicef.org/media/126821/file/Promoting%20and%20protecting%20mental%20health%20in%20schools%20and%20learning%20environments.pdf

UNICEF. (2022). Promoting and Protecting Mental Health in Schools and Learning Environments. Retrieved from https://www.unicef.org/media/126821/file/Promoting%20and%20protecting%20mental%20health%20in%20schools%20and%20learning%20environments.pdf

United Nations Children's Fund. (2021). [*On my mind. Promoting, protecting and caring for children's mental health.* UNICEF Office of Global Insight and Policy.]. *The State of the World's Children*, 2021.

Van Camp, A. M., Wehby, J. H., Copeland, B. A., & Bruhn, A. L. (2021). Building from the bottom up: The importance of Tier 1 supports in the context of Tier 2 interventions. *Journal of Positive Behavior Interventions*, 23(1), 53–64. DOI: 10.1177/1098300720916716

Van de Weijer-Bergsma, E., Langenberg, G., Brandsma, R., Oort, F. J., & Bögels, S. M. (2014). The effectiveness of a school-based mindfulness training as a program to prevent stress in elementary school children. *Mindfulness*, 5(3), 238–248. DOI: 10.1007/s12671-012-0171-9

Van Houtte, M. (2005). Climate or culture? A plea for conceptual clarity in school effectiveness research. *School Effectiveness and School Improvement*, 16(1), 71–89. DOI: 10.1080/09243450500113977

Van Westrhenen, N., & Fritz, E. (2014). Creative arts therapy as treatment for child trauma: An overview. *The Arts in Psychotherapy*, 41(5), 527–534. DOI: 10.1016/j.aip.2014.10.004

Verduyn, C., Rogers, J., & Wood, A. (2009). *Depression: cognitive behavior therapy with children and young people*. Routledge. DOI: 10.4324/9780203879894

Verhoog, S., Eijgermans, D. G. M., Fang, Y., Bramer, W. M., Raat, H., & Jansen, W. (2022). Contextual determinants associated with children's and adolescents' mental health care utilization: A systematic review. *European Child & Adolescent Psychiatry*, 1–15. PMID: 36129544

Vieira, A. P. A., Peng, P., Antoniuk, A., DeVries, J., Rothou, K., Parrila, R., & Georgiou, G. (2024). Internalizing problems in individuals with reading, mathematics and unspecified learning difficulties: A systematic review and meta-analysis. *Annals of Dyslexia*, 74(1), 4–26. DOI: 10.1007/s11881-023-00294-4 PMID: 38135829

Villegas, A. M., & Lucas, T. (2002). Preparing culturally responsive teachers: Rethinking the curriculum. *Journal of Teacher Education*, 53(1), 20–32. DOI: 10.1177/0022487102053001003

Vincent, K. (2017). "It's small steps, but that leads to bigger changes:" Evaluation of a Nurture Group intervention. *Emotional & Behavioural Difficulties*, 22(4), 303–316. DOI: 10.1080/13632752.2017.1290882

Vogiatzoglou, P., & Galanaki, E. (2011). Classroom life of children with behavioral problems. *Proceedings of the 2nd Panhellenic Conference of Special Education: "Special Education as a starting point for developments in science and practice".* Greek Society of Special Education - University of Athens. (in Greek)

Voight, A., & Nation, M. (2016). Practices for improving secondary school climate: A Systematic review of the research literature. *American Journal of Community Psychology,* 58(1-2), 174–191. DOI: 10.1002/ajcp.12074 PMID: 27535489

von Bertalanffy, L. (2013). *General system theory: Foundations, development, applications* (rev. ed.). Braziller. (Original work published 1968)

Vygotsky, L. S. (1978). *Mind in society: The development of higher psychological processes.* Harvard University Press.

Waasdorp, T., Bradshaw, C., & Leaf, P. (2012). The impact of School-wide Positive Behavioral Interventions and Supports on bullying and peer rejection: A randomized controlled effectiveness trial. *Archives of Pediatrics & Adolescent Medicine,* 166(2), 149–156. DOI: 10.1001/archpediatrics.2011.755 PMID: 22312173

Wagnild, G. M., & Young, H. M. (1993). Development and psychometric evaluation of the Resilience Scale. *Journal of Nursing Measurement,* 1(2), 165–178. PMID: 7850498

Walker, H. M., Horner, R. H., Sugai, G., Bullis, M., Sprague, J. R., Bricker, D., & Kaufman, M.

Walker, H. M., Horner, R. H., Sugai, G., Bullis, M., Sprague, J. R., Bricker, D., & Kaufman, M. J. (1996). Integrated approaches to preventing antisocial behavior patterns among school-age children and youth. *Journal of Emotional and Behavioral Disorders,* 4(4), 194–209.

Walker, K., Myers-Bowman, K. S., & Myers-Walls, J. A. (2003). Understanding war, visualizing peace: Children draw what they know. *Art Therapy: Journal of the American Art Therapy Association,* 20(4), 191–200. DOI: 10.1080/07421656.2003.10129605

Walker, V. L., & Loman, S. L. (2022). Strategies for including students with extensive support needs in SWPBIS. *In Practice,* 1(1), 23–32.

Walsh, F. (2015). *Strengthening family resilience.* Guilford Press.

Wang, C., Berry, B., & Swearer, S. M. (2013). The critical role of school climate in effective bullying prevention. *Theory into Practice,* 52(4), 296–302. DOI: 10.1080/00405841.2013.829735

Wang, M.-T., & Degol, J. L. (2016). School climate: A review of the construct, measurement, and impact on student outcomes. *Educational Psychology Review*, 28(2), 315–352. DOI: 10.1007/s10648-015-9319-1

Wang, M.-T., Degol, J. L., Amemiya, J., Parr, A., & Guo, J. (2020). Classroom climate and children's academic and psychological wellbeing: A systematic review and meta-analysis. *Developmental Review*, 57, 100912. DOI: 10.1016/j.dr.2020.100912

Wang, W., Vaillancourt, T., Brittain, H. L., McDougall, P., Krygsman, A., Smith, D., Cunningham, C. E., Haltigan, J. D., & Hymel, S. (2014). School climate, peer victimization, and academic achievement: Results from a multi-informant study. *School Psychology Quarterly: The Official Journal of the Division of School Psychology, American Psychological Association*, 29(3), 360–377. DOI: 10.1037/spq0000084 PMID: 25198617

Wannarka, R., & Ruhl, K. (2008). Seating arrangements that promote positive academic and behavioural outcomes: A review of empirical research. *Support for Learning*, 23(2), 89–93. DOI: 10.1111/j.1467-9604.2008.00375.x

Watkins, D. C., Hunt, J. B., & Eisenberg, D. (2012). Increased demand for mental health services on college campuses: Perspectives from administrators. *Qualitative Social Work: Research and Practice*, 11(3), 319–337. DOI: 10.1177/1473325011401468

Watson, J. B. (1914). *Behavior: An introduction to comparative psychology*. Henry Holtand., DOI: 10.1037/10868-000

Watzlawick, P. (1981). *The language of change: Elements of therapeutic communication*. Basic Books.

Weaver, C., Kutcher, S., Wei, Y., & Mcluckie, A. (2014). Sustained improvements in students' mental health literacy with use of a mental health curriculum in Canadian schools. *BMC Psychiatry*, 14(1), 1–6. DOI: 10.1186/s12888-014-0379-4 PMID: 25551789

Weisgram, E. S., & Dinella, L. M. (Eds.). (2018). *Gender typing of children's toys: How early play experiences impact development*. American Psychological Association., DOI: 10.1037/0000077-000

Weissberg, R. P., Durlak, J. A., Domitrovich, C. E., & Gullotta, T. P. (2015). Social and emotional learning: Past, present, and future. In Durlak, J. A., Domitrovich, C. E., Weissberg, R. P., & Gullotta, T. P. (Eds.), *Handbook of social and emotional learning: Research and practice* (pp. 3–19). The Guilford Press.

Weissberg, R. P., Durlak, J. A., Domitrovich, C. E., & Gulotta, T. P. (2017). Social emotional learning: Past, present, and future. In Durlak, J. A., Domitrovich, C. E., Weissberg, R. P., & Gullotta, T. P. (Eds.), *Handbook of Social and Emotional Learning: Research and Practice* (pp. 3–19). The Guildford Press.

Weiss, H. B., Lopez, M. E., & Caspe, M. (2018). *Joining Together to Create a Bold Vision for Next Generation Family Engagement: Engaging Families to Transform Education.* Global Family Research Project.

Weist, M. D., Evans, S. W., & Lever, N. A. (Eds.). (2000). *Handbook of school mental health: Advancing practice and research.* Springer Science & Business Media.

Weist, M. D., Splett, J. W., Halliday, C. A., Gage, N. A., Seaman, M. A., Perkins, K. A., Perales, K., Miller, E., Collins, D., & DiStefano, C. (2022). A randomized controlled trial on the interconnected systems framework for school mental health and PBIS: Focus on proximal variables and school discipline. *Journal of School Psychology*, 94, 49–65. DOI: 10.1016/j.jsp.2022.08.002 PMID: 36064215

Wentzel, K. R., & Muenks, K. (2016). Peer influence on students' motivation, academic achievement, and social behavior. In *Handbook of social influences in school contexts* (pp. 13–30). Routledge. DOI: 10.4324/9781315769929

Weyandt, L., & Dupaul, G. J. (2013). *Students with ADHD.* Business Media. DOI: 10.1007/978-1-4614-5345-1

Whaley, A. L. (2001). Cultural mistrust: An important psychological construct for diagnosis and treatment of African Americans. *Professional Psychology: Research and Practice, 32*(6), 555.

Whittingham, K., & Coyne, L. W. (2019). Values and proto-values. In Whittingham, K., & Coyne, L. W. (Eds.), *Acceptance and commitment therapy: The clinician's guide for supporting parents* (pp. 153–186). Academic Press. DOI: 10.1016/B978-0-12-814669-9.00007-2

Wilkinson, C., & Wilkinson, S. (2022). Using Persona Dolls in research with children to combat the insider/ outsider researcher status dilemma. *Children's Geographies*, 20(3), 375–380. DOI: 10.1080/14733285.2022.2051433

Willemse, T. M., Goei, S. L., Boei, F., & de Bruïne, E. J. (2022). School-wide positive behaviour interventions and support in Dutch schools for special education. *European Journal of Special Needs Education*, 38(3), 424–443. DOI: 10.1080/08856257.2022.2120331

Winner, E., Goldstein, T. R., & Vincent-Lancrin, S. (2013). Art for art's sake. The impact of arts education. doi, 10.

Worsley, J. D., Pennington, A., & Corcoran, R. (2022). Supporting mental health and wellbeing of university and college students: A systematic review of review-level evidence of interventions. *PLoS One*, 17(7), e0266725. Advance online publication. DOI: 10.1371/journal.pone.0266725 PMID: 35905058

Yager, Z. (2009). Exploring young people's digital lives: From theory to practice. *Australian Journal of Education*, 53(2), 177–191.

Yang, C., Chan, M. K., Nickerson, A. B., Jenkins, L., Xie, J. S., & Fredrick, S. S. (2022). Teacher victimization and teachers' subjective well-being: Does school climate matter? *Aggressive Behavior*, 48(4), 379–392. DOI: 10.1002/ab.22030 PMID: 35383978

Yang, W., Datu, J. A. D., Lin, X., Lau, M. M., & Li, H. (2019). Can early childhood curriculum enhance social-emotional competence in low-income children? A meta-analysis of the educational effects. *Early Education and Development*, 30(1), 36–59. DOI: 10.1080/10409289.2018.1539557

Yusufov, M., Nicoloro-SantaBarbara, J., Grey, N. E., Moyer, A., & Lobel, M. (2019). Meta-analytic evaluation of stress reduction interventions for undergraduate and graduate students. *International Journal of Stress Management*, 26(2), 132–145. DOI: 10.1037/str0000099

Zacharia, M. G., & Yablon, Y. B. (2021). School bullying and students' sense of safety in school: The moderating role of school climate. *European Journal of Psychology of Education*, 37(3), 903–919. DOI: 10.1007/s10212-021-00567-9

Zafiropoulou, M. (2000). *Understanding our behavior: The role of learning in the acquisition and development of behavior*. Kastaniotis. (in Greek)

Zafiropoulou, M. (2004). Cognitive-behavioral interventions at school. In Kalantzi-Azizi, A., & Zafiropoulou, M. (Eds.), *Adaptation to school prevention and coping with difficulties* (pp. 26–50). Ellinika Grammata. (in Greek)

Zagona, A. L., Hara, M., Loman, S., Kurth, J. A., & Walker, V. L. (2024). Educators' perceptions on the involvement of students with complex support needs in PBIS: The role of educational placement. *Research and Practice for Persons with Severe Disabilities : the Journal of TASH*, •••, 15407969241263515. DOI: 10.1177/15407969241263515

Zenner, C., Herrnleben-Kurz, S., & Walach, H. (2014). Mindfulness-based interventions in schools—A systematic review and meta-analysis. *Frontiers in Psychology*, 5, 603. DOI: 10.3389/fpsyg.2014.00603 PMID: 25071620

Zhang, Q., Wang, J., & Neitzel, A. (2022). School-based mental health interventions targeting depression or anxiety: A meta-analysis of rigorous randomized controlled trials for school-aged children and adolescents. *Journal of Youth and Adolescence: A Multidisciplinary Research Publication, 52*(1), 195–217. https://doi.org/DOI: 10.1007/s10964-022-01684-4

Zimmer-Gembeck, M. J., & Skinner, E. A. (2016). The development of coping: Implications for psychopathology and resilience. *Development and Psychopathology*, 1–61.

Zinsser, K. M. (2015). Promoting positive classroom climates: What can we learn from the research on social and emotional learning? *Psychology in the Schools*, 52(2), 2–20. DOI: 10.1002/pits.21829

Zoogman, S., Goldberg, S. B., Hoyt, W. T., & Miller, L. (2015). Mindfulness interventions with youth: A meta-analysis. *Mindfulness*, 6(2), 290–302. DOI: 10.1007/s12671-013-0260-4

Zullig, K. J., Ward, R. M., Huebner, S. E., & Daily, S. M. (2018). Association between adolescent school climate and perceived quality of life. *Child Indicators Research*, 11(6), 1737–1753. DOI: 10.1007/s12187-017-9521-4

About the Contributors

Louiza Ioannidou is an Assistant Professor in Children and Adolescent Mental Health at the European University Cyprus and a Registered School Psychologist. Dr Ioannidou has obtained her PhD in Psychology, her MA in School Psychology (applied program), and her BA in Psychology, all from the University of Cyprus. Dr. Ioannidou has also trained in the field of Cognitive - Behavioural Therapy, Positive Psychology, Mindfulness, Solution Focused Therapy, and Business - Team Coaching. She has also a diploma in the Master Practitioner in Eating Disorders and Obesity. Her teaching and research experience focuses on school bullying, children and adolescents' mental health and resilience, and parental involvement. Her research interests also focus on developing, implementing, and evaluating psychoeducational programs to promote children's and adolescents' mental health, well-being, resilience, and a safe school climate. Her research findings are published in scientific journals and presented in scientific conferences. Finally, Dr. Ioannidou is the author and editor of the book "Building Mental Resilience: Positive Psychology, Emotional Intelligence, and Play" (2024) published by IGI Global.

Agathi Argyriadi is a Psychologist with specialization on Cognitive – Behavioral Psychotherapy and Developmental Psychology. Her PhD thesis is entitled "The effects of "Aesthetic flow experiences" in school's environment of first graders. A psycho-educational approach". She also holds a M.Ed. on Special Education. She is a Lecturer in the Department of Education at Frederick University, teaching developmental and cognitive psychology. In the past she has also taught at Cyprus University of Technology (Therapeutic communication), at the East London University (Research Methods and Statistics) and at the Technological Educational Institute of Peloponnese at the department of Speech Pathology (teaching Developmental Psychology and Clinical Neuropsychology), for 3 years. She has acted as a self- employed Psychologist and for a 3-year project against violence at the Ministry of Internal Affairs of the Hellenic Republic. She has also acted for two years, as an external associate at a private school in Greece, with the aim of monitoring and supporting students with learning difficulties, psychological problems and counseling of parents. Agathi Argyriadi was also a professor at the Foundation for Youth and Lifelong Learning and specifically at the Institute for Vocational Training of the Ministry of Education. She has published articles in international journals and she has participated in numerous of training seminars. She is the writer of 10 scientific books in the field of psychology. Her research interests focus on optimizing learning environments using positive psychology and aesthetic theories, developmental psychological issues, special education field, social inclusion issues. She teaches in the Distance Learning Program of Special Education.

* * *

Jehan Abdulla is pursuing a Ph.D. in the Department of Special Education at the College of Education, United Arab Emirates University (UAEU). She has conducted seminars on social-emotional learning at both UAEU and Fredrik University. Additionally, she presented an oral poster at the UAE GSRC 2024 conference, discussing "Teachers' Emotional Intelligence and Social-Emotional Learning in the United Arab Emirates: Integrating Artificial Intelligence." Her research is focused on improving teaching methods within the special needs sector, drawing from her extensive experience in education and assistive technology.

Sandro Anella holds a degree in philosophy with a focus on psycholinguistics and philosophical-scientific studies. He has participated in post-graduate research on Office Automation. An expert trainer in the Pedagogy for the Third Millennium method, he is a member of the Education and Teaching Department of the research institute of the Patrizio Paoletti Foundation. He designs, creates, and disseminates scientific content and participates as a trainer in various educational and teaching contexts.

Alexandros Argyriadis is an Assistant Professor at Frederick University, in the domain of Mental Health and Learning Disabilities. He coordinates the Distance Learning Master's Program in Community Health Care and the Practicum of the MEd in Special Education. He has authored numerous scholarly books and high impact factor articles.

Tania di Giuseppe is a psychologist, a psychotherapist, and the director of the Department of Psychological Research and Didactics at Fondazione Patrizio Paoletti's RINED institute. She is an expert in resilience, hope, and projects to help individuals and communities facing emergencies. She is head of the project Envisioning the Future targeted at sharing knowledge about human functioning to help individuals face stress, gain awareness, and acquire the ability to reprogram the future.

Maria Efstratopoulou, Ph.D., is an associate professor at the Department of Special Education, College of Education, United Arab Emirates University. Her research interests are the assessment and diagnosis of children with emotional, behavioral, and developmental disorders and intervention strategies for professionals and families. She is a member of The European Framework on Psycho-motor Therapy for Children (EFP), and she is the author of 4 books on Children's behavior, education, and health.

Argyro Fella is an Assistant Professor at the Department of Education, University of Nicosia. She pursued her graduate studies (M.A. in 2010 and Ph.D. in 2017) at the University of Cyprus in Psychology, where she also worked as a Research Associate at the Center for Applied Neuroscience, specifically in the Learning Disabilities group. Her research interests focus on studying, diagnosing, and treating learning and individual differences, emphasizing cognitive and linguistic factors associated with specific learning disabilities. Specifically, her research employs eye-tracking and electroencephalography (EEG, ERP) methodologies for studying reading development and related difficulties. She has participated in the consortiums of international projects funded by both international and national agencies from the European Union (e.g., COST MultiplEYE), or Cyprus (e.g., Youth Board of Cyprus). Dr. Fella publishes her work in scientific journals and routinely presents at national and international conferences.

Hawraa Habeeb is a Ph.D. candidate specializing in special education at the College of Education, United Arab Emirates University. She had worked in Kuwait and Qatar as a teacher of children with moderate and severe autism and intellectual disabilities. Her research interests include interventions for challenging behavior and sensory processing disorder in children with autism spectrum disorders. Awarded a certificate for completing an autism spectrum disorder course (by the University of California, Davis). Her Latest article publication was in 2022, titled "Emerging Themes on Factors Influencing Career and Employment Decisions".

Lefki Kourea, PhD, is an Associate Professor in Special/Inclusive Education and Applied Behavior Analysis at the Department of Education of the University of Nicosia. Her research interests focus on prevention and early intervention through designing and implementing behavioral and academic interventions for students with mild to moderate disabilities and at-risk students. Dr. Kourea worked as a teacher in public primary schools in Cyprus.

Carmela Lillo has a degree in Philosophy. She is an expert trainer of the Pedagogy for the Third Millennium method. She is a member of the Education and Didactics Department of the Research Institute of the Patrizio Paoletti Foundation. She designs, realises and disseminates scientific content in educational and scholastic contexts, aimed at individuals and groups.

Fotini Lytra, M.Sc., is a psychologist specializing in child and adolescent psychology. She has worked as a scientific and research associate at the "Attention Deficit Hyperactivity Disorder and Learning Disorders Unit" at P&A Kyriakou Children's Hospital, as well as in the child psychiatry department of Agia Sofia Children's Hospital. She has extensive clinical and consultation practice with primary and secondary school students. Her research interests focus on designing and implementing interventions for children and adolescents with neurodevelopmental disorders and learning disabilities.

Katerina Michael is a Visiting Lecturer in Health Education at the Frederick University (Cyprus). Her research interests include developing, implementing, and evaluating health promotion programs in various settings and populations. She has published numerous journal articles and presented his research at many international conferences.

Georgia Panayiotou is the Dean of the Graduate School and a Professor of Clinical Psychology at the University of Cyprus. She holds a BA in Psychology and Sociology from New College of Florida, as well as a Master's and Ph.D. in Clinical Psychology from Purdue University, Indiana. She completed her Doctoral Internship at McLean Hospital/Harvard Medical School. Her research primarily focuses on emotions and emotional processes in mental health, particularly their interaction with coping mechanisms. She is especially interested in how individuals experience, process, and regulate emotions, and how these factors relate to mental health and overall well-being. She has served as Principal Investigator (PI) or co-PI on numerous nationally and internationally funded projects, including Marie Curie ETN and Erasmus+ KA2. Additionally, she is a founding member of Center for Applied Neuroscience at University of Cyprus. She sits on editorial boards of international journals.

Giulia Perasso has a Ph.D. in Psychology, Neuroscience and Data Science at University of Pavia (Italy), completed in 2020. Nowadays she is a post-doc fellow at univesity of Genoa (Italy). Her main research interests are: developmental psychology, resilience, attachment.

Matilde Pisano is a student, with a bachelor's degree in social work completed in February 2024 with a thesis titled "How to talk to children about war: promoting empathy and coping in families in conflict areas." She is currently pursuing her master's degree at Alma Mater Studiorum: University of Bologna.

Erika Salemi holds a BA in Social Work. Her dissertation, titled "Parental Burnout and Vulnerable Families: The Role of Social Service in Child Protection," focuses on parenting and intervention programs that prevent forced separation between children and their biological families. She currently works in a residential service for minors and is deeply interested in the child protection system.

Dingfei Shen is a Ph.D. candidate in Special Education at the College of Education, United Arab Emirates University. He also works as a coordinator of the Chinese Language Expansion Program in the UAE. He has experience teaching Chinese as a foreign language for eight years, including in the United States, Thailand, and UAE. He has interests in researching special and inclusive education, and comparative studies of education. He published The Overview of ASIAN Education as the second editor in China in 2015.

Marios Theodorou is a Lecturer of Clinical Psychology at Frederick University and a researcher at the Frederick Research Center. He holds a Ph.D. in Clinical Psychology from the University of Cyprus. Dr. Theodorou is currently involved as a co-Principal Investigator (co-PI) in pilot feasibility randomized controlled trials (RCTs) focused on building transversal skills as a form of mental health promotion for higher education students. His previous research primarily centered on correlational studies and laboratory experiments, employing physiological methodologies.

Potheini Vaiouli is a postdoctoral fellow at the University of Luxembourg and a licensed music therapist. She holds a Ph.D. in Special Education from Indiana University Bloomington and an MA in Music Therapy from New York University. Her research interests focus on the social, emotional, and academic development of individuals with autism and other neurodevelopmental disabilities, with her work published in both national and international peer-reviewed journals. Potheini has extensive experience in participating in multi-site, interdisciplinary research projects in the EU and US, including those funded by the Creative Europe grant and Swedish Erasmus+ (E+ NA, E+ KA2). She also brings over ten years of teaching experience at both undergraduate and graduate levels, alongside clinical work with youth with disabilities and their families.

Elena Vigogna is currently a master's student in social sciences, she completed a bachelor's thesis entitled: 'Culture and child development, a comparison between Africa and the West'.

Giulia Viviano is a student in the Master's degree program in Social Policies and Services at the University of Turin. She earned her Bachelor's degree in Social Work at the University of Genoa, with a thesis in developmental psychology entitled "The Consequences of Maltreatment Trauma on the Life Cycle from a Contemporary Perspective".

Index

A

academic achievement 2, 3, 4, 5, 10, 17, 18, 21, 24, 25, 26, 30, 57, 60, 80, 137, 147, 150, 153, 179, 187, 196, 197, 220, 271, 297

academic performance 5, 6, 8, 18, 28, 57, 58, 61, 77, 79, 141, 159, 161, 162, 164, 170, 171, 172, 173, 174, 183, 186, 187, 191, 194, 195, 197, 208, 210, 226, 227, 232, 233, 235, 236, 237, 239, 249, 250, 251, 253, 261, 287, 291

adolescents 5, 6, 53, 54, 55, 56, 57, 59, 60, 75, 76, 77, 79, 126, 127, 131, 135, 136, 137, 138, 140, 143, 144, 151, 152, 153, 154, 155, 156, 176, 191, 192, 199, 202, 206, 208, 209, 210, 211, 217, 221, 223, 229, 231, 244, 270, 289, 290, 293, 294, 300, 314, 324, 332, 333, 337, 338, 339, 340, 346, 347

at-risk students 56, 65, 66, 74, 80

attention deficit hyperactivity disorder 141, 270, 277, 278, 280, 286, 295

autism spectrum disorder 56, 141, 142, 148, 151, 153, 269, 274, 275, 276, 277, 278, 279, 281, 282, 283, 285, 286, 294

B

Behaviour problems 29, 85

C

Children 19, 21, 22, 23, 25, 26, 27, 29, 33, 34, 35, 36, 37, 38, 39, 40, 41, 42, 43, 44, 45, 46, 47, 48, 49, 50, 51, 52, 53, 54, 55, 56, 75, 76, 77, 78, 79, 80, 81, 82, 83, 85, 86, 87, 93, 95, 102, 105, 106, 107, 108, 109, 110, 115, 116, 117, 118, 121, 122, 123, 124, 126, 127, 128, 129, 130, 131, 132, 133, 135, 136, 137, 138, 139, 140, 141, 142, 143, 144, 145, 146, 148, 149,

151, 152, 153, 154, 155, 156, 160, 170, 176, 177, 178, 190, 192, 199, 201, 202, 203, 205, 206, 207, 208, 210, 211, 212, 213, 214, 215, 216, 217, 218, 220, 221, 222, 223, 225, 226, 227, 228, 229, 231, 232, 233, 234, 235, 236, 237, 238, 239, 240, 242, 243, 244, 247, 248, 249, 250, 251, 252, 253, 254, 255, 258, 259, 260, 261, 262, 263, 264, 265, 266, 269, 270, 271, 272, 273, 274, 275, 276, 277, 278, 279, 280, 281, 282, 283, 284, 285, 286, 287, 288, 289, 290, 291, 292, 293, 294, 295, 301, 321, 327, 328, 329, 331, 332, 333, 334, 335, 336, 337, 338, 339, 340, 341, 342, 343, 344, 345, 346, 347, 348, 349, 350, 351

chronic health conditions 225, 226, 227, 228, 229, 231, 232, 233, 234, 235, 236, 237, 238, 239, 240, 242, 244

college 20, 151, 244, 264, 265, 293, 321, 322, 324, 325

communication 14, 16, 33, 37, 39, 42, 45, 58, 73, 101, 107, 110, 112, 133, 141, 162, 163, 167, 170, 184, 191, 199, 208, 211, 212, 215, 228, 249, 250, 251, 255, 256, 258, 259, 270, 284, 286, 301, 310, 327, 328, 340, 343, 346, 348, 350

cultural diversity 226, 227, 228, 229, 230, 232, 239, 240, 247, 248, 250, 251, 255, 257, 258, 261, 262, 263, 266

D

depression 41, 56, 57, 59, 60, 72, 87, 136, 139, 140, 143, 144, 146, 148, 154, 156, 166, 185, 186, 188, 191, 209, 210, 220, 223, 226, 238, 243, 250, 269, 270, 271, 272, 273, 274, 275, 282, 289, 290, 291, 292, 293, 294, 295, 307, 323, 324

developmental psychology 123, 265, 291, 328, 346, 347

dyslexia 82, 269, 274, 275, 276, 277, 278, 279, 280, 281, 283, 284, 285, 286,

291, 293

E

ecosystemic model 91, 92, 99
education 4, 6, 19, 20, 21, 22, 23, 24, 25,
26, 27, 28, 29, 30, 31, 34, 35, 37, 40,
49, 52, 53, 62, 65, 67, 68, 70, 77, 78,
79, 80, 81, 87, 92, 93, 95, 116, 124,
125, 127, 129, 130, 131, 133, 136,
137, 143, 147, 149, 150, 152, 154,
156, 158, 159, 160, 161, 165, 167,
168, 169, 170, 172, 173, 174, 176,
177, 178, 179, 181, 182, 187, 189,
191, 192, 193, 194, 195, 196, 197,
198, 200, 201, 202, 203, 206, 208,
209, 210, 216, 223, 225, 227, 232,
233, 235, 236, 237, 238, 239, 242,
245, 247, 249, 251, 254, 262, 263,
265, 267, 290, 297, 298, 303, 306,
308, 311, 314, 318, 322, 325, 328,
331, 334, 342, 343, 345, 346, 348, 350
educational environments 26, 136, 142,
144, 158, 164, 227, 261
educators 83, 85, 95, 110, 122, 127, 130,
136, 137, 149, 150, 158, 160, 161,
165, 170, 171, 172, 173, 174, 177,
182, 188, 189, 193, 194, 195, 196,
198, 199, 200, 217, 225, 227, 234,
236, 237, 239, 240, 243, 248, 250,
251, 255, 261, 262, 287, 319, 322,
324, 325, 328, 334, 338, 341, 344, 345
Effectiveness 8, 9, 19, 27, 29, 30, 33, 36,
40, 41, 47, 68, 77, 80, 81, 85, 94, 98,
109, 122, 127, 128, 129, 132, 135,
138, 141, 147, 148, 149, 151, 152,
153, 154, 155, 160, 163, 176, 181,
186, 191, 192, 193, 201, 203, 210,
215, 217, 221, 227, 233, 234, 239,
242, 251, 252, 253, 254, 255, 257,
260, 261, 263, 289, 298, 299, 300,
301, 304, 305, 307, 309, 315, 316,
319, 320, 323
emotional regulation 57, 141, 144, 146,
148, 159, 161, 162, 164, 166, 169,
170, 171, 172, 174, 186, 187, 188,
191, 192, 193, 194, 196, 197, 202,

206, 207, 208, 210, 227, 232, 233,
237, 238, 240, 248, 254
Evidence-Based Strategies 128

H

humanistic model 92, 93

I

inclusive education 27, 237, 238
inclusive practices 227, 235
intervention 9, 11, 13, 14, 15, 17, 19, 20,
27, 40, 47, 53, 54, 61, 66, 67, 68, 69,
72, 73, 76, 77, 79, 80, 82, 85, 86, 95,
100, 101, 102, 109, 111, 112, 114,
115, 116, 117, 118, 120, 121, 122,
123, 126, 127, 137, 138, 139, 140,
141, 142, 143, 144, 145, 146, 147,
148, 149, 151, 152, 154, 155, 156,
157, 165, 166, 168, 170, 176, 188,
199, 200, 203, 205, 209, 210, 211,
212, 215, 216, 217, 218, 220, 221,
227, 228, 229, 232, 239, 240, 241,
242, 244, 252, 253, 254, 263, 266,
287, 298, 299, 307, 312, 317, 319,
320, 338, 346, 350
intervention models 227, 228, 232, 239

L

learning experiences 157, 250, 320

M

Mental flow 157, 158, 164
mental health 3, 5, 8, 12, 18, 21, 22, 24,
30, 33, 34, 35, 37, 38, 39, 41, 42, 43,
47, 48, 49, 50, 51, 52, 53, 54, 55, 56,
57, 58, 59, 60, 61, 71, 72, 73, 74, 75,
76, 77, 78, 79, 80, 81, 82, 87, 124,
125, 127, 135, 136, 137, 138, 140,
142, 143, 144, 146, 147, 148, 149,
150, 151, 152, 153, 154, 155, 156,
157, 158, 159, 160, 162, 165, 166,
167, 168, 169, 170, 171, 172, 173,
174, 175, 176, 177, 178, 179, 182,

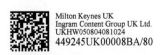

Milton Keynes UK
Ingram Content Group UK Ltd.
UKHW050804081024
449245UK00008BA/80